PAIN
FROM SYMPTOM TO TREATMENT

Manuel M. Villaverde, M.D.

C. Wright MacMillan, M.D.

VNR **VAN NOSTRAND REINHOLD COMPANY**
NEW YORK   CINCINNATI   ATLANTA   DALLAS   SAN FRANCISCO
LONDON   TORONTO   MELBOURNE

Van Nostrand Reinhold Company Regional Offices:
New York   Cincinanti   Atlanta   Dallas   San Francisco

Van Nostrand Reinhold Company International Offices:
London   Toronto   Melbourne

Copyright © 1977 by Litton Educational Publishing, Inc.

Library of Congress Catalog Card Number: 76-53754
ISBN: 0-442-25107-6

All rights reserved. No part of this work covered by the copyright hereon may be reproduced or used in any form or by any means—graphic, electronic, or mechanical, including photocopying, recording, taping, or information storage and retrieval systems—without permission of the publisher.

Manufactured in the United States of America

Published by Van Nostrand Reinhold Company
450 West 33rd Street, New York, N.Y. 10001

Published simultaneously in Canada by Van Nostrand Reinhold Ltd.

15 14 13 12 11 10 9 8 7 6 5 4 3 2

Library of Congress Cataloging in Publication Data

Villaverde, Manuel Maria, 1905–
  Pain : from symptom to treatment.

  1. Pain. 2. Analgesics. I. MacMillan, Charles Wright, 1895–   joint author. II. Title.
[DNLM: 1. Pain.   WL700 V727p]
RB127.V54   616'.047   76-53754
ISBN 0-442-25107-6

Preface

In the first quarter of this century, a very successful book was published called *Du Symptôme a la Maladie* ("From the Symptom to the Disease"), which, in its time, summarized a good philosophic approach for the medical profession. From the patient's standpoint this thinking fell short: a sick person may be interested in knowing what the disease is, but the truly urgent need is to be cured. Therefore, the guiding thought, in our new presentation has to be "From Symptom to Treatment," since the one suffering an agonizing abdominal pain (or any other distressing symptom, be it fever, fear, or the like) is not primarily concerned with whether it is acute appendicitis, biliary colic, or any other medical puzzle of which the symptom is only a small part of the clinical edifice called disease; pain is the demon to him, and to get rid of it is his overwhelming obsession. Without any false steps, the physician, with dignity and assurance, must hasten from the symptom to the treatment.

To work correctly, the physician must know the nature of the disease giving rise to the symptom, so as to be able to remove the basic cause. He then plunges into the mazes of science where he must travel a lonely journey, the course taken with each individual patient being different because it depends on the patient's own peculiar reactions to the familiar disease and the familiar drugs. Thus, in treating each case a doctor must travel a lonely road, never traveled before and never exactly to be traveled again. In an attempt to help, we plan to give some quickly read signposts on this road of patient management.

Years ago, it was said that "the medical profession as a whole has been criticized for being fully ignorant of matters pertaining to prescription drugs." The response of the American Medical Association has been the publication of *AMA Drug Evaluation*, providing information on the vast field of modern Materia Medica. Nevertheless, the efforts of scientists and pharmaceutical manufacturers, commendable as they are, offering the medical practitioner an ever increasing number of active and effective drugs, put the doctor in a difficult position: that of choosing the suitable medication. In this volume we present groups of drugs according to action and use, together with illustrations of the graphic formulae, which explain many of the drug's relationships and actions. We present an analysis of each particular situation: how to diagnose, and thereafter how to treat, the annoying symptom. The unique emphasis of our volume is that it respects the frantic need of the doctor on the firing line for a thumbnail answer to the hot question from his office line up. He who is not a specialist—the one who teaches the rest of us which one is the selected drug for a selected patient—has to be led firmly away from the unintelligible cacophony of fanciful names of the drugs on the market. In trying to stumble through our heap of bottles and boxes, we think with melancholy of the remarks of Oliver Wendell Holmes when he said: "—if the whole materia medica, as now used, could be sunk to the bottom of the sea, it would be all the better for mankind—and the worse for fish!" He tried to make a selection of a few useful drugs, but was too selective. More generous was the French doctor who accepted "Therapeutics in Twenty Medicaments". But more than twenty medicaments are needed.

Consistent with the above thoughts, our program "From Symptom to Treatment" offers this book on "Pain." Its purpose is not the treatment of a number of diseases (though a reasonable summary is given in each instance), but only the treatment of pain, just stepping from the evaluation of a symptom to the next category, which is the treatment. The book is divided into two main parts: a review of the pharmacology of drugs used to treat pain, and a section on the diagnosis and treatment of diseases presenting pain as an annoying symptom. The anatomical location of pain determines the designation of the topical paragraph, for easy reference. Of course, diseases which may provoke pain on different sites are, at times, described at these different locations. In general, the book is designed to enable the practitioner to see the symptom quickly, isolate the significant and characteristic features, eliminate the unlike causes, and give proper priority to the causes under suspicion. With the diagnosis made, the principles and method of the control of pain in mind, and the drugs to be used briefly presented, many problems should be simplified.

If our readers think this initial volume facilitates their help to their patients, we commend to their attention the further books in this series.

MANUEL M. VILLAVERDE, M.D.
C. WRIGHT MACMILLAN, M.D.

Contents

Part I   PHARMACOLOGY OF DRUGS USED TO COMBAT PAIN

I	Narcotic Analgesics	2
II	Salicylates	23
III	Coal-Tar Derivatives	29
IV	Pyrazolon Derivatives	31
V	Phenylquinolines	34
VI	Colchicum Derivatives	36
VII	Antimalarials	38
VIII	Local Anesthetics	41
IX	Vasodilators	56
X	Vasoconstrictors	59
XI	Corticoids	61
XII	Other Drugs Used in Conditions Causing Pain	68

Part II   DIAGNOSIS AND TREATMENT

I	Headache	75
II	Pain in the Face	117
III	Stomatalgia	123
IV	Opthalmodynia	131
V	Otalgia	139
VI	Dysphagia	145
VII	Pain in the Neck	149
VIII	Pain along the Spine and Lower Back	153
IX	Thoracodynia	170
X	Acute Abdomen	187
XI	Chronic Abdominal Pain	223
XII	Limbs	261
XIII	Muscles	303

XIV	Pain in the Perineum, Rectum, and Sex Organs	310
XV	Pain in the Skin	329

Index 339

Part One

Pharmacology of Drugs Used to Combat Pain

The history of man is the history of pain. Since the first wound after an accidental trauma, or the first gastrointestinal colic after trying a new indigestible morsel, man has attempted to soothe his sufferings. And from his efforts were born first magic and then medicine.

Pain is still the most frequent complaint physicians hear about from their patients. These patients may stay at home and try some popular remedies—or nothing—when coughing or presenting other supposed minor symptoms; but as soon as pain becomes only a little bothersome, they will immediately resort to the physician.

Analgesics are in constant medical or surgical use. The election of the best adequate one for a specific pain is not always easily accomplished: some are of weak potency, some may provoke important side effects. The *ideal analgesic* should be effective when given orally, rapidly active after ingestion, and sufficiently strong for an appropriate analgesia; it should not be prone to tolerance, addiction, or respiratory depression; it should show few side effects or specific effects on high nervous centers; its action should be controllable; and, finally, an antidote must be available when needed. In other words, the ideal analgesic will effectively control pain and will not provide undesirable reactions from the central nervous, respiratory, cardiovascular, genitourinary, dermal, or musculoskeletal systems or any other parts of the body.

Let us stress now that, under special circumstances, particular side effects may be considered "ideal," such as anti-inflammatory properties of a substance used against pain provoked by inflammation (aspirin in rheumatic diseases), or depression of the nervous system by a substance used against pain in terminal diseases (morphine in cancer).

I. NARCOTIC ANALGESICS

Narcotic analgesics, as implied by their name, are those that, together with the pain-relief effect, also show sleep-inducing properties. Because of the induction of sleep, mostly accompanied by euphoric sensations and dreams, the narcotic analgesics may induce addiction and are subject to restrictive ordinances and laws. Nevertheless, because they are powerful analgesics, they are unsurpassed by any others for the relief of severe pain, as occurs in biliary colic or cancer. Most of them are opium derivatives; others are semisynthetic or synthetic products. Morphine and meperidine are the principal members of the group.

Morphine

Morphine is one of the several alkaloids extracted from opium, a phenanthrene derivative which occurs as a soluble, bitter white powder. Its structural formula is as follows:

The two hydroxy groups (OH) are of paramount importance regarding the pharmacologic properties of the drug: they are a phenolic group and an alcoholic hydroxy group, with the analgesic properties of morphine depending on the phenolic group.

Its powerful analgesic action is probably due to its ability to depress the afterdischarge following afferent nociceptive stimuli; but at the same time it appears to enhance reflex responses to nonnociceptive stimuli, thus giving a possible explanation why its analgesic effect is not accompanied by anesthesia or paralysis. Analgesia is particularly produced when the pain is dull and continuous rather than of sharp, intermittent character, not only when it arises from viscera but also from other body structures. The threshold for pain is increased, and its reactions (alertness for pain, anxiety, fear) are decreased under the action of morphine.

Other effects of the drug upon the central nervous system are sleepiness and depression, including slowing of respiration (which affects metabolism indirectly), and gastrointestinal, biliary and pancreatic secretions. It also checks cough and diarrhea, and induces euphoria. Miosis is a characteristic effect of opiates, particularly morphine. In an opposite way, this alkaloid increases the tone of smooth muscle in the biliary tract, ureters, and urinary bladder.

Morphine is rapidly absorbed from the gastrointestinal tract and from the subcutaneous tissue, but not from the oral mucosa or the intact skin. About 10% of an administered dose is destroyed in the body; most of the rest is conjugated in the liver and perhaps the kidney, and involves the phenolic hydroxyl radical of the molecule. The portion not destroyed is mainly eliminated in the urine, with smaller amounts in the feces and sweat. The analgesic effect lasts for about 4 hours.

After the administration of morphine for several days, tolerance develops, which extends (cross-tolerance) to codeine and the other natural or semisynthetic opium alkaloids. Tolerance seems to develop when certain cells of the central nervous system become able to perform normal functions in the presence of the drug, by a mechanism still not well-known.

Besides the control of pain, morphine can cause other reactions, some of them considered undesirable side effects. Sleepiness may be helpful in some occasions of severe pain; rarely, insomnia may occur instead. Nausea and vomiting are frequent responses. Respiratory depression may be a serious problem, especially among the elderly, the very young, the debilitated, and those suffering from certain diseases (respiratory, convulsive, delirium tremens, alcoholism, cerebral edema, gastrointestinal hemorrhage, asthma, prostatism, diabetic acidosis, anemia, and others).

The drug may provoke very serious reactions, either acute (morphine poisoning) or chronic (morphine addiction). In acute poisoning, the three symptoms coma, shallow respiration, and pinpoint pupils are almost pathognomonic, particularly if knowledge of previous use of morphine is obtained. The treatment for acute morphine poisoning is to be carried out as soon as possible. A patent air-way should be maintained, and the specific antidote, either nalorphine or levallorphan, given immediately in adequate dosage, namely:

Nalorphine HCl (Nalline), 5 mg per ml in 2-ml ampuls

given at rate of 5 to 10 mg, intramusuclarly, repeated after 10 to 15 minutes if not effective, provided that a total of 40 mg is not exceeded over a 3-hour period. It may be repeated at 3–4-hour intervals; or:

Levallorphan tartrate (Lorfan), 1 mg per ml in 1-ml ampuls

given at a dose of 1 mg intravenously, followed by 0.5 mg at 3-minute intervals, for one or two consecutive injections.

Morphine addiction is not easily diagnosed by any symptomatological complex. It can be proved by the administration of either nalorphine or levallorphan, which will bring on withdrawal symptoms manifested by a craving for the drug, tremor, irritability, lacrimation, sneezing, etc. The treatment of morphine addiction should be carried on in specialized clinics and by specialized personnel. Treatment centers for narcotic addiction now base their plan of therapy largely on the substitution of methadone (q.v.), for the opium-derived drugs. The methadone addiction which often results has been easier to overcome. Addiction, which requires progressively increasing doses of the drug, also develops among patients treated for long-standing pain, as in terminal cancer. In these instances, progressive increase of dosage is required.

The principal use of morphine is for the treatment of severe pain when it cannot be alleviated by other analgesics, as in cancer, visceral infarction, pneumothorax, pleurisy, pericarditis, and some traumatic accidents, such as burns and fractures. In cases of biliary or renal colic, morphine will be employed only after failure of other antispasmodic drugs (atropine, theophylline, and even papaverine). It is also used in cases of insomnia, particularly if due to pain or cough, and in psychoses, delirium, mania, heart failure, internal hemorrhage, thyrotoxicosis, and some encephalopathies which interfere with sleep. When used in obstetrics it should never be given within 2 hours before delivery is expected because of possible depression of respiration in the newborn. Good effects are also produced in acute vascular occlusion (coronary, peripheral, pulmonary), particularly if given together with papaverine.

In surgery, morphine is employed together with scopolamine or atropine, but only 2 hours before starting anesthesia.

In most cases, the regular dosages range from 10 to 20 mg every 4 hours, subcutaneously. For rapid action, in severe hepatic or renal colic, the dose may be slowly injected intravenously, dissolved in 5 ml of saline. Children should not receive morphine before 1 year of age (formerly, before 6 months), and then only very small amounts: 1 mg up to 3 years; 1.5 mg up to 6 years; 2 mg up to 9 years; and 4 mg up to 12 years.

Morphine is available for prescription in the following pharmaceutical preparations:

> Morphine sulfate, hypodermic tablets, containing 5, 8, 10, 15, or 30 mg per tablet;

> Morphine sulfate, capsules, containing 15, 30, or 60 mg per capsule;

> Morphine sulfate, injectable, containing 8, 10, 15, 20, or 30 mg per ml in 1-ml ampuls and 10- or 20-ml vials.

Pantopon

Pantopon, also called Pantopium and Omnopon, is a mixture of purified opium alkaloids derived from waxes, gums, and resins, in about the same proportions as found in the plant, morphine being some five times more concentrated.

The effects of Pantopon are mainly due to its content of morphine; 20 mg of Pantopon contains 10 mg of morphine. Also, the side effects are substantially the same as those of an equal amount of pure morphine.

The indications and contraindications for the use of Pantopon are the same as previously discussed for morphine.

The drug is available as:

> Pantopon, injectable, 20 mg of opium alkaloids, with 10 mg morphine in 10 ml ampuls;

> Pantopon, hypodermic tablets, 20 mg of opium alkaloids, with 10 mg morphine per tablet.

The manufacturers of Pantopon claim that the combination of morphine with the other opium alkaloids enhances its activity and lessens the side effects. They recommend Pantopon for the relief of severe pain in lieu of morphine.

Opium Preparations

In wide medical use, up to the first half of this century, were several opium preparations, the following being the most frequently prescribed:

Paregoric elixir, or camphorated tincture of opium, was indicated particularly for the relief of intestinal colic. The regular dose is 4 ml to be repeated several times a day.

Laudanum, or tincture of opium, is also used for gastrointestinal pain or diarrhea, at a dosage of 0.5 ml several times a day.

Powdered opium has also been used for diarrhea, at a dose of 50 mg several times a day. Powdered opium with extract of belladonna plus tannic acid are used in suppositories for hemorrhoids.

Not so widely used at the present time, are *cough preparations*, most of them containing a dose equivalent to 1 mg of morphine or dihydromorphinone (Dilacol, Dilaudid Cough Syrup, and others).

Methyldihydromorphinone (Metopon)

Metopon is methyldihydromorphinone, a semisynthetic morphine derivative, closely related to dihydromorphinone, with an added methyl group (CH_3) in the phenanthrene ring, which occurs in needles, is slightly soluble in organic solvents, and corresponds to the structural formula:

The hydrochloride is freely soluble in water, and slightly soluble in alcohol or chloroform.

The analgesic effect of methyldihydromorphinone is about twice as potent as that of morphine, and its duration, about the same. Nausea and vomiting are not too frequent, and other side effects are also less marked, particularly repiratory depression. When used in the treatment of severe pain in cancer and similar terminal diseases, it may show some advantages as an active oral medication with a slower development of dependence and tolerance. When it is used for nonterminal diseases, its withdrawal symptoms disappear more rapidly than those caused by morphine. However, it cannot be used for preanesthesia in surgery, because it is poorly hypnotic and might induce unpredictable and dangerous respiratory depression when given with inhalation anesthetics. In general, the drug is somewhat safer than morphine, but the disadvantages are of almost the same nature and it should not be given in status asthmaticus or in increased intracranial pressure.

The regular dose is 6 mg by the oral route, repeated only when its analgesia begins to vanish. Somewhat larger doses should be given to patients who have previously become tolerant to morphine (cross-tolerance).

The drug is available for prescription only for oral administration, as follows:

Methyldihydromorphinone hydrochloride, capsules, containing 3 mg.

Dihydromorphinone (Dilaudid)

Dihydromorphinone is a semisynthetic morphine derivative in which an oxygen atom substitutes for the alcohol hydroxy group;

It occurs in crystals soluble in three parts of water, and very slightly soluble in alcohol.

The therapeutic indications for dihydromorphinone are essentially the same as for morphine: acute or chronic pain from myocardial infarction, hepatic or renal colic, cancer, and trauma (surgery included). Its potency is greater than that of morphine, but the duration of its analgesia is not so prolonged. Action may be extended by rectal administration with suppositories. Side effects, like hypnosis and constipation, are less marked, but are also of the same nature as those caused by morphine, including tolerance and addiction.

As with methyldihydromorphinone, dihydromorphinone might bring on dangerous respiratory depression, which could even require the administration of morphine antidotes, and should not be given to patients with status asthmaticus or increased intracranial pressure.

The usual dosage is 1 to 4 mg and can be given by any of the common routes, namely, oral, subcutaneous, intravenous, or rectal. The administration of 2 mg equals 8 to 10 mg of morphine; the effect is also rapidly obtained (10 to 20 minutes) and lasts some hours. The dose by the rectal route is 3 mg. When administered intravenously, the injection should be given very slowly.

The medication is available for prescription under the following forms:

> Dihydromorphinone hydrochloride, tablets, containing 1, 2, 3, or 4 mg per tablet.
>
> Dihydromorphinone hydrochloride, injectables, containing 2, 3, or 4 mg per 1-ml ampul. Also, disposable syringe containing 2 mg and vials containing 10 or 20 ml (2 mg per ml) are available.
>
> Dihydromorphinone hydrochloride, suppositories, containing 3 mg per suppository.

Oxymorphone (Numorphan)

A synthetic narcotic analgesic, chemically related to dihydromorphinone, is 1-14-hydroxydihydromorphinone, a water-soluble, white crystalline powder corresponding to the structural formula, as the hydrochloride:

[structural formula of oxymorphone hydrochloride]

It is more potent than morphine; since it is absorbed rapidly, the analgesic effect starts about 5 to 10 minutes after injection, and lasts from 3 to 6 hours. Little or no sedation is obtained, nor does depression of cough reflex occur. Side effects are similar to those of dihydromorphinone.

The drug is recommended for the same purposes as morphine or dihydromorphinone, at a dosage of 10 mg every 4 to 6 hours by mouth; or 2 to 5 mg in suppositories, also every 4 to 6 hours; or by intramuscular or subcutaneous injection, 1 to 1.5 mg every 4 to 6 hours; or intravenously, 0.5 mg as initial dose. Contraindications are essentially the same as with similar drugs.

Oxymorphone is available in the following forms:

Oxymorphone, tablets, containing 10 mg;

Oxymorphone, suppositories, containing 2 or 5 mg;

Oxymorphone, injectable, containing 1 mg per ml in 1- and 1.5-ml ampuls or 15-ml vials;

Oxymorphone, injectable, containing 1.5 mg per ml in 1- and 2-ml ampuls or 10-ml vials.

Codeine (Methylmorphine)

Codeine is closely related to morphine, and is obtained by methylation of the drug. It is used in the form of the free alkaloid or its phosphate or sulfate salts, the phosphate being more soluble and more suitable for pharmacological preparations. The structural formula is:

10 PHARMACOLOGY OF DRUGS USED TO COMBAT PAIN

$$CH_3N \quad CH_2 \quad CH_2$$

$$OCH_3$$

$$OH \qquad H_3PO_4$$

Codeine is similar to morphine, but markedly weaker and less habit-forming (not used by addicts). It is mainly used as an antitussive medicament and, together with nonnarcotic analgesics, is used for the treatment of mild to moderate pain. For this purpose, a dose of 15 to 60 mg is usually effective (if a dose of 60 mg does not allay pain, larger doses will also fail). The route of administration may be either the oral or the parenteral. As morphine, it is rapidly absorbed by any route, but the analgesic effect only lasts for 3 to 4 hours. As with morphine, codeine causes addiction, though its toxicity is much less.

For therapeutic purposes, small, repeated doses, of 15 to 30 mg, are recommended. Infants (6–12 months of age) will take less than 15 mg; up to 3 years, 15 mg; up to 12 years, 30 mg. The treatment of cough requires even smaller doses—from 5 to 10 mg.

The available preparations for medical prescription are the following:

Codeine phosphate, tablets, containing 15, 30, or 60 mg.

Codeine phosphate, capsules, containing 15, 30, or 60 mg.

Codeine phosphate, injectables, containing 15 mg, 30, or 60 mg in 1-ml ampuls, or 30 mg per ml in 20-ml vials.

Papaverine

Just as morphine is the representative opium alkaloid pertaining to the phenanthrene group, papaverine is the principal benzylisoquinoline. It is a white powder, without odor but slightly bitter. Its crystals are soluble in water, and correspond to the following structural formula:

[Chemical structure of papaverine: dimethoxyisoquinoline connected via CH₂ to a dimethoxybenzene ring]

The absorption of papaverine seems to be relatively rapid, though there is very little known about its metabolism and excretion; on the other hand, its toxicity appears to be low, since doses several times the therapeutic range can be given without provoking undesirable effects. Nevertheless, the rapid administration of the drug by the intravenous route may result in cardiac arrhythmias and even death. Other side effects may include gastrointestinal distress, drowsiness, malaise, sweating, and headache, which may force the patient to stop the medication. To minimize the untoward reactions to injected papaverine, it should be diluted (isotonic saline or glucose) and forced very slowly into the vein (100 mg in 5 to 10 minutes).

The principal pharmacological effects of papaverine are exerted on the smooth muscle (including the heart). On the heart, it depresses conduction and prolongs the refractory time. In general, all smooth muscles are relaxed by the drug (antispasmodic direct effect). Papaverine does not produce analgesia, but it may alleviate pain indirectly by relaxation of contracted muscles in cases of colic (biliary, urinary, gastrointestinal) or relaxation of contracted blood vessels (myocardial infarction, mesenteric thrombosis, pulmonary infarction, peripheral arterial embolism).

Papaverine has been recommended for the treatment of biliary and renal colic, and for the treatment of asthma, but it has not gained wide acceptance in these fields. Its main use refers to the treatment of angina pectoris and myocardial infarction, peripheral arterial embolism, pulmonary embolism, mesenteric thrombosis, cerebral thrombosis, and impaired circulation to the brain (vascular encephalopathy associated with vasopasm).

The usual dose is 100 mg to be repeated three to five times a day, or even more (with due caution) if required. The oral dose may reach 200 mg, also three to five times a day. The injected dosage should not exceed 100 mg per dose. We repeat that the intravenous administration should be slow, using a dilute solution.

Better results are said to be obtained with the addition of atropine (1 mg) in cases of pulmonary embolism, and in association with digitalis and quinidine whenever these drugs are indicated.

Papaverine is available for therapeutic use under the following pharmaceutical forms:

> Papaverine hydrochloride, tablets, containing 30, 60, 90, 100, 180, or 200 mg per tablet;
>
> Papaverine hydrochloride, capsules (Cerespan), containing 150 mg in each sustained-release capsule;
>
> Papaverine hydrochloride, injectable, containing 30 mg per ml in 1- or 2-ml ampuls, or 10-ml vials; or 60 mg per ml in 2-ml ampuls;
>
> Papaverine hydrochloride, powder, in bottles containing 1, 4, or 5 oz, for individualized prescriptions.

Dioxyline (Paveril)

Dioxyline, 6,7-dimethoxy-1-(4'-ethoxy-3'-methoxybenzyl)-3-methylisoquinoline, is a derivative of papaverine corresponding to the formula:

Both the phosphate and the hydrochloride occur in crystals soluble in water (the phosphate is more soluble).

The absorption seems to be rapid, as with papaverine, but it is known that it is degraded in the liver, mainly, and excreted in the urine.

The effects of dioxyline are identical with papaverine, though the drug appears to be less toxic and to provoke milder and less frequent side effects of the same nature as with papaverine.

It is recommended for the treatment of angina pectoris and myocardial infarction, arterial thrombosis (pulmonary and peripheral) and other arterial diseases due to vasospasm.

The suggested dosage is 200 to 300 mg per dose, three to four times a day, by the oral route. The pharmaceutical forms available are:

> Dioxyline phosphate, tablets, containing 100 or 200 mg per tablet.

Meperidine (Demerol)

Meperidine is ethyl-1-methyl-4-phenylpiperidine-4-carboxylate, crystalline white powder, slightly bitter to taste, soluble in water as the hydrochloride, which shares pharmaceutical properties corresponding to both morphine and atropine, and corresponds to the structural formula (as the hydrochloride):

$$\text{structure} \quad COOC_2H_5 \quad \cdot HCl \quad CH_3$$

The main effects of meperidine are analgesic and antispasmodic, useful principally against pain of spastic origin. It has also some euphoric and sedative effects, and may lead to addiction.

Absorption from the gastrointestinal tract and the subcutaneous tissues is rapid; its effects are noted in from 20 to 60 minutes (oral) or 15 minutes (subcutaneous injection), lasting for only 3 hours since the drug is rapidly metabolized (particularly in the liver) and excreted, thus causing few accumulation symptoms.

Dizziness is the most important side effect, and frequently, dryness of the mouth, sweating, and flushing of the face. Most of these side reactions are minor and transient, and occur more frequently in the ambulatory patient. Nausea, vomiting, respiratory depression, tremors, incoordination, blurring of vision, and syncope rarely occur. Overdosage may provoke cerebral excitation. Because of its vasodilating effect, it may exaggerate symptoms of hypotension and shock.

Prolonged administration may cause tolerance and addiction.

Both effects are by far less marked than with morphine and other opiates.

The pharmacological effects of meperidine are relaxation of the smooth muscle of the lower gastrointestinal tract, the bronchi, the urinary bladder, and the uterus. Contrariwise, it may provoke contraction of the upper gastrointestinal tract and the gall bladder. On account of these effects, meperidine is recommended for the treatment of pain of the lower gastrointestinal tract, the urinary bladder, or the uterus, when it is due to spasm of the smooth musculature of these organs. Also, it is used before and after surgery, and to induce obstetrical analgesia. Meperidine very rarely provokes respiratory depression, but if this occurs, particularly in the newborn, the use of nalorphine as an antidote is indicated.

The administration of meperidine may be by either the oral, the parenteral, and even the intravenous route. Usually, a dose of 100 mg is effective, but it may range from 50 to 150 mg. A dose of 25 mg may be useful in some instances. Infants should receive 1.5 mg per kg. Amounts over 200 mg per dose should not be used.

The drug is available for prescription in the following forms:

Meperidine hydrochloride, tablets, containing 50 or 100 mg per tablet;

Meperidine hydrochloride, elixir, containing 50 mg per teaspoonful;

Meperidine hydrochloride, powder, in bottles containing 15 g, for individual prescriptions;

Meperidine hydrochloride, injectables, containing 50 mg per ml, in ampuls of 1, 1½, and 2 ml, and in 10-, 20-, or 30-ml vials;

Meperidine hydrochloride, injectable, containing 75 mg per ml, in disposable units;

Meperidine hydrochloride, injectable, containing 100 mg in 1-ml ampuls or disposable units, and in 10- or 20-ml vials.

Meperidine is marketed in combination with other medications, as tablets also containing acetylsalicylic acid, acetophenetidin, and caffeine; and in injectables containing atropine or scopolamine.

Methadone (Dolophine)

Methadone is 4,4-diphenyl-6-dimethylamino-3-heptanone, a crystalline white powder, bitter to taste and soluble in water and alcohol. The structural formula of its hydrochloride is:

$$\text{(C}_6\text{H}_5\text{)}_2\text{C}(\text{COC}_2\text{H}_5)\text{CH}_2\text{—CH(CH}_3\text{)—N(CH}_3\text{)}_2 \cdot \text{HCl}$$

The effects of methadone are essentially similar to those of morphine, the differences being only quantitative, which fact is the basis for its therapeutic applications.

Absorption is rapid from tissues, but less complete from the gastrointestinal tract. It is also rapidly degraded and excreted. Analgesia is obtained in less than 15 minutes (injection) or 30 minutes (oral), and lasts as much as with morphine.

The pharmacological action is entirely similar to that of morphine, as are also the side effects and toxicity (q.v.).

Methadone is recommended in painful, chronic conditions. It is less effective than morphine for the induction of sedation, for which reason it is not so widely recommended for preanesthetic medication. It is also a good antitussive medication.

Methadone has been in wide use recently in the treatment of drug addiction. Since it has an action similar to that of morphine, it is satisfying to the addict and can be substituted for a narcotic drug. Although it has similar addictive properties, it appears easier to break the habit. Substitute doses should start at the minimum acceptable amount and be steadily reduced.

The dosage is 5 to 15 mg per dose by the oral route, and a little less when given by injection. Doses may be repeated three or four times a day, only when needed. Large doses given by injection are irritating.

The medication is available for prescription under the following forms:

Methadone hydrochloride, tablets, containing 2.5, 5, 7.5, and 10 mg;

Methadone hydrochloride, elixir, containing 5 mg per teaspoonful in 4 cc;

Methadone hydrochloride, syrup, containing 1.7 mg in 4 cc;

Methadone hydrochloride, injectable, containing 10 mg per ml, in 1-ml ampuls and 20-ml vials;

Methadone hydrochloride, suppositories, containing 10 mg.

Alphaprodine (Nisentil)

Closely related to meperidine, alphaprodine is 1,3-dimethyl-4-phenyl-4-propionoxypiperidine, a crystalline white powder, bitter to taste, freely soluble in water, and corresponding to the following structural formula (as the hydrochloride):

Its analgesic power is intermediate between morphine and meperidine, its onset of action is relatively rapid, but the duration of effect is shorter than with other analgesics.

Alphaprodine is particularly used for analgesia in obstetrics, surgery, and minor procedures in surgical specialties (diagnostic and therapeutic procedures). It is contraindicated in status asthmaticus and in injuries to the head. Respiratory depression and other morphine side effects may occur with alphaprodine.

Regular dosages are 40 to 60 mg by injection, the dose repeated every 2 hours if needed. By the intravenous route, smaller doses are given (20 to 30 mg).

The medication is available for prescription in the following preparations:

Alphaprodine hydrochloride, injectable, containing 40 or 60 mg per ml in 1-ml ampuls. There are 10-ml vials with 60 mg per ml.

Anileridine (Leritine)

Anileridine dihydrochloride occurs in crystals that are freely soluble in water and less soluble in ethanol or methanol, and corresponds to the formula:

$$H_2N-\text{C}_6H_4-CH_2CH_2-N\underset{\diagdown}{\overset{\diagup}{\text{C}_5H_9N}}\Big\langle \begin{array}{l} COOC_2H_5 \\ C_6H_5 \end{array} \cdot 2HCl$$

This derivative of meperidine has only one-fourth of the analgesic potency of morphine; the effect is manifest in 10 to 30 minutes and lasts about 2 hours after intramuscular injection. In all other respects, the similarities of morphine and anileridine are about the same.

Anileridine is recommended in angina pectoris, colic (biliary and renal), cancer, trauma, and surgery. Also, it is used in pre- and postsurgery, in obstetrics (labor analgesia), and for the relief of apprehension in acute congestive heart failure. Cautions and contraindications are as with other narcotic analgesics.

The oral dose is 25 to 50 mg every 6 hours. By injection, 25 to 75 mg may be given every 4 to 6 hours by the intramuscular route. For surgery and obstetrics special dosages are recommended.

The medication is available for prescription in the following preparations:

> Anileridine dihydrochloride, tablets, containing 25 mg;
>
> Anileridine phosphate, injectable, containing 25 mg per ml in 1- or 2-ml ampuls, and in 30-ml vials.

Phenazocine (Primadol)

Phenazocine is also a benzomorphan derivative, 1,2,3,4,5,6-hexahydro-6,11-dimethyl-3-phenthyl-2,6-methano-3-benzazocin-8-ol; a white powder soluble in alcohol and only slightly soluble in water. It corresponds to the following structural formula:

Subject to narcotic regulations, it is used for injection as the hydrobromide.

On a weight basis, as an analgesic, it appears to be more potent than morphine (three or four times), but produces only light sedation. It is rapidly absorbed, the onset of action being apparent within 15 minutes (or less if injected intravenously), and the effects last for about 4 hours. It causes less addiction and less side effects than morphine, but respiratory depression, hypotension, bradycardia, headache, and gastrointestinal symptoms may appear. Toxic symptoms of the narcotic type are antagonized by levallorphan and by nalorphine.

Phenazocine has been advised as a substitute for morphine in acute or chronic pain; also, pre-operatively, in obstetrics, and for lessening withdrawal symptoms in the treatment of narcotic addiction. It is contraindicated in patients with central nervous system depression (coma included), intracranial hyperpressure, hepatic insufficiency, alcoholism, and symptoms due to other depressant drugs.

The recommended dosage is from 1 to 3 mg (average, 2 mg), by intramuscular injection, repeated every 4 to 6 hours. The daily total dosage should not be over 12 mg. It can be used preoperatively and in obstetrics or anesthetic procedures. The drug is available as:

Pentazocine hydrobromide, injection, containing 2 mg per ml, in 1-ml ampuls and 10-ml vials.

Analgesics Not Requiring Narcotic Prescription

Propoxyphene Hydrochloride (Darvon). A synthetic, nonnarcotic (that is, not requiring the official narcotic prescription) related to methadone. It is 4-dimethylamino-3-methyl-1,2-diphenyl-2-butanol propionate hydrochloride and occurs as a white crystalline powder, slightly bitter, soluble in water, and corresponds to the formula:

$$\left[\text{C}_6\text{H}_5\text{—CH}_2\text{—}\underset{\underset{\text{C}_6\text{H}_5}{|}}{\overset{\overset{\text{OOC—CH}_2\text{CH}_3}{|}}{\text{C}}}\text{—CH(CH}_3)\text{—CH}_2\text{—NH(CH}_3)_2 \right] \text{Cl}$$

Propoxyphene is easily and rapidly absorbed from the gastrointestinal tract; once passed into the blood it is demethylated in the liver, and excreted in the urine.

A regular dose of propoxyphene produces analgesic effects for about 6 hours. The principal charcteristic of the drug is that it does not cause respiratory depression or tolerance, but it can cause addiction.

Side effects are ordinarily mild and of little consequence. Nausea, vomiting, drowsiness, dizziness, or hypersensitivity reactions can occur. Only the ingestion of large amounts will cause coma, circulatory and respiratory depression, or convulsions. The remedy would be morphine antidotes (levallorphan and nalorphine) and supportive therapy (gastric lavage, oxygen inhalation).

Propoxyphene is an analgesic somewhat less potent than codeine (65 mg equals 30 to 45 mg of codeine, or 325 to 650 mg (one or two tablets) of acetyl salicylic acid) but also less inductive of side effects than codeine when given at low dosages. It is recommended for the treatment of aches and pains, such as headache, migraine, toothache, dysmenorrhea, arthritis, fibrositis, hemorrhoidal, and postpartum discomfort.

Because it is irritant to the subcutaneous and muscular tissues, propoxyphene is only given by mouth at a dosage of 65 mg four times a day. The 32-mg dose is not constantly better than a placebo, in well-controlled trials.

It is to be noted that the combination of propoxyphene with acetylsalicylic acid may show a greater analgesic potency than either drug alone. It can be tried when the usual doses of acetylsalicylic acid or acetaminophen are not tolerated or are not effective.

The available pharmaceutical preparation for use in prescriptions is:

Propoxyphene capsules, containing 32 or 65 mg.

There are also available other pharmaceutical forms in which propoxyphene is used together with acetylsalicylic acid, alone or with acetophenetidin and caffeine.

Pentazocine (Talwin) is a benzazocine or benzomorphan, namely, 1,2,3,4,5,6-hexahydro-*cis*-6,11-dimethyl-3-(3-methyl-2-butenyl)-2,6-methano-3-benzazocin-8-ol, a white crystalline substance soluble in acid water solutions, which corresponds to the structural formula:

$$\text{[aromatic bicyclic ring with OH, CH}_3\text{, CH}_3\text{]}-N-CH_2-CH=C\begin{cases}CH_3\\CH_3\end{cases}$$
with $-CH_3$ on N

It is used as the lactate for injections, and as the hydrochloride in tablets.

The absorption of the drug is very rapid, analgesia being obtained within 3 minutes after intravenous injection, or within 15 to 20 minutes following intramuscular or subcutaneous injection. When it is given by the oral route, the analgesic effect is manifest in 15 to 30 minutes. It is rapidly excreted in the urine and feces. Analgesia lasts for about 3 hours.

According to most authorities, the analgesic potency of pentazocine is not superior to other analgesics when the medications are given at their own adequate dosage (50 mg pentazocine, 60 mg codeine, 600 mg acetylsalicylic acid). It is listed as a nonnarcotic drug, but in some instances it may cause addiction and may also induce withdrawal symptoms.

No matter that the depression of the central nervous system, particularly respiratory, is slight, its use should be followed with caution in cases of head injury, increased intracranial pressure, or any brain condition in which clouding of the sensorium could lead to dangerous situations. Care should be taken if the patient drives a car, works with dangerous machinery, suffers from respiratory depression or obstruction, as in asthma, has myocardial injury, or is contemplating surgery.

The manufacturers recommend the drug for the treatment of all types and degrees of pain, and as a substitute for morphine or its analogues. Nevertheless, medical authorities state that it is only advisable in cases of chronic pain not relieved by codeine or nonnarcotic analgesics. On the other hand, it has a shorter duration of action than other analgesics, and the side effects, though milder, are like those produced by codeine or other narcotic analgesics. Consequently, it is used for pain due to trauma, acute and chronic medical and surgical conditions, obstetrical discomfort, urological procedures, and the like.

The available pharmaceutical preparations for prescription are the following:

Pentazocine lactate, injectable, containing 30 mg per ml in ampuls of 1, 1½ or 2 ml, or in 10-ml vials;

Pentazocine hydrochloride, tablets, containing 50 mg per tablet.

Ethoheptazine (Zactane) is used as the ethylhexahydro-1-methyl-4-phenylazeptine-4-carboxylate citrate, and corresponds to the structural formula:

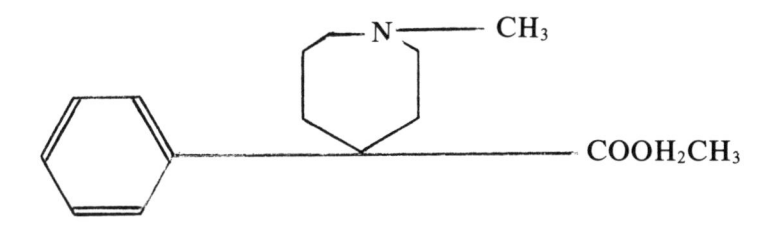

$$\text{Structure: phenyl—azepane ring with N—CH}_3\text{ and COOH}_2\text{CH}_3$$

This drug possesses a weaker analgesic action than codeine, but does not suppress cough. Both absorption and excretion are rapid, and the side effects are almost negligible.

As with the weaker analgesics, it may be used alone, but preferably is used in combination with acetylsalicylic acid, for the treatment of mild to moderate pain, low back pain, bursitis, dental, and other moderate pains. The usual dosage is 150 mg three or four times a day. The drug is available as:

Ethoheptazine, tablets, containing 75 mg;

Ethoheptazine with acetylsalicylic acid, tablets, containing 75 mg of the former and 325 mg of the latter.

Indomethacin (Indocin). Chemically, indomethacin differs from both corticoids and salicylates in spite of its possessing antiinflammatory, antipyretic, and analgesic properties. Its formula is:

Absorption is prompt from the gastrointestinal tract, and when it is given at the recommended dosage, it will not accumulate in tissues. The drug has been advised for the treatment of patients with rheumatoid arthritis, ankylosing spondylitis, osteoarthritis of the hip, and gout. According to some authorities, it is no more effective than acetylsalicylic acid when given at comparative doses, and should be reserved for those who do not tolerate acetylsalicylic acid. In some patients a combination of acetylsalicylic acid with indomethacin proved to be better than either drug alone. On the other hand, it has been stated that indomethacin is equally effective and less risky than phenylbutazone for the treatment of ankylosing spondylitis. Also, it seems to be less hazardous than corticoids, gold, and other drugs used for the treatment of rheumatic diseases. The control of gout attacks is said to be rapid and often dramatic (pain controlled in 2 to 4 hours). It can be used for the treatment of chronic gout, together with a uricosuric agent.

Children should not be treated with indomethacin, nor should patients with active or latent peptic ulcer, ulcerative colitis, regional enteritis, asthma sensitive to acetylsalicylic acid, epilepsy, parkinsonism, nervous diseases that could cause dizziness, and other conditions in which corticoids are contraindicated. Side effects are about the same as those caused by the aforementioned drugs.

The recommended dosage varies from 25 mg two or three times a day, up to a total of 200 mg a day. Larger doses will not be more effective. In all instances, the amount of medication to be given should be adjusted to each particular patient. Prolonged medication with 25 mg twice a day is usually well tolerated.

Indomethacin is available under the following pharmaceutical form:

Indomethacin, capsules, containing 25 or 50 mg.

II. SALICYLATES

Acetylsalicylic Acid (Aspirin)

The acetic acid ester of salicylic acid occurs as a crystalline powder, little soluble in water, odorless but acid in taste. It is not totally stable (hydrolyzes to salicylic and acetic acids) and corresponds to the following structural formula:

The absorption of acetylsalicylic acid is very rapid, though less rapid than for other salicylates. It is also rapidly excreted in the urine, the analgesic and antipyretic effects lasting for only 4 hours.

It has an antipyretic effect when the body temperature is elevated, because of some sort of "resetting" to normal of the regulatory nervous mechanism of temperature in the hypothalamus. It has little or no action on normal body temperature. Also, because of a central depressed activity, the drug has a notable analgesic effect, more marked against integumental than against visceral pain. It does not cause any anesthesia or other mental change when given at therapeutic dosages. Of course, the analgesic effect is inferior to that of codeine. When given in large doses, as those used in rheumatic fever, it may cause hyperventilatòjn, thus leading to alkalosis first, and then to acidosis. It has also an action upon gout pain, because of its uricosuric effect, but large doses are required for a useful treatment of gout. An antiinflammatory effect, in addition to analgesia, may explain the good therapeutic activity of acetylsalicylic acid against rheumatic fever.

Because of the above reasons, acetylsalicylic acid is recommended for the treatment of headache, arthritis, dysmenorrhea, neuralgia, and other painful conditions, as well as for the symptomatic relief of fever and the miseries of a common cold (which course it cannot modify). Only large amounts, if tolerated, are effective for the treatment of rheumatic fever and gout.

Intolerance to acetylsalicylic acid is frequently found among patients taking the medication: gastrointestinal upsets (nausea and even vomiting), urticaria, and edema. Salicylism is the intoxication produced by salicylates, including acetylsalicylic acid. The well-known symptoms of salicylism are ringing of the ears, gastrointestinal distress, sweating, and, on some occasions, mental confusion. The administration of sodium lactate may allay the symptoms of salicylism, and at the same time decreases the concentration of salicylate in the blood.

The usual dose of acetylsalicylic acid is 300 to 600 mg by mouth, repeated every 2 to 4 hours. Children should receive 80 mg per kg per day, in four or more divided doses. This dosage schedule covers the treatment of moderate pain. In case of gout or acute rheumatic fever the dose may be increased to 5, 10, or even more g a day to start with, and then reduced for maintenance, to 6 g a day, in divided doses, always given after meals. The concomitant administration of sodium bicarbonate (to counter the drug's acidity) requires the use of larger doses to compensate for the increased excretion. Tablets containing buffers, or coated for intestinal release of the drug, are also recommended to avoid gastric irritation.

The medication may be prescribed in any of the following preparations:

> Acetylsalicylic acid, tablets, containing 60, 75, or 300 mg;
>
> Acetylsalicylic acid, buffered tablets, containing 300 mg;
>
> Acetylsalicylic acid, enteric coated tablets, containing 300 or 600 mg;
>
> Acetylsalicylic acid, capsules, containing 300 or 600 mg;
>
> Acetylsalicylic acid, suppositories, containing 60, 200, 300, or 600 mg.

Compounds of acetylsalicylic acid containing other medications are innumerable, and perhaps represent item number one of over-the-counter (OTC) preparations. They are not to be disregarded, because some benefit might be obtained from them in special instances. The combination of acetylsalicylic acid (ASA) with caffeine is well known. There are also other familiar combinations, such as ASA with acetophenetidin, or codeine, or even meperidine. As a general indication of the broad purpose of these preparations, we will mention a few:

> ASA, 300 mg with chloropheniramine maleate, 2 mg and caffeine, 30 mg (Coricidin, Schering, tablets), to take four tablets a day;

> ASA, 325 mg together with propoxyphene hydrochloride, 65 mg (Darvon with ASA, Lilly), pulvules, to take three or four a day;

> ASA, 300 mg together with prednisolone, 0.5 mg (Cordex, Upjohn) or prednisolone, 1.5 mg (Cordex-Forte), both either in plain tablets or buffered, to take one or two tablets, four times a day;

> ASA, 200 mg together with peperidine hydrochloride, 30 mg, phenacetin, 150 mg, and caffeine, 30 mg (APC with Demerol tablets, Winthrop), take one or two tablets, three or four times a day.

Sodium Salicylate

The sodium salt of salicylic acid occurs as a white powder, or crystals (becomes pinkish when exposed to light for a long period of time), readily soluble in water, and a little less in alcohol and in glycerol, and corresponds to the structural formula:

This salt is rapidly absorbed from the gastrointestinal tract, reaching high blood concentration in less than 2 hours. It is widely distributed in the body to all tissues, and binds to plasma proteins in a considerable proportion. Excretion occurs rapidly, principally in the urine, but also in sweat and saliva, and is hastened by alkalies, such as sodium bicarbonate, which also lowers its blood concentration.

Intolerance to sodium salicylate is mainly shown by gastric distress, which may be due to the local action of the drug when it closely follows its administration, or to a central effect, when the distress is delayed. Salicylism may also occur with sodium salicylate, provoking the habitual symptomatology (nausea, vomiting, ringing in the ears, sweating, and even psychoneurological complaints).

For analgesia in common pain, the usual dosage is 300 mg orally, every 3 or 4 hours. In cases of more severe pain the dosage may be increased to 1 g every 3 or 4 hours.

For the treatment of acute rheumatic fever, the dosage is up to 15 g a day, also orally, in divided doses every 4 hours. The drug may be given by injection, a route rarely employed. Tolerance to salicylates is probably increased by giving small doses of thyroid extract (30 mg) at the same time.

To obtain a better tolerance of this irritant drug, sodium bicarbonate or aluminum hydroxide gel should be used concommitantly. Enteric coated tablets may also be given. When the intolerance is central, the local acting antacids or coating are useless.

Because of the tendency of salicylates to reduce blood prothrombin after prolonged use, menadione (1 mg per g of sodium salicylate) should be added to avoid hemorrhagic complications.

The prescription of sodium salicylate may follow the following suggestions:

> Sodium salicylate, tablets, containing 300, 500, or 600 mg;
>
> Sodium salicylate, enteric coated tablets, containing 300, 500, or 600 mg;
>
> Sodium salicylate, injection, containing 200 mg per ml in 5-ml ampuls or 10-ml vials.

Methylsalicylate (Oil of Wintergreen)

Methylsalicylate is an oily liquid, colorless, reddish, or yellowish, with odor and taste of gaultheria, the wintergreen plant. It is only slightly soluble in ether and miscible with alcohol. The structural formula is:

$$\text{methyl salicylate: benzene ring with COOCH}_3 \text{ and OH ortho substituents}$$

For pains of muscles and joints, methylsalicylate is used topically as a counterirritant, diluted in olive oil or incorporated in salves, ointments, and liniments. Most probably it acts locally rather than systemically, even though there is a substantial absorption of the drug.

The drug is obtainable as:

> Methylsalicylate (oil of wintergreen), liquid, in bottles containing 500 cc or 2.5 liters for individualized prescriptions.

Salicylamide

Salicylamide is a salicylate derivative which occurs as a crystalline powder, white or slightly pink, with bitter taste and a sensation of warmth on the tongue, soluble in water and other solvents, and corresponding to the following structural formula:

$$\text{salicylamide: benzene ring with CONH}_2 \text{ and OH ortho substituents}$$

It is said that its analgesic and antipyretic properties are at least equal to if not greater than those of other salicylates. The absorption from the gastrointestinal tract is rapid; also, it is rapidly bound to plasma proteins and thereafter excreted in the urine, the effects lasting 6 hours or less. The toxic effects are similar to those of other salicylates, causing death by depression of the central nervous system with stoppage of respiration or cardiac. On the other hand, it is less irritant to the gastrointestinal mucosa.

Doses of 2 g every 4 to 8 hours are recommended for rheumatic conditions, including rheumatic fever.

Salicylamide is available for prescription in the following forms:

Salicylamide, tablets, containing 300 mg;

Salicylamide, powder, in bottles containing 120 g;

0.5 or 2.5 kg for individualized prescriptions.

Salicylsalicylic Acid

Salicylsalicylic acid is a white crystalline powder, soluble in alcohol and in alkaline solutions, but not in water, corresponding to the structural formula:

It is absorbed in the form of salicylic acid, two molecules formed from each one of salicylsalicylic acid. The change occurs mainly in the intestines, not in the stomach, because of its poor solubility in water or in acid media. It is slowly hydrolyzed, for which reason salicylsalicylic acid shows retarded and prolonged action. Also, its excretion is slow.

The average dosage is 300 to 600 mg twice or three times a day. Except rarely, it is given together with aspirin, as in the formula below, one tablet after each meal and at bedtime, for patients weighing up to 80 kg; and the same daily dosage with two tablets at night for patients over 80 kg. For night pains, three tablets are recommended.

The drug is available in the following form:

Salicylsalicylic acid, tablets, containing 485 mg together with 160 mg acetylsalicylic acid.

III. COAL-TAR DERIVATIVES

Acetophenetidin (Phenacetin)

Acetophenetidin is a white crystalline powder; almost insoluble in water, and has the following structural formula:

$$\underset{\text{NHCOCH}_3}{\overset{\text{OC}_2\text{H}_5}{\text{C}_6\text{H}_4}}$$

Taken by mouth, acetophenetidin is rapidly absorbed from the gastrointestinal tract. Peak concentrations in the blood occur 1 to 2 hours after ingestion, and the drug is metabolized in about 5 hours, conjugated with glucuronic and sulfuric acids, and oxidized to acetylparaaminophenol, in which form it is excreted in the urine, giving it a dark brown or wine color. The effects last for about 3 hours.

Antipyresis and analgesia are the main pharmacological activities of acetophenetidin, the latter probably due to its metabolite, acetylparaaminophenol. The drug is not frequently recommended for elevated temperature, but is useful for headache, migraine, dysmenorrhea, joint and muscle pains, peripheral nerve irritation, and other mild discomforts. It is not the best remedy for pains due to smooth muscle spasm such as intestinal, biliary, or renal colic.

Every 3 hours, a dose of 300 mg is given according to the average practice, but smaller doses at shorter intervals may be equally effective and less toxic. Larger doses of 600 mg may be given, but only for short periods of time; otherwise, intoxication might occur. In acute poisoning, there is a cyanotic color due to the formation of methemoglobin and sulfhemoglobin, dyspnea, vertigo, and anginal pain, progressing to circulatory failure, collapse, shock, coma, and death. Chronic poisoning also results in cyanosis and dyspnea. In acute poisoning the treatment consists of stomach lavage, blood transfusion, and inhalation of oxygen. In chronic poisoning, stop the drug and give supportive therapy.

Acetophenetidin is available for prescription in the following preparations, and also in innumerable over-the-counter remedies.

Acetophenetidin, tablets, containing 120, 200, or 300 mg;

Acetophenetidin, tablets, containing 150 mg together with acetylsalicylic acid, 230 mg and caffeine, 30 mg.

Acetaminophen

Several manufacturers market acetaminophen under different trade names (Tempra, Tylenol, Apamide, etc.). Acetaminophen is acetylparaaminophenol, a synthetic product closely related to acetophenetidin; it occurs as colorless crystals or a white powder, slightly bitter to taste, soluble in hot water and in alcohol, and corresponds to the structural formula:

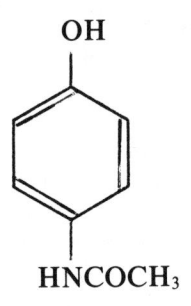

OH

HNCOCH$_3$

The absorption of acetaminophen is rapid from the gastrointestinal tract, exerting its analgesic and antipyretic action in 15 to 30 minutes. The analgesic and antipyretic action of acetophenetidin and acetanilid seems to be due to their metabolic conversion to acetylparaaminophenol (acetaminophen). When it is given as acetaminophen, the effects last for 2 to 3 hours, and the final excretion occurs in the urine, mainly conjugated with glucuronic or sulfuric acid.

Only moderate pain will respond to acetaminophen, such as headache, migraine, dysmenorrhea, myalgia, arthralgia, and similar discomforts.

Rarely, the drug is used as such. Then, the dosage is 60 mg for infants; up to 250 mg for older children; and 300 to 600 mg for adults, always every 4 hours. Each trade name requires a dosage schedule in accordance with the manufacturer's instructions.

Acetaminophen is available as tablets and oral liquid:

Acetaminophen, tablets, containing 300 mg (also, effervescent tablets of same dosage);

Acetaminophen, liquid, containing 120 mg per 5 ml (1 teaspoonful), or as solution of 100 mg per ml.

IV. PYRAZOLON DERIVATIVES

Antipyrine

Antipyrine is a pyrazolon derivative, soluble in water, and occurs as an odorless white powder. It was widely used in the past but is not so frequently used now. Its structural formula is:

$$\text{structural formula of antipyrine}$$

It is rapidly absorbed from the gastrointestinal tract, attaining its maximal blood concentration in 2 hours. Slowly metabolized, it changes into hydroxyantipyrine, which is conjugated with glucuronic acid for its excretion in the urine, which becomes red. Analgesia is maintained for at least 4 hours after an average dose.

Analgesia and antipyresis are the main effects of antipyrin, in which respects the drug resembles the salicylates. It has other effects, such as to induce a mild local anesthesia and antisepsis as a gargle, but these effects are almost useless for therapeutic purposes. With antipyrine, analgesia seems to be somewhat more prolonged than with salicylates (?).

Skin eruptions are frequent with antipyrine, but only rarely does it affect the blood.

Average doses are 300 mg once or twice every 4 hours, under the following form:

Antipyrine, tablets, containing 300 mg.

Aminopyrine (Pyramidon)

A dimethylamino derivative of antipyrine, aminopyrine occurs as a white, odorless, crystalline powder, soluble in water. Its structural formula is:

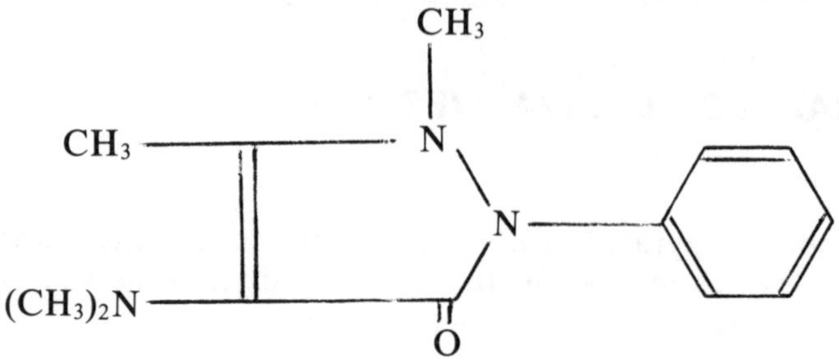

The properties of aminopyrine are almost identical with those of antipyrine (q.v.), the principal difference and the more important disadvantage being its agranulocytic effect, though it is only rarely encountered in medical practice.

Dosage is the same, namely, 300 to 600 mg every 4 hours. It is available as:

Aminopyrine, tablets, containing 300 mg.

Phenylbutazone (Butazolidin)

This pyrazol derivative, 4-butyl-1,2-diphenyl-3,5-pyrazolidinedione, occurs as a bitter powder, white or yellowish, with a slight aromatic odor, soluble in alcohol, only slightly soluble in water (more soluble, the sodium salt), and corresponds to the formula:

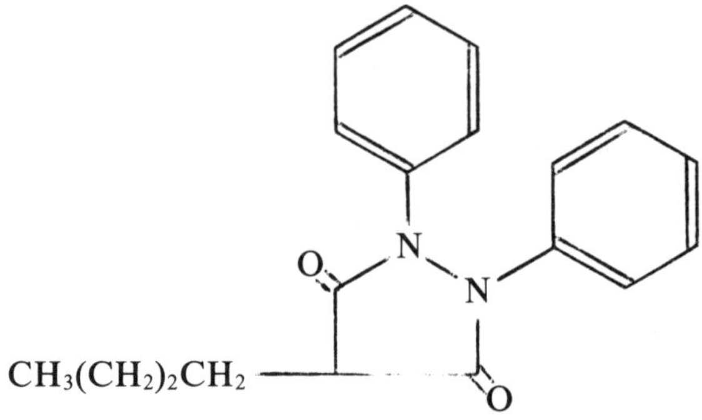

Phenylbutazone is rapidly absorbed from the gastrointestinal tract (it is not used by injection), but its blood concentration only increases over a period of about 3 days, until it reaches a stable level. It is bound to plasma proteins to a considerable extent. The metabolism is slow, and so is the excretion in the urine, in which different metabolites are found. Detectable pyrazolon remains in the blood until 1 week after its intake is discontinued.

The main pharmacologic effects of phenylbutazone are anti-inflammatory, analgesic, and antipyretic; consequently, the principal uses are for the treatment of arthritis, particularly of the gouty or rheumatoid variety, ankylosing spondylitis, psoriatic arthritis, and osteoarthritis. In osteoarthritis, phenylbutazone is used only for acute exacerbations not responsive to other adequate medication. The drug has also been employed for the treatment of post-traumatic inflammations (including surgery), acute superficial thrombophlebitis, cancer, Hodgkin's disease, inflammatory ocular conditions, and other conditions on an experimental basis.

Because phenylbutazone may cause severe blood dyscrasias (thrombocytopenic purpura, leukopenia, or agranulocytosis) or less severe complications (gastrointestinal distress, and even hepatitis, rashes, pruritus, polyuria, nervous symptoms, and so forth) following its use, it should be reserved only for selected cases not responding to usual therapy.

Care should be taken when giving the drug to patients with gastric ulcer (reactivation), hypertension, drug allergy, blood dyscrasia, or cardiac, hepatic, or renal disease, particularly when there is a suspicious tendency or an actual edematous condition.

It is preferable to give the medication with milk or after meals, and to use sodium-free antacids or belladona alkaloids, or both, to avoid local irritation. The dose should be from 300 to 600 mg a day in divided doses, to start, and if there is some improvement after 1 week of treatment, to resort to the minimal maintenance dosage (not exceeding 400 mg a day, always in three or four divided doses) or to discontinue it if there is no noticeable improvement. A slightly higher schedule of dosage could be followed in cases of gouty arthritis (400 mg initially, followed by 100 mg every 4 hours, not to exceed 1 week of treatment).

The drug is available for prescription in the following forms:

Phenylbutazone, tablets, containing 100 mg;

Phenylbutazone, 100 mg together with dried aluminum hydroxide gel, 100 mg, magnesium trisilicate, 150 mg, and homatropine methylbromide, 1.25 mg in capsules (Butazolidin Alka, Geigy).

V. PHENYLQUINOLINES

Phenylcinchoninic Acid or Cinchophen (Atophan)

Cinchophen is a bitter white powder, insoluble in water, deteriorating quickly in light and air, and corresponds to the structural formula:

Absorption from the gastrointestinal tract is rapid, the metabolism leaves unchanged only 2% of the total amount ingested, and the excretion of the drug and its metabolites occurs in the urine (which turns red). The analgesic effect lasts for 3 or 4 hours, starting 3 hours after ingestion. Cinchophen is not used by injection.

Because of its acidity, cinchophen may cause burning sensations in the stomach, and even encourage the development of peptic ulcers. Large quantities of water and sodium bicarbonate (which should not be combined with cinchophen) may prevent gastric irritation and the precipitation of urates in the urine. Toxic symptoms are similar to those produced by salicylates, particularly allergic reactions (skin allergy, angioneurotic edema) and hepatotoxic effects, which could be fatal. Important toxic reactions are rare when the drug is given judiciously and avoided in patients with liver or kidney damage.

Pharmacologically, cinchophen exerts the same effects as salicylates. Nevertheless, its diuretic effect is greater, for which reason the drug is particularly advised for the treatment of gout. It is also used in other rheumatic conditions, including rheumatic fever, but because of its hepatic toxicity, other drugs are ordinarily preferred.

Cinchophen is administered by the oral route, 300 mg to 1 g every 3 to 4 hours. In the acute attack of gout, the suggested dosage is 500 mg every 3 hours, for four or five doses; in chronic cases, 500 mg every 8 hours for only 5 days each week. Some patients respond better to a combination of cinchophen and colchicin than to either drug alone.

Cinchophen is available for prescription in the following forms:

Cinchophen, tablets, containing 300 or 500 mg.

Neocinchophen

Neocinchophen is the ethyl ester of 6-methyl-2-phenylquinoline-4-carboxilic acid, a crystalline powder almost insoluble in water. Its color is pale yellow, which changes if it is left exposed to air and light, and it has the structural formula:

$$\text{structure: 6-methyl-2-phenylquinoline-4-carboxylic acid ethyl ester (COOC}_2\text{H}_5\text{)}$$

Because of its poor solubility in water, the gastrointestinal absorption may be incomplete. It is excreted in the urine.

Pharmacologically, the actions of neocinchophen are identical with those of cinchophen, but it is practically nonirritating to the gastrointestinal tract, its diuretic activity is less marked, and it seems to be less toxic.

It may be used in the same way as the salicylates, but its main indication is for the treatment of gout. By the oral route, 300 mg to 1 g is given every 3 to 4 hours; and in acute gout, 500 mg every 3 hours up to a total of four or five doses. In chronic cases, give 500 mg every 8 hours, 5 days a week.

Neocinchophen is available in the following preparations:

Neocinchophen, tablets, containing 300 or 500 mg.

Hydroxyphenylcinchoninic Acid (Oxinophen, Fenidrone)

Hydroxyphenylcinchoninic acid forms very small, deep yellow prisms, very slightly soluble in water, and more soluble in acetic acid, hot alcohol and other solvents. It corresponds to the structural formula:

$$\text{[structure: 4-ethoxycarbonyl-3-hydroxy-2-phenylquinoline]}$$

The drug is well absorbed from the gastrointestinal tract, but it builds up its blood concentration very slowly as it is bound by plasma proteins. The drug is degraded slowly, and only a very small amount is recovered in the urine.

It is used for the treatment of rheumatic fever, rheumatoid arthritis, scleroderma, and gout. Gastrointestinal side effects are the most frequently encountered, but there are also skin rashes, drug fever, and others.

The dosage generally advised ranges from 10 to 20 mg per kg of body weight per day, the total daily amount always given in four or five divided doses.

> Hydroxyphenylcinchoninic acid is sold under the trade names Oxinophen and Fenidrone, but is not available in the United States.

It is to be noted that this is not a drug in general use, because except for some promising results in the treatment of gout and scleroderma, it has not proved superior to salicylates in the treatment of rheumatism, and is poorly tolerated (particularly during prolonged therapy) in most cases.

VI. COLCHICUM DERIVATIVES

Colchicine

The alkaloid obtained from *Colchicum autumnale* (meadow saffron) is a pale yellow powder, soluble in water, probably corresponding to the following structural formula:

The absorption of the drug is rapid, but it stays in the body for prolonged periods of time, probably being changed to a more toxic metabolite. The excretion takes place in the bile and through the small intestine. Colchicine is highly toxic, the first symptoms being gastrointestinal in nature.

Therapeutically, colchicine has been used as an antimitotic agent, but its main indication is for the treatment of the acute gouty attack, for which it seems to be the drug of choice, though it should be given together with ACTH.

The recommended oral schedule is 1 mg every 2 to 3 hours, for no more than five doses, and to stop at the first gastrointestinal warning. If it is given by strictly intravenous injection (very irritant to tissues when extravasated), no more than 4 mg should be given, 1 mg initially and 0.5 mg in subsequent injections every 6 hours. The combined administration of ACTH and colchicine requires continuing with colchicine after withdrawal of ACTH. For prolonged treatment, the dosage is 0.5 mg to 2 mg daily or every other day (better given at night), adjusting the amount to the patient's need.

Colchicine is available for prescription in the following forms:

Colchicine, tablets, containing 0.5 or 0.6 mg.

Colchicine, injectable, containing 0.5 mg per ml in 1-ml ampuls.

Colchicum Official Preparations

Colchicine is to be preferred to any of the several colchicum official preparations, because the latter do not offer a constant potency in

38 PHARMACOLOGY OF DRUGS USED TO COMBAT PAIN

each of its forms, nor do they offer equally effective therapeutic applications. They are available as follows:

Colchicum corm, fluid extract, in bottles of 500 ml for individualized prescriptions;

Colchicum corm, strong tincture, in bottles of 500 ml for individualized prescriptions;

Colchicum seed, fluid extract, in bottles of 500 ml and of 4 liters for individualized prescriptions;

Colchicum seed, tincture, in bottles of 500 ml and of 4 liters for individualized prescriptions.

Colchicum may be prescribed as follows:

Colchicum corm, fluid extract may be given at dosages of 0.25 cc;

Colchicum seed, tincture, 10%, 0.6–2 cc;

Colchicum seed, fluid extract, 0.12–0.25 cc;

Colchicum corm, tincture, 40%, 0.3–1.0 cc.

VII. ANTIMALARIALS

Quinine

Among the many alkaloids obtained from the bark of trees belonging to the rubiaceous genera, particularly *Cinchona ledgeriana*, one is of great importance in medicine, namely, quinine. It is a microcrystalline, white powder, odorless and with an intense bitterness, and soluble in water and alcohol. Its structural formula is:

Several salts of quinine are soluble and used instead of pure quinine. All of them, as well as quinine, are rapidly absorbed from the gastrointestinal tract and pass into the blood in 1 to 3 hours. Blood concentration is not more rapid after injection, and is almost negligible when the drug is given by the rectal route. Quinine is rapidly metabolized and eliminated from the bloodstream (no accumulation), and finally excreted in the urine (only minor amounts in other liquids), also very rapidly, particularly in an acid urine.

The pharmacological actions of quinine are manifold, but its main use is for the treatment of malaria. It also produces analgesia and antipyresis, in a way similar to that of salicylates. It is useless in severe pain, but shows good effects for the treatment of pain in muscles or in joints. Regarding antipyresis, it is remarkable in the case of fever of malarial origin, but almost negligible in other fevers. Other pharmacological actions of quinine are of great importance (cardiovascular, oxytocic, muscular, and so on), but are of little interest in our review.

The average dose of quinine is 300 to 600 mg, not to exceed 2 g in 24 hours. Quinine salts, e.g., quinine dihydrochloride or quinine sulfate, are given in identical amounts. The treatment of malaria requires a special dosage, i.e., 600 mg a day, for suppression of either Plasmodium vivax, P. malaria or P. falciparum, or 1 g three times a day for 2 days, before the chill, and then 600 mg three times a day for 5 days (but other agents are preferred).

Overdosage or idiosyncrasy will produce cinchonism, a clinical syndrome similar to salicylism (q.v.), particularly distressing in hearing and vision. Treatment of cinchonism includes stomach lavage, the use of alkaloid precipitants (tannic acid), cardiotonics, oxygen, blood transfusion, and other symptomatic measures. The drug should be avoided for patients sensitive to it (skin rashes), pregnant women, and patients with tinnitus or optic neuritis.

As said before, the main indication for the use of quinine or its salts is the treatment of malaria; also, the treatment of certain myopathies, night cramps, headaches, neuralgias, and pains of muscles or joints. As an analgesic, its effects are perhaps weaker than those of the salicylates.

Quinine and its salts are available in the following preparations:

Quinine capsules, containing 180 or 300 mg;

Quinine powder, in bottles containing 30 or 150 g for individualized prescriptions;

Quinine dihydrochloride, powder, in bottles containing 30 or 150 g for individualized prescriptions;

Quinine dihydrochloride, injectable, containing 500 mg in 2-ml ampuls and 1000 mg in 5-ml ampuls;

Quinine sulfate, tablets, containing 120 or 300 mg;

Quinine sulfate, capsules, containing 120, 180, 200, or 300 mg.

Other quinine preparations, all dispensed in bottles containing 30 or 150 g of the powder, are: ethylcarbonate, glycerophosphate, hypophosphite, hydrochloride, phosphate, salicylate, and hydrobromide.

Other Antimalarials

Nowadays other antimalarials are used for the treatment of paludism, which are by far more effective for prophylaxis, suppression, control of the clinical attack, gametocidal therapy, or radical cure. Chloroquine, quinacrine, primaquine, pamaquine, chloroguanidine, and pyrimethamine are the drugs principally employed. They are not truly analgesics or antipyretics, but are mentioned here because by their antimalarial effects they will relieve the miseries and pains of patients with malaria.

Chloroquine phosphate (Aralen, Resochin) is given at a dose of 500 mg once a week, for suppression; 1 g, as the initial dose, and then 500 mg after 8 hours and finally 500 mg daily for 3 days, for control of the attack of malaria; and the same schedule for either gametocidal therapy in cases of P. vivax or P. malariae or for radical cure in cases of P. falciparum. It is available as:

Chloroquine phosphate, tablets, containing 125 or 200 mg.

Quinacrine hydrochloride (Atabrine, Mepacrine) is used for the same purposes as chloroquine, but at a dose one-fifth the size, more frequent and administered for longer periods.

Drug preparations available are:

Quinacrine hydrochloride, tablets, containing 50 or 100 mg;

Quinacrine hydrochloride, injectable, a powder for solution, 200 mg in 7 ml of sterile, distilled water, for intramuscular injection.

Primaquine phosphate is the most effective antimalarial for radical cure (P. vivax, P. malaria, or P. falciparum) when given at a dosage of one tablet (26.3 mg) daily for 2 weeks. It is recommended to take primaquine together with chloroquine phosphate, available as:

Primaquine phosphate, tablets, containing 26.3 mg;

Chloroquine phosphate tablets, 26.3 mg.

Pamaquine, chloroguanidine, and *pyrimethamine* are also effectively used for the treatment of malaria, chloroguanidine being perhaps the most versatile of the three, and probably of all others, since it is useful in prophylaxis, suppression, and control of the attack by gametocidal therapy and radical cure. Dosage ranges from 100 to 300 mg a week, and more frequently for control of the attack. It is marketed under the brand names of Paludrine, Proguanil, and Guanatol, and is available as:

Chloroguanidine hydrochloride, tablets, containing 25, 50, 100, or 300 mg per tablet.

VIII. LOCAL ANESTHETICS

Cocaine

Cocaine, an alkaloid obtained from the leaves of *Erythroxylon coca*, a tree from Peru and Bolivia, is benzoylmethylecgonine, a white crystalline powder with a hydrochloride salt soluble in water; the base is soluble only in organic solvents. Its structural formula is:

$$\begin{array}{c} H_2C \longrightarrow \quad\quad\quad COOCH_3 \\ | \quad\quad\quad\quad | \\ N-CH_3 \quad HC \longrightarrow OOC \\ | \quad\quad\quad\quad | \\ H_2C \longrightarrow CH_2 \end{array}$$

Cocaine is absorbed slowly because of the vasoconstriction that it induces. Excretion and detoxification are still slower, thus easily allowing drug intoxication. It is not active when given by mouth because of hydrolysis in the gastrointestinal tract. Detoxification occurs in the liver at a slower pace than for synthetic local anesthetics.

A dose of 20 mg may cause serious toxic symptoms, and over 1 g is ordinarily fatal. The initial toxic symptoms are nervous irritability, restlessness, anxiety, confusion and headache, rapidly leading to delirium, convulsions, and final respiratory arrest. Sometimes death occurs instantaneously. The treatment of choice for cocaine intoxication is the intravenous administration of a short-acting barbiturate (sodium pentobarbital, for instance). Other helpful measures are artificial respiration and the application if possible of a tourniquet, proximal to the site of injection. Cocaine may induce tolerance and addiction. (See p. 51 for recommendations on the use of cocaine.)

The pharmacological effects are particularly marked on nerve conduction, which is blocked; on the central nervous system, which is stimulated (first the cortex and later the medulla); and on the cardiovascular system, in which it provokes bradycardia followed by tachycardia and vasoconstriction accompanied by hypertension. In the eye, cocaine induces local anesthesia, vasoconstriction, and mydriasis, and may cause corneal ulceration.

Cocaine is not intended for systemic administration (either oral or parenteral). The drug is available in the following preparations for surface anesthesia:

> Cocaine, powder or crystals, in bottles containing 4, 8, 30, or 150 g;

> Cocaine, granules, in bottles containing 4, 8, or, for individualized prescriptions, 30 g;

> Cocaine hydrochloride, to prepare solutions, in bottles containing 4, 8, 30, or 150 g.

Procaine (Novocaine)

Procaine is a synthetic white crystalline powder, mainly used as the hydrochloride salt, which is freely soluble in water and corresponds to the following structural formula:

$$\text{H}_2\text{N-C}_6\text{H}_4\text{-COOCH}_2\text{CH}_2\text{N}(\text{C}_2\text{H}_5)_2 \cdot \text{HCl}$$

After injection, procaine is very rapidly absorbed from the injected site (a vasoconstrictor, epinephrine, is usually added to retard absorption), and once absorbed is also rapidly hydrolyzed to paraaminobenzoic acid (PABA) and diethylaminoethanol, both excreted in the urine (but the greater amount of diethylaminoethanol is metabolized to other products).

Toxicity is less than with cocaine, and much less than with butacaine and dibucaine; and when it is given together with a vasoconstrictor (epinephrine), toxic reactions are rare. Death, probably due to idiosyncrasy, is very rare but may occur with 10 to 100 mg of the drug (circulatory collapse).

Blocking of sensitive nerves is the most important pharmacological action of procaine, but some generalized analgesia, maximal in 20 minutes and lasting for about 1 hour, may follow systemic administration. The well-known procaine–sulfonamide antagonism should be kept in mind.

Therapeutically, procaine is perhaps the most widely used local anesthetic; but it has also been recommended for the treatment of urticaria, delayed serum sickness, and cardiac arrhythmia, but not always with better results than with more appropriate drugs.

Procaine is available in the following preparations:

Procaine, powder, in bottles containing 30 or 120 g, or 2, 10, or 20 kg;

Procaine, tablets, N.F. preparations;

Procaine, solution, at a concentration of 1 or 2% in vials containing 30 or 100 ml;

Procaine, injectable, 1 or 2% solution, in ampuls or vials containing 1, 5, 10, 30, 50, or 100 ml;

Procaine, solution, at a concentration of 2%, together with epinephrine, in vials containing 30 ml;

Procaine, injectable, at a concentration of 1 or 2%, together with epinephrine, in vials containing 30 ml and ampuls containing 2.3 ml;

Procaine, injectable, at a concentration of 4%, in ampuls containing 2.3 ml.

Tetracaine (Pontocaine)

Tetracaine is related to paraaminobenzoic acid (PABA), and corresponds to the following structural formula:

$$\underset{\text{COOCH}_2\text{CH}_2\text{N}}{\overset{\text{N}\begin{smallmatrix}\text{C}_4\text{H}_9\\ \text{H}\end{smallmatrix}}{\underset{}{\bigcirc}}}\begin{smallmatrix}\text{CH}_3\\ \text{CH}_3\end{smallmatrix}$$

Its disadvantage of a higher toxicity (ten times greater than procaine) is compensated for by the equal activity of weaker concentrations. It has the remarkable advantage of absorption through mucous membranes, making it useful for surface anesthesia instead of the more toxic cocaine. It is rapidly absorbed on injection and the effects are somewhat more prolonged than with procaine. The therapeutic usage is the same as with other local anesthetics.

The drug is available in the following preparations:

Tetracaine, ophthalmic solution, in bottles containing 15 ml;

Tetracaine, base, in bottles containing 10 g, for individualized prescriptions;

Tetracaine hydrochloride, ophthalmic solution, at a concentration of 0.5% in bottles of 1 ml or 15 ml;

Tetracaine hydrochloride, injectable, containing 500 ml in 2 ml or in 7.5 ml;

Tetracaine, injectable, 0.15% solution;

Tetracaine hydrochloride, containing 250 mg together with zinc sulfate, 100 mg in 7.5-ml vials;

Tetracaine hydrochloride, powder, in bottles containing 15 or 30 g;

Tetracaine, 1% cream and ointment, and 0.5% ophthalmic ointment;

Tetracaine, tablets, containing 100 mg.

Dibucaine (Nupercaine)

Dibucaine, a quinoline derivative, occurs in colorless crystals soluble in water and alcohol, and corresponds to the structural formula:

$$\text{CONHCH}_2\text{CH}_2\text{N} \begin{matrix} \diagup \text{C}_2\text{H}_5 \\ \diagdown \text{C}_2\text{H}_5 \end{matrix}$$

$$\text{OC}_4\text{H}_9$$

Dibucaine is a potent local anesthetic, but is also very toxic. Nevertheless, toxicity is low when the drug is used in high dilution, which, however, does not impair adequate and prolonged activity. It has been used for all types of local anesthesia, but because some vasodilation occurs from the injection of low concentrations, epinephrine should be added for vasoconstriction.

Dubucaine is available in the following preparations:

Dibucaine, ointment, at a concentration of 1%, in jars of 2.2 kg;

Dibucaine, cream, at a concentration of 0.5% in tubes of 30 g;

Dibucaine hydrochloride, suppositories, containing 20 mg;

Dibucaine hydrochloride powder, in bottles containing 10, 25, 30, or 120 g;

Dibucaine hydrochloride, injectable, containing 5 mg in 2-ml ampuls (0.25%).

Dibucaine, lozenges, for oral use, containing 1 mg per lozenge.

Lidocaine (Xylocaine)

An aminoacyl amide, lidocaine corresponds to the structural formula:

$$\text{CH}_3-\underset{\underset{\text{NHCOCH}_2\text{N}(C_2H_5)_2}{|}}{\bigcirc}-\text{CH}_3$$

Both surface and deep anesthesia are well obtained with lidocaine. It may be used without a vasoconstrictor, but the effects are less prolonged and the toxicity increases; nevertheless, lidocaine should be used when epinephrine is contraindicated (hypersensitivity).

Pharmaceutical preparations available are the following:

> Lidocaine, viscous, an aqueous solution, at 2% concentration for oral administration, in bottles containing 100 or 450 ml (average dose, 1 tablespoonful for adults, 1 teaspoonful for children, not to exceed eight doses in a day);
>
> Lidocaine, jelly, at a 2% concentration, in 30-ml tubes, for mucous membranes;
>
> Lidocaine, ointment, at a concentration of 2.5 or 5%, in 15- or 35-g collapsible tubes;
>
> Lidocaine, suppositories, containing 100 mg;
>
> Lidocaine, injectable, at concentrations from 0.5 to 1, 1½, and 2%, in ampuls or vials, 2, 5, 10, 20, 30, 50, or 100 ml [available either plain or with epinephrine, the latter 1:50,000 (for dental use), 1:100,000, or 1:200,000];
>
> Lidocaine, solution, 4%, in 5-ml ampuls or 50-ml bottles;
>
> Lidocaine, for spinal anesthesia, at a concentration of 5%, containing 50 mg per ml, in 2-ml ampuls.

Diperodon (Diothane)

A phenyluretane derivative, diperodon corresponds to the following structural formula:

$$\text{C}_6\text{H}_5\text{-NHCOOCH}_2$$

$$\text{C}_6\text{H}_5\text{-NHCOOCH-CH}_2\text{-N}\begin{Bmatrix}\text{CH}_2\text{-CH}_2\\\text{CH}_2\text{-CH}_2\end{Bmatrix}\text{CH}_2$$

Diperodon is a toxic, long-acting local anesthetic, used mainly in suppositories or ointment for hemorrhoidal pain.

The drug is available in the following forms:

Diperodon, powder, in 5-g bottles;

Diperodon, ointment, 1%, in 30-g tubes of 2.2-kg jars;

Diperodon, 1%, suppositories.

Alcohol

Ethanol, or ethyl alcohol, is a colorless, volatile liquid, corresponding to the formula:

$$\text{H}-\underset{\underset{\text{H}}{|}}{\overset{\overset{\text{H}}{|}}{\text{C}}}-\underset{\underset{\text{H}}{|}}{\overset{\overset{\text{H}}{|}}{\text{C}}}-\text{OH}$$

Alcohol is highly hygroscopic, which makes it almost impossible to use absolute alcohol; only 95% by volume alcohol is practical for clinical purposes.

For pain relief, alcohol has been used by injection, intravenously, by which route it also acts as a sedative and a nutrient. It is also a vasodilating agent, so that care should be taken in cases of impending or actual shock. Nerve injection block is carried out for the treatment of trigeminal neuralgia, sciatica, cancer, or even in cases of angina pectoris, thromboangiitis obliterans, or lumbar paravertebral block.

The average dosage used, for relieving pain, is 2 to 4 ml of alcohol injected around the involved nerve. If used intravenously, no more than 10 ml of alcohol per hour should be given (200 ml of a 5% solution). It is available as:

Alcohol, 95% by volume, in vials containing 5 or 50 ml;

Alcohol, solution, containing 5% alcohol and 5% glucose, in 1000-ml bottles;

Dehydrated alcohol, 100% by volume, in 2-ml amupls.

Other Local Anesthetics

Butamben picrate (Butesin picrate) is a yellow amorphous powder, poorly soluble in water, closely related to procaine, and corresponding to the structural formula:

$$\left[\begin{array}{c} NH_2 \\ \\ \\ COOC_4H_9 \end{array} \right]_2 \quad C_6H_2OH(NO_2)_3$$

The drug is a long-acting surface anesthetic, because of its poor absorption from the site of application. Also, because of the picric acid content it shows some antiseptic properties.

For minor burns and abrasions, butamben picrate is a useful drug. Only in rare cases, it may cause dermatitis, and it should not be given to patients sensitive to procaine and its analogues.

Butamben picrate ointment (with Metaphen) in tubes;

Butamben picrate ointment, in 30- or 60-g jars.

Ethylaminobenzoate (Benzocaine) is a white, crystalline substance, insoluble in water, also closely related to procaine and its analogues. Its structural formula is:

$$\underset{COOC_2H_5}{\overset{NH_2}{C_6H_4}}$$

Because of its poor absorption, ethylaminobenzoate is indicated for surface anesthesia, either as a dusting powder or incorporated in ointments or in suppositories. It is also recommended for superficial abrasions or minor burns. It is available as:

Ethylaminobenzoate, crystals, for individualized prescriptions;

Ethylaminobenzoate, 1% otic solution, in bottles containing 15 or 30 ml;

Ethylaminobenzoate, ointment, in 5% concentration (also, 20% in water-soluble base);

Ethylaminobenzoate, suppositories, containing 120, 180, or 500 mg.

In contrast to the yellow butamben picrate, ethylaminobenzoate ointment is white and does not stain the skin.

Guaiacol may be obtained either as a natural derivative of hardwood tar or synthetically. It occurs as a white (or pale yellow) crystalline mass, or liquid, soluble in water and miscible with alcohol and other solvents, and corresponds to the formula:

$$\underset{}{\overset{OH}{C_6H_4}}\text{—}OCH_3$$

For topical anesthesia, 12 ml of guaiacol mixed with 18 ml of olive oil is used. It is available as:

Guaiacol, liquid, in bottles containing 30, 120, or 500 ml or 2.5 liters.

Eugenol, eugenic or caryophyllic acid, is a colorless (or pale yellow) liquid obtained from oil of clove, has a pungent taste, is insoluble in water but soluble in fat solvents, and corresponds to the structural formula:

$$\text{benzene ring with OH, OCH}_3\text{, and CH}_2\text{CH}=\text{CH}_2 \text{ substituents}$$

It is employed in dentistry as an antiseptic and weak anesthetic, for the treatment of caries. It is available as:

Eugenol, liquid, in bottles containing 30, 120, or 500 ml.

Chlorobutanol (Chloretone) is a colorless crystalline substance, soluble in water and alcohol, corresponding to the structural formula:

$$\text{CCl}_3-\text{C(CH}_3\text{)(OH)}-\text{CH}_3$$

It possesses a local anesthetic effect and is not irritant to the gastric mucosa. For this reason, the drug is recommended for gastralgia and for vomiting. Also, dentists use chlorobutanol as a surface anesthetic in "toothache drops." The drug is available as:

Chlorobutanol, powder, 1 or 5%, for prescription;

Chlorobutanol, substance, anhydrous or hydrous, in bottles containing 120 or 500 g for individualized prescriptions;

Chlorobutanol, 10% ointment;

Chlorobutanol, 25% in olive oil, for toothache.

Pyridium is recommended by the manufacturers as a mild analgesic to the urinary tract, for the relief of symptoms of pain, burning, and urgency, particularly in cases of cystitis. It is available as:

Pyridium, tablets, containing 100 mg.

Technic for the Use of Local Anesthetics

Strictly speaking, except for a few selected instances, the use of local anesthetics falls within the domain of the anesthetist, who is familiar with the many preparations marketed. Other physicians or surgeons should become familiar with only a few of the better known and more widely used agents, and should follow the advice of the American Medical Association recommending that: (1) very special care be taken not to confuse cocaine and procaine, an error which has caused fatalities, since cocaine is much more toxic than procaine; (2) cocaine not be used for purposes other than surface anesthesia; (3) butacaine not be used except for surface anesthesia; (4) the user not exceed a total amount of 100 mg of cocaine, that is, 0.5 ml of a 20% solution, 1 ml of a 10% solution, or 10 ml of a 1% solution, and one should use only solutions containing 1 or 2% procaine for injection; and (5) there should not be passed into the urethra any anesthetic solution if there is inflammation, stricture, or trauma.

Local surface anesthesia may be used on wounded skin or intact, diseased mucosae; also, for instrumentation or surgery of the latter. Cocaine preparations include:

Cocaine, 1 to 4% solutions, preferable with
epinephrine (1:100,000) for use on the cornea;

Cocaine, 10 or 20% solutions, also with epinephrine, for use in the nose or throat;

Cocaine, 4% solution, which is the surface anesthesia of choice for many European authors.

As a general rule, aqueous solutions of local anesthetics do not pass through intact skin, but are absorbed by eroded skin and mucous membranes. Cocaine should be used accordingly.

An available procaine preparation is:

Procaine, tablets, for use on the mucosa of the mouth or the throat.

Procaine is probably the most widely used local anesthetic, but because the easily soluble procaine hydrochloride is not absorbed by mucous membrane, it is not adequate for surface anesthesia. More toxic, and absorbable, anesthetics must be used on the surface of mucous membranes, but necessary precautions should be kept in mind. Preparations available:

Dibucaine, 1% ointment, for use on the skin or rectal mucosa;

Dibucaine, 0.5% cream, for more prolonged or more extensive surface applications;

Dubucaine, 20% suppositories, for rectal use;

Dibucaine, 1-mg lozenges, for anesthesia of the mouth or throat.

In spite of its high toxicity, dibucaine is well tolerated for the above-mentioned surface anesthesia.

Lidocaine preparations include:

Lidocaine, viscous, to use 1 tablespoonful (adults) or 1 teaspoonful (children), not to exceed 8 in a day, for surface anesthesia of the proximal parts of the digestive system (pharynx, esophagus, stomach);

Lidocaine, 2.5 or 5% ointment, to use on the skin, on rectal mucosa, and as anesthetic lubricant for instrumentation of body cavities;

Lidocaine, 2% jelly, for mucous membranes and instrumentation, particularly of the urethra, nose, throat, and ears;

Lidocaine, suppositories, for rectal application.

Lidocaine is widely used for surface anesthesia because it is more potent than procaine, and of about the same toxicity when used topically or in low concentrations.

Tetracaine preparations include:

> Tetracaine, either base or hydrochloride, in ophthalmic solutions; also, in ophthalmic ointment for use on the cornea;

> Tetracaine, cream and ointment, to use in the skin and on the rectal mucosa;

> Tetracaine, 2% solution (extemporaneous preparation), to use on the mucosa of the nose or the throat.

The advantage of tetracaine consists of its longer duration of effects, but its high toxicity must be taken into consideration.

Among diperodon preparations are:

> Diperodon, 1% ointment, preferably recommended for rectal use;

> Diperodon, 1% suppositories, for the relief of hemorrhoidal pain.

Diperodon is employed when a prolonged effect is the most desirable action of an anesthetic preparation.

Infiltration and block anesthesia are the most frequently used forms for local anesthesia. Infiltration of the intradermal tissues is almost immediately followed by superficial anesthesia; subcutaneous injection exerts its effects upon more extensive areas of the skin or the adjacent mucosae. In block anesthesia, the local effect is obtained by interruption of nerve transmission from the affected area when the anesthetic solution is injected in the vicinity of a nerve. Different technics are employed according to the nerve involved, and are best handled by specialists in such procedures.

Infiltration is the procedure of choice for minor operations, including suturing of wounds. The slow introduction of the needle preceded by instillation of a drop of the anesthetic at the site of injection is practically painless. Then, the amount of solution to be introduced depends on the extent of the area to be manipulated, about 1 ml per each 2 square centimeters (average concentrations). Injecting a circle around the operative area (ring block) and a quantity at a deeper level may spare anesthetic solution. Care should be taken, always, not to inject into a blood vessel (frequent suction with the syringe!).

As said before, nerve block is a technic for the specialist. Nevertheless, some simple procedures may be carried out by any skilled physician. A *finger* is anesthetized by injecting on each side of the corresponding metacarpal, at its midpoint, and then advancing the needle to the interdigital web. The *hand* is anesthetized by blocking the median, the ulnar, and the radial nerves at the wrist. A needle inserted between the palmaris longus and the flexor carpi ulnaria (the tendons at the middle of the palmar side of the wrist, and the following one at the radial side) will meet the median nerve. If inserted at the radial side of the flexor carpi ulnaris tendon (the first tendon at the ulnar side of the wrist), it will meet the ulnar nerve. The radial nerve is met by a needle inserted in the anatomic snuffbox. To block the brachial plexus, for anesthesia of both *arm* and *forearm*, the supraclavicular or the axillary route is followed. The first is risky; the second, somewhat easier: a point is marked bisecting a vertical line drawn between the humeral insertions of the pectoralis major and the latissimus dorsi; the needle is inserted, and maintained always at a right angle to the shaft of the humerus. The brachial artery is under the marked point, and should be retracted with the finger to insert the needle towards the median nerve; then, the needle is withdrawn, almost to the skin, and re-inserted at a 45° angle anterior to the first injection, to meet the musculocutaneous nerve; it is withdrawn again, and re-inserted at a 45° angle posterior to the first injection, retracting the artery anteriorly, to meet the ulnar nerve; finally, at 45° angle anterior to the former (90° anterior to the insertion required to meet the median nerve) will lead to the radial nerve. The *foot* is anesthetized by injecting around the posterior tibial nerve just on the medial aspect of the tendon of Achilles at the level of the internal malleolus of the tibia. The *leg* is anesthetized by injecting around the sciatic nerve 3 cm below the middle point between the great trochanter of the femur and the posterosuperior iliac spinous process. The *thigh* is anesthetized by injecting around the femoral nerve at a point external to the femoral artery at the midpoint of the inguinal ligaments. Blocking both the sciatic and the femoral nerves gives good anesthesia for operations from *below the knee* to the foot.

Procaine preparations include:

Procaine, 1 or 2% solution for injection, in ampuls or vials containing 1, 5, 10, 30, 50, or 100 ml;

Procaine, 1 or 2% solution also containing epinephrine, in 2.3-ml ampuls or 30-ml vials;

Procaine, 4% solution, for injection, in ampuls containing 2.3 ml.

Procaine 2% solution is, perhaps, the most frequently used local anesthetic, injected at doses ranging from 20 to 25 ml. For small nerves, namely, infiltration of digits, 1% solution may suffice; large nerves, namely, the sciatic nerve, may require 4% solution. It is to be noted that 0.5% solutions are also frequently recommended for infiltration.

Dibucaine is available as:

Dibucaine hydrochloride, 0.25% solution, for injection, in 2-ml ampuls.

Dibucaine is not recommended for infiltration or nerve block, because of its high toxicity. Only those familiar with the drug will take advantage of the long duration of the anesthesia it produces. Because low dilutions may provoke vasodilation, they should be given together with vasoconstrictors (epinephrine).

Lidocaine preparations available are:

Lidocaine, 0.5, 1, 1.5, and 2% solutions, for injection, in ampuls or vials containing 2, 5, 10, 30, 50, or 100 ml;

Lidocaine, same as above but with epinephrine 1:50,000 (for dental use), 1:100,000, or 1:200,000.

Lidocaine is effective in low concentrations, and is a versatile local anesthetic, effective for infiltration and for nerve block. For infiltration, 0.5% solution is used; for nerve block, 1 or 2% solution. The addition of epinephrine is not needed for prolonged anesthesia; so lidocaine is advised for those sensitive to epinephrine. Also, it is recommended for patients sensitive to procaine.

Also available for nerve block is:

Alcohol, 95% by volume, in vials containing 5 or 50 ml.

Prolonged relief, even for months, is obtained in some patients with neuralgia after injection of alcohol around the affected nerve (2 to 4 ml per injection).

Spinal anesthesia and other forms of local anesthesia, such as paravertebral, epidural, and caudal, are extremely useful in surgery, but are better carried out by anesthetists who are familiar with the advantages and the risks in each particular case.

IX. VASODILATORS

Nitrates

Nitroglycerin is a highly explosive liquid, insoluble in water but miscible with most fat solvents. It has the structural formula:

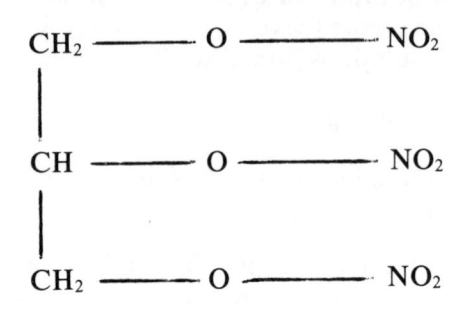

$$\begin{array}{c} CH_2 - O - NO_2 \\ | \\ CH - O - NO_2 \\ | \\ CH_2 - O - NO_2 \end{array}$$

The basic action of nitroglycerin is its ability to relax smooth muscle by direct action, that is, independently of innervation, particularly in small blood vessels. This reduces blood pressure, but increases the rate of capillary flow. A deep flush from the clavicles upward is noted, together with vasodilation of the retinal, meningeal, splanchnic, and coronary blood vessels. There is also a relaxation of the smooth muscle of the bronchial, biliary, gastrointestinal, and genito-urinary tract.

Absorption occurs very rapidly from the mouth (under the tongue), the stomach, and the rest of the gastrointestinal tract.

Continuous use develops some tolerance, but activity is restored after a few days without taking the drug. Side effects are: headache (because of dilation of intracranial vessels), syncope, and methemoglobinemia. Intraocular pressure may increase, contraindicating the use of nitroglycerin in glaucoma; also, the drug is contraindicated in marked anemia and in patients with increased intracranial pressure.

The main indication for nitroglycerin is for the treatment of angina pectoris, both as a preventive and for relief of the acute attack. Other uses of nitroglycerin, as for hypertension or gastrointestinal spasm, have become obsolete.

Nitroglycerin is available in the following forms, and it should be always kept in mind that it deteriorates very easily when exposed to air:

Nitroglycerin, granules, containing 0.25 mg;

Nitroglycerin, tablets, containing 0.15, 0.3, 0.4, or 0.6 mg.

Other nitrates are also used for the treatment of angina pectoris. Amyl nitrite may relieve an attack within 30 seconds after inhalation of its vapors. It is a volatile, clear yellow liquid unpleasant to smell. Sodium nitrite, a yellow powder soluble in water giving unstable solutions, is used orally for the preventive treatment of angina. Also explosive substances are erythrityl tetranitrate (Erythrol), mannitol hexanitrate, and pentaerythritol tetranitrate (Peritrate), all used for the preventive treatment of angina. The therapeutic dosages for almost all the above-mentioned nitrates are from 15 to 60 mg every 3 to 6 hours, excepting for amyl nitrite, the dosage 0.2 ml, and pentaerythritol tetranitrate, the dosage 10 to 20 mg, 6 to 8 hours. These nitrates are available in the following forms:

Amyl nitrite, pearls, containing 0.2 ml;

Sodium nitrite, granules or tablets, 60 mg;

Erythrityl tetranitrate, tablets, 5, 10, or 15 mg; also chewable tablets containing 10 mg;

Mannitol hexanitrate, tablets containing 30 mg;

Pentaerythritol tetranitrate, tablets, containing 10 or 20 mg; also, sustained-action tablets containing 80 mg.

Peripheral Vasodilators

Drugs which act directly on the smooth muscle of the blood vessels that supply the skin or the skeletal muscles are considered peripheral vasodilators.

Nicotinic acid or niacin provokes a flushing from the clavicles upwards, and perhaps other skin rashes.

Nicotinyl alcohol (Roniacol) shows the same skin vasodilation as its congener nicotinic acid.

Cyclandelate (Cyclospasmol) dilates the vessels of most areas of the skin, frequently including the fingers and toes.

Tolazoline hydrochloride (Priscoline) also exerts a powerful action on the skin vessels, including fingers and toes, and also to a limited extent the skeletal muscle circulation.

Phenoxybenzamine hydrochloride (Dibenzyline) increases blood flow, mainly to the skin, thus supplying an agent for skin temperature regulation. It also lowers blood pressure.

These peripheral vasodilators have been recommended for the treatment of acrocyanosis, acroparesthesia, Buerguer's disease, vascular spasm, skin ulcers, chilblains, intermittent claudication, cramps,

Raynaud's disease and Raynaud's phenomenon, Meniere's syndrome, arteriosclerosis, thrombophlebitis, thromboangiitis obliterans, causalgia, endarteritis, gangrene, and many other diseases in which a deficit of blood supply is either proved or assumed. It is problematic if their action helps those diseases in which a deficit of blood supply to skeletal muscles is the substratum. On the other hand, they seem to be of some help when the defect mainly concerns skin circulation, namely, ulcers, chilblains, Raynaud's disease and phenomenon, acrocyanosis, acroparesthesia, and similar derangements.

Isoxsuprine hydrochloride (Vasodilan) is being recommended as a vasodilator in peripheral vascular disease and cerebral insufficiency. It acts directly on the circulation to muscle tissue, and its use is advised in arteriosclerosis obliterans, thromboangiitis obliterans, arterial occlusion, and thrombophlebitis, and even in impaired cerebral circulation.

Nylidrin (Arlidin) is recommended for the same uses as isoxsuprine, and also in cases of impaired circulation to the eye and the ear and in angina inversa (attacks occur at rest). Perhaps an added advantage is the simultaneous increase in cardiac output, which makes more efficient the subsequent vasodilation for a better blood supply to ischemic areas.

Both nylidrin and isoxsuprine hydrochloride seem to be especially effective in all forms of occlusion of those vessels supplying the extremities and the endocranial structures.

The peripheral vasodilators are available in the following forms:

Nicotinic acid, tablets, containing 25, 50, or 100 mg;

Nicotinic acid, capsules, containing 25, 50, or 100 mg;

Nicotinyl alcohol, tablets, containing 50 mg per tablet;

Nicotinyl alcohol, elixir, containing 50 mg per teaspoonful in bottles of 500 cc or 4 liters;

Nicotinyl alcohol, sustained-release action tablets (Timespan tablets), containing 150 mg;

Cyclandelate, tablets, containing 100 mg;

Cyclandelate, capsules, containing 200 mg;

Tolazoline hydrochloride, tablets, containing 25 mg;

Tolazoline hycrochloride, sustained-release action tablets (Lontabs), containing 80 mg;

Tolazoline hydrochloride, injectable, containing 25 mg per ml in 10-ml vials;

Phenoxybenzamine hydrochloride, capsules, containing 10 mg;

Isoxsuprine hydrochloride, tablets, containing 10 mg;

Isoxsuprine hydrochloride, injectable, containing 5 mg per ml in 2-ml ampuls;

Nylidrin, tablets, containing 6 mg per tablet;

Nylidrin, injectable, containing 5 mg per ml in 1-ml ampuls and 10-ml vials.

X. VASOCONSTRICTORS

Ergotamine Tartrate (Gynergen)

Ergotamine tartrate occurs as a crystalline powder, colorless or white, slightly soluble in alcohol, and corresponds to the following structural formula:

Little is known about the metabolic fate of ergotamine after a dose is given. The drug disappears rapidly from the blood, and seemingly is detoxified by the liver.

The principal use of ergotamine tartrate is for the treatment of migrane, but not for other forms of headache. It is also used as an oxytocic, and has been recommended in a miscellaneous group of diseases or symptoms (itching, thyrotoxicosis, hypertension, neuroses) not always substantiated after a careful investigation.

Ergotamine is contraindicated in pregnancy, and in those patients with sepsis, toxemia, coronary heart disease, obliterative vascular disease, and impaired function of the liver or kidney.

Dosage is 0.5 to 1 mg by injection, or 1 mg per tablet. Tablets may be repeated up to six times in each migraine attack; by injection no more than 2 ml per week may be given. Dosage should be adjusted for each patient.

The medication is available in the following forms:

Ergotamine tartrate, tablets containing 1 mg;

Ergotamine tartrate, injectable, containing 0.5 mg/ml in ½-ml and 1-ml ampuls.

Dihydroergotamine Mesylate (D.H.E. 45)

Dihydroergotamine is obtained by hydrogenation of ergotamine, which is said to reduce the likelihood of side effects without impairment of the ability of the drug to control the vascular-type headaches. The drug is recommended for those patients who do not tolerate ergotamine, and is contraindicated in the same cases as is ergotamine. The specific recommendations for dihydroergotamine are vascular headache, postlumbar-puncture headache, and herpes zoster or other neuritic pains. Dosage is adjusted for each particular patient, the average dose being similar to that used with ergotamine.

Dihydroergotamine is available as:

Dihydroergotamine mesylate, injectable, containing 1 mg per ml in 1-ml ampuls.

Ergonovine Maleate (Ergotrate Maleate)

Ergonovine is the hydroxyisopropylamide of lysergic acid, a white or yellowish crystalline powder, soluble in water and sensitive to light. Its structural formula is supposed to be the following:

This drug is mainly used as an oxytocic, but it may also relieve migraine headache. Of course, it should be avoided in pregnant women. It is available as:

Ergotrate maleate, tablets, containing 0.2 mg.

XI. CORTICOIDS

Cortisone, hydrocortisone, and similar steroids are not only glycogenic (in contrast to desoxycorticosterone, which is salt-retaining), but possess a powerful anti-inflammatory activity, which indirectly is analgesic after reduction of inflammation in rheumatic and other painful diseases. But hydrocortisone also has some salt-retaining action, for which reason equally effective anti-inflammatory steroids have been developed with very little or no salt-retaining activity.

All of these steroids are derivatives of the basic cyclopentenophenanthrene structure:

and have in common the presence of OH in the 17th position.

The absorption of corticoids following parenteral administration is excellent for all, but not so the gastrointestinal absorption, which is limited for some, like desoxycorticosterone. Once in the body, all are largely degraded, and finally excreted mainly in the urine.

The physiologic effects are noted on the carbohydrate metabolism, thus worsening diabetes mellitus, particularly when the cortisone group is considered. Desoxycorticosterone has little action upon glucose levels in the blood. There are also marked effects upon protein and fat metabolism, increasing protein catabolism and causing fat deposition in certain areas of the body.

Aldosterone, particularly, and also desoxycorticosterone provoke a marked sodium retention, leading to the production of edema. Other corticoids also enhance sodium retention, but to a lesser extent.

Additional corticoid effects are the maintenance of muscle capacity, particularly of the striated muscles, increased irritability of the central nervous system, depression of lymphoid tissues and of circulating eosinophils in the blood, augmentation of the androgenic effect of the testicular hormones, and, of the greatest interest for our purpose, the anti-inflammatory effect on mesenchymal tissues. The response to injuries of connective tissues is so altered that the normal hypersensitivity reaction is almost suppressed, thus producing the control of symptoms in rheumatic disease, inflammatory diseases of the eye, the bowel, and skin, and also acute gouty arthritis.

Side effects are important, and may force the withdrawal of the corticosteroids. Increased fat deposition with plethoric appearance is perhaps the most frequently encountered, together with the production of ankle edema due to sodium retention. Hypertension is extremely frequent, and so are sex disturbances, like menstrual disorders and hirsutism. Headache, skin striae, mental symptoms, acne, hyperpigmentation, peptic ulcer, glycosuria, osteoporosis, and purpura may also be important side effects.

These hormones are indicated in the treatment of Addison's disease, hypopituitarism, allergic diseases, lupus erythematosus, periarteritis nodosa, dermatomyositis, scleroderma, sarcoidosis, pemphigus, atopic dermatitis, psoriasis, pulmonary fibrosis, nephrosis, hepatitis, multiple sclerosis, and Sjögren's syndrome.

Rheumatoid arthritis and gouty symptoms respond to corticoid therapy rapidly (in a few hours) and effectively (control of lesions), though the basic process of the disease is not modified and the recurrence of symptoms follows withdrawal of the medication. It also controls all clinical manifestations of rheumatic fever (including carditis). Bursitis is equally controlled by corticoids.

Similar effects are found in the treatment of inflammatory diseases of the eye, including iritis, iridocyclitis, keratitis, retinitis, optic neuritis, and choroiditis.

Comparative activity of the corticosteroids that will be studied in the following pages can be graded as follows to obtain same results:

Hydrocortisone	20
Cortisone	25
Prednisone	5
Prednisolone	4
Dexamethasone	0.75

Cortisone

Cortisone has a powerful action upon inflammation, but also powerfully affects carbohydrate metabolism and electrolyte balance. It provokes sodium retention, edema, and hyperglycemia and other undesirable side effects on osteoporosis, peptic ulcer, hypertension, acne, hirsutism, cutaneous striae, cervicothoracic hump, rounded facies, and others.

It is recommended for the treatment of rheumatoid arthritis, rheumatic fever, and inflammatory eye diseases, but its main indication is for the treatment of Addison's disease and perhaps some allergic diseases, such as asthma.

Initial dosage schedule may range from 30 to 300 mg a day, if severity deserves the risk of elevated doses, such as may be the case in some inflammatory diseases of the eye. As soon as symptoms are under control, the dosage should be adjusted to the lowest effective amount.

Cortisone is available in the following forms:

Cortisone, tablets, containing 5, 10, or 25 mg.

Cortisone, injectable, in solution containing 25 mg per ml in 20-ml vials.

Hydrocortisone (Cortef)

More powerful than cortisone is hydrocortisone, but its actions and effects are essentially the same as those of cortisone. Consequently, more care should be exerted when using this hormone, and patients must always be under very close medical control. As with cortisone, the main use for hydrocortisone is replacement therapy for Addison's disease; it is also used for suppressive therapy in adrenocortical syndrome. It is recommended as well for ulcerative colitis, some allergic diseases, neoplastic diseases, and pulmonary or meningeal tuberculosis.

In all other instances, hydrocortisone should be reserved for diseases resistant to cortisone or any other less active corticosteroid. Such may be the case in inflammatory eye diseases and some collagenoses, but only rarely in rheumatic diseases, except for the injection of the hormone into the diseased joints or bursae.

Side effects may reach undesirable levels, particularly sodium retention, for which condition sodium intake should be restricted to minimal amounts (no more than 0.5 g a day), at the same time that potassium is added to the diet (about 10 g a day). Diabetes, hypertension, or heart failure may be aggravated or induced. Cataracts may appear after long-term therapy with hydrocortisone. Also, signs of infection may be masked; and its spreading, enhanced.

Effective dosage may vary with the involved disease; initial daily doses range from 20 to 500 mg (100 or 200 mg, average); and maintenance doses, from 10 to 60 mg. It will always be kept in mind that stoppage of the drug should be followed very closely because of the suppression of activity of the adrenal glands in those receiving corticosteroids, particularly hydrocortisone.

Hydrocortisone is available as the following pharmaceutical preparations:

Hydrocortisone, tablets, containing, 5, 10, or 20 mg;

Hydrocortisone, oral suspension, containing 10 mg per teaspoonful (5 ml);

Hydrocortisone, ointment, 1 or 2.5%;

Hydrocortisone, injectable, containing 50 mg per ml.

Prednisone (Deltasone)

Prednisone is also more potent than cortisone, but its mineralocorticoid activity is much lower, producing little or no retention of sodium, and thus making easier the handling of patients, except in adrenal insufficiency, in which case prednisone is undesirable.

Prednisone is indicated in rheumatoid arthritis, inflammatory diseases of the eye, collagen diseases, and in all other illnesses in which cortisone or hydrocortisone is of good effect. The dosage varies from 10 to 80 mg a day, initially, to be reduced as soon as

66 PHARMACOLOGY OF DRUGS USED TO COMBAT PAIN

possible to lower, effective levels (2.5 to 20 mg a day), except for nephrosis and tuberculosis, which require higher maintenance doses.
Prednisone is available as:

Prednisone, tablets, containing 2.5 or 5 mg.

Prednisolone (Delta-Cortef)

This corticoid is in the same category as prednisone, but is somewhat more active.
The following forms are available:

Prednisolone, tablets, containing 1, 2.5, or 5 mg.

Dexamethasone (Hexadrol, Decadron)

Still stronger than prednisolone, but also possessing the same type of activity, dexamethasone can be used at very low pharmacological dosages, which make almost negligible the risk of sodium retention and blood glucose imbalance.

As with all other corticosteroids, the dose is individualized at levels about one-half of those corresponding to prednisolone (35 times as potent as cortisone).

Dexamethasone is available in the following forms:

Dexamethasone, tablets, containing 0.25, 0.5, 0.75, or 1.25 mg;

Dexamethasone elixir, containing 0.5 mg per teaspoonful (5 ml);

Dexamethasone, ophthalmic solution, at 0.1% concentration;

Dexamethasone, ophthalmic ointment, at 0.05% concentration;

Dexamethasone, injectable, containing 4 mg per ml in 1-ml ampuls or 5-ml vials.

Other Corticoids

Many synthetic corticosteroids have been developed, but they do not differ essentially from those mentioned above, excepting for the different potency, which ranges between the most active betamethasone (0.6 mg equivalent to 0.75 mg of dexamethasone) and triamcinolone and methylprednisolone (about 4 mg equivalent to 5 mg prednisone).

A few of these corticosteroids are available in the following forms:

Methylprednisolone, tablets, containing 2, 4, or 16 mg;

Methylprednisolone, cream, at 0.25 or 1% concentration:

Methylprednisolone, sustained-action capsules, containing 2 or 4 mg;

Paramethasone, tablets, containing 1 or 2 mg;

Triamcinolone, tablets, containing 1, 2, 4, or 8 mg;

Triamcinolone, syrup, containing 4 mg per teaspoonful (5 ml).

XII. OTHER DRUGS USED IN CONDITIONS CAUSING PAIN

Drugs reviewed in the foregoing pages are not the only ones used for the treatment of diseases in which pain is an important, distressing symptom. Antibiotics and muscle-relaxant drugs may also be advantageously administered. Because these drugs are not essential for the relief of pain, in spite of the fact that they may be fundamental for the basic treatment of a given disease, they will be considered here only in an abridged form.

Muscle Relaxants

From the pharmacological group of tranquilizing drugs, some exert a marked activity for the control of muscle spasm, relieving pain and disability through their action on the central nervous system, which induces a decrease of skeletal muscle tone. Among the tranquilizers, meprobamate also presents muscle-relaxant activity. More specifically designed for muscle relaxation are mephenesin, methocarbamol, carisoprodol, chlorzoxazone, chlormezazone, orphenadrine, phenyramidol, metaxalone, and, perhaps, others.

Curare and curariform drugs block nerve impulses, thus decreasing or even paralyzing muscle contractility and tonicity.

Meprobamate is recommended for the treatment of muscle spasm

$$H_2NCOO-CH_2-\underset{\underset{CH_2CH_2CH_3}{|}}{\overset{\overset{CH_3}{|}}{C}}-CH_2-OOCNH_2$$

in rheumatic diseases or following trauma. It can cause drowsiness, allergic reactions and, very rarely, aplastic anemia. The average dosage is 400 mg, three or four times a day. It is available as:

Meprobamate, tablets, containing 200 or 400 mg;

Meprobamate, sustained effect, in capsules, containing 400 mg;

Meprobamate, suspension, containing 200 mg per teaspoonful (5 ml).

Mephenesin is used to induce muscular relaxation in rheumatic

$$\text{benzene ring with } CH_3 \text{ and } O\text{—}CH_2CHOHCH_2OH$$

diseases and other spastic conditions, whenever abnormal hypertonicity is present. Parenterally, it has been used as an adjuvant to general anesthesia. Side effects are of little importance in most cases; but intravenous administration of solutions of over 2% concentration may cause thrombosis. It is available as:

Mephenesin, tablets, containing 250 or 500 mg per tablet;

Mephenesin, capsules, containing 250 or 500 mg;

Mephenesin, elixir, containing 100 mg per ml (500 mg per teaspoonful, 5 ml);

Mephenesin, injectable, containing 20 mg per ml, in 50-ml or 100-ml ampuls.

Carisoprodol has some analgesic effect as well as its muscle-relaxant activity. It has been recommended for the treatment of muscle spasm and stiffness with pain, occurring in musculoskeletal dyskinesias (traumatic, inflammatory, or degenerative), neurologic disturbances; or muscular dyskinesias. Side effects are of minor importance when the drug is given in proper dosage, namely 350 mg four times a day. It is available as:

Carisoprodol, tablets, containing 250 or 350 mg.

Chlormezazone exerts also some tranquilizing effect, and is recommended for the treatment of skeletal muscle spasm, particularly in rheumatic diseases, low back pain, disc syndrome, torticollis, bursitis, and the like. Side effects may occur in a few cases, drowsiness being the most important. Adequate dose is 200 mg three or four times a day. It is available as:

Chlormezazone, tablets, containing 100 mg or 200 mg

Methocarbamol possesses a marked relaxing action upon the skeletal muscle, and is recommended for the treatment of skeletal muscle hyperactivity in disc syndrome, sprains, strains, and other traumatic conditions, rheumatic diseases, low back pain, and other acute or chronic disorders involving reactional muscle spasm. The injectable is contraindicated in kidney diseases. The adequate dosage is up to 2000 mg four times a day (average 1500 mg q.i.d.) reducing to 1000 mg. q.i.d. for maintenance. Available forms are:

Methocarbamol, tablets, containing 500 or 750 mg per tablet;

Methocarbamol, injectable, containing 1000 mg in a 10-ml ampul.

Phenyramidol produces muscle relaxation and analgesia. Gastrointestinal side effects may occur. It has been recommended as an analgesic for common pains. The dosage is 200 to 400 mg every four hours. Available forms are:

Phenyramidol, tablets, containing 200 or 400 mg;

Phenyramidol, elixir, containing 100 mg per teaspoonful (5 ml).

Orphenadrine shows long-lasting effects in the treatment of muscle spasm. It should not be given to patients with glaucoma, prostatism, or gastrointestinal obstruction. The dosage is 200 mg a day, by mouth; or 60 mg once or twice a day, by the parenteral route. Available forms are:

Orphenadrine, tablets, containing 100 mg;

Orphenadrine, injectable, containing 60 mg in a 2-ml ampul.

Metaxalone should not be given to patients with a tendency to hemolytic or any other form of anemia. It is recommended as a muscle relaxant, at a dosage of 800 mg three or four times a day. It is available as:

Metaxalone, tablets, containing 400 mg.

Chlorzoxazone reduces muscle spasm and pain when given at a dosage of 250 to 500 mg, three or four times a day. Maintenance dosage is smaller. It is available as:

Chlorzoxazone, tablets, containing 250 mg.

Curare has no chemical relationship with the above-mentioned muscle relaxants. It induces a selective paralysis of motor-end plates in skeletal muscle, which finally abolishes all movement. When given in proper dosage, curare will produce only a relaxation, not a paralysis, of muscles, for which reason the drug is employed as an adjuvant in anesthesia, for the prevention of fractures in shock therapy, for the treatment of muscle spasm that follows rheumatic or similar illnesses, and also for the treatment of spastic or convulsive disorders. It is contraindicated in patients with myasthenia gravis, and others with allergic disorders; but, generally speaking, the drug should be reserved for those familiarized with its use. Because it is used only by injection, a closer supervision of patients is needed, even when it is given only at amounts of 3 mg per 20 kg of body wieght by the intramuscular route. It is available as:

Curare (dimethyltubocurarine or similar salts), injectable, containing 1 mg per ml in 10-ml vials.

Decamethonium is one of the methonium agents derived from curare, but its mechanism of action is somewhat different; and its effects are about four times more potent. It is mainly used to facilitate surgical, therapeutic, and diagnostic procedures.

Antibiotics and Sulfas

The management of infections, including the painful local ones, has greatly improved after the general use of sulfas and antibiotics, which not only control the multiplication of causative germs, but also the subsequent symptoms, pain included. They are not adequate for the treatment of pain, per se, but at long range they will relieve pain by healing inflammation.

The choice of an adequate antibiotic depends on the nature of the infective agent, the sensitivity or resistance of the agent, and the severity of the infection. The choice of a sulfa drug is easier. But because of the intricacies of good selection in this area, we refer our reader to any authoritative book. Here, we will only present a cursory review of indications and dosages for some of the more popular anti-infective agents.

Penicillin is the best choice for the treatment of streptococcal infections (both alpha and beta), gonococcal infection, anthrax, syphilis, yaws, and Vincent's angina; it may be excellent or may show lesser efficiency in the treatment of staphylococcal infections, depending on the sensitivity of the infecting organism. It is better to combine penicillin with sulfadiazine for the treatment of meningococcal meningitis and actinomycosis; it should be used together with antitoxin therapy in cases of tetanus and gas gangrene; and it may be good, but it is not always as good as desired, in diphtheria, anaerobic infections, Weil's disease, psittacosis, ornithosis, and lymphogranuloma inguinale.

Streptomycin and its analogues are the best choice for the treatment of tuberculosis, Friedlander's pneumonia, granuloma inguinale, and plague (together with sulfadiazine), and a fairly good choice for coli infections, infections by Proteus, A. aerogenes, Pseudomonas aeruginosa, brucellosis (better together with sulfadiazine), tularemia, Hemophylus influenzae meningitis (better together with sulfadiazine), chancroid, leprosy, and granuloma inguinale. They may be of some help in streptococcal, staphylococcal, pneumonococcal, gonococcal, and paratyphoidal infections, bacillary dysentery, cholera, pertussis, and actinomycosis.

The tetracyclines are the best choice in tularemia, chancroid, rickettsial infections, psittacosis, ornithosis, lymphogranuloma and granuloma inguinales, and intestinal amebiasis. They are better used together with streptomycin for the treatment of brucellosis (the treatment of choice) and together with sulfadiazine for the treatment of Hemophylus influenzae meningitis (the treatment of choice). Acceptable results are obtained in the treatment of streptococcal, staphylococcal, pneumococcal, gonococcal, meningococcal, and anaerobic infections, in anthrax, infections from coli, Proteus, A. aerogenes, Ps. aeruginosa, Friedlander's pneumonia, syphilis, bacillary dysentery, pertussis, yaws, Weil's disease, actinomyces, Vincent's angina, trachoma, atypical pneumonia, and herpes zoster.

Sulfas are still drugs of choice for the treatment of trachoma and chancroid, and together with penicillin in coccal meningitis. They are good alternates in bacillary dysentery, cholera, gonorrhea; and together with penicillin or streptomycin in pneumococcal infections, plague, psittacosis, ornithosis, lymphogranuloma inguinale, and actinomucosis. They can be tried in granuloma inguinale, staphylococcal infections, diphtheria, clostridial infections, urinary infections, and brucellosis.

Part Two

Diagnosis and Treatment

Pain, the distressful sensation of discomfort or even agony, may be felt in any part of the body, wherever specialized nerve endings are found. It relates to almost all types of pathologic disturbances, either medical, surgical, or environmental, and is, perhaps, the symptom that forces most patients to seek medical advice. Regardless of its frequency as a sympton, pain serves adequately to point out a diseased organ, not only when directly related to that particular organ, but also when it constitutes heterotopic or "referred pain," distant from the affected part of the body.

Pain may be divided into several categories, according to its character, intensity, and so forth; but the most practical approach will be to consider pain in accordance with its anatomical location, which is the pattern to be followed in our study.

Consistent with this purpose, it will be classed in these categories:
1. Headache or cephalalgia.
2. Pain in the face.
3. Ophthalmodynia, or pain in the eyes, including pain related to the eyes.
4. Otalgia, or pain in the ears, including the mastoid area.
5. Stomatalgia, or pain in the mouth, including the pharyngeal area.

6. Dysphagia.
7. Pain in the neck.
8. Rachialgia, or pain in the spine, including low back pain.
9. Thoracodynia, or pain in the thorax, including shoulder pain.
10. Acute abdomen.
11. Chronic abdominal pain.
12. Pain in the extremities; arms, legs, hands, and feet.
13. Pain in the muscles.
14. Pain in the perineum, rectum, and sex organs.
15. Pain in the skin.

It must be kept in mind that the diagnosis of pain is merely one of the many steps towards a complete diagnosis, and includes detection of the causal factor, because knowing the etiology is indispensable to the institution of effective treatment: the treatment of pain itself is only a small part of the complete management of the case.

In the following lines we will try to present a practical approach to the path that should be trod from the symptom, pain, to the diagnosis of the causal disease, the indispensable steps before treatment is begun.

We shall remind our readers, once more, about the purpose of this book, namely, the treatment of pain; that is to say, not the treatment of a number of diseases, but only the treatment of pain, whenever it is present among other symptoms during the course of these illnesses.

As already stated, pain is among the principal motivations forcing patients to consult their physicians, seeking its relief, no matter how small a part it might be in the whole treatment of a given disease. But it is always a very important part for the person who suffers it.

The best approach to an adequate treatment depends, primarily, on a good diagnosis of the basic medical problem, which might be either organic or merely psychological. The fundamental treatment of the disease will be carried out immediately, irrespective of the urgency of analgesia, though analgesia will be the main subject dealt with in the following pages.

Mild to moderate pain only requires mild analgesics of the type of salicylates, coal-tar derivatives, and similar drugs. Pain due to specific causes, like gout, requires specific analgesics. Pain of a more severe nature may force the use of morphine when other narcotic drugs, such as codeine, have failed. Extremely severe pain in terminal diseases, like cancer, may require drastic measures, including the continuous use of narcotics, the use of surgery, or whatever is needed.

I. HEADACHE

Headache (cephalalgia) is the most common of all pains, not only when it appears sporadically from emotional or psychological causes, but also when it is due to organic diseases, the list being notably long. In the following pages we will review for treatment the majority of organic causes of headache.

Many patients with a disease that presents symptoms characteristic enough for an accurate diagnosis will give special emphasis to the headache. For instance, it is not rare that a particular person with glaucoma, instead of pointing out the excruciating ocular pain, will tell the physician about a killing headache. This is one of the reasons why our following review of causes of headache might seem somewhat extensive for the main purpose of this book.

The character of a particular headache, mild or severe, localized or generalized, in one side of the vertex, intermittent or continuous, sudden or slowly progressive, throbbing or dull, may be distinctive in some conditions, though any disease might cause any particular type of headache. For this reason, we cannot rely on the type of headache entirely to decide a diagnosis, but can only consider it as an important clue leading to the search for other important symptoms.

Headache and Fever

Fever, by itself, can provoke cephalalgia; and the great majority of infections, particularly systemic infections with fever, cause headache. Coinciding with the peak of hyperthermia, there is a pounding, constant headache, in most instances a severe one, either limited to the frontal area, the base, or more frequently generalized to all the head. Probably it is due to intracranial vascular changes, particularly of the hypertensive type. Ordinarily, it is resistant to analgesics, and may respond better to an ice bag, or in extreme cases to lumbar puncture.

An infectious disease is the most frequent cause of fever accompanied with headache; but no special characteristic of the headache will reveal the nature of the infection, though some instances of extremely violent cephalalgia will arouse great suspicion of meningitis or smallpox.

Now, we will try to give some hints to help the physician find an acceptable way to establish a final diagnosis, starting with the consideration of other specific symptoms that may also be present.

Temperature Curve. At times, the nature of the disease could be strongly suspected because of the type of the curve. A sustained temperature, above normal during the entire course of the disease, is the usual pattern for infections; hectic or septic fever, with marked ups and downs above the normal line and frequently accompanied by chills and sweating, is characteristic of bacteria entering the bloodstream (bacteremia, osteomyelitis, certain forms of pulmonary tuberculosis, etc.); remittent daily ups and downs above normal may also be a modification of the sustained type of hyperthermia (typhoid fever, paratyphoid fever, etc.); and recurrent fever after periods of normal temperature gives the name to some spirochetoses, such as "relapsing fever." The regularly recurrent paroxysms of chills, fever, and sweats is dramatically suggestive of malaria, especially when characterized by days of normal temperature. These afebrile intervals occur typically every 24 hours in tertian (vivax) malaria, and every 48 hours in quartan malaria. In estivo-atumnal (falciparum) malaria, the temperature tends to be irregular and sustained with shorter periods of remittance.

Chills. Chills are present in almost all patients with an elevated temperature, but are more conspicuous in the following diseases: variola, influenza, dengue, bacteremia, scarlet fever, typhoid fever and other salmonelloses, malaria, plague, glanders, tularemia, brucellosis, and encephalitis.

Tachycardia. Tachycardia is a common accompanying symptom of fever. In some conditions it may be more marked, as in variola, influenza, dengue, bacteremia, scarlet fever, typhoid fever (in this case it may be slower starting than expected), malaria, plague, rickettsial infection, and meningitis. In yellow fever, there is a frequent lack of parallelism between pulse and temperature.

Rash. The eruptive diseases will show a characteristic rash in each particular case; variola, varicella, rubella, scarlet fever, and the rickettsial diseases. Also other diseases may occur associated with some sort of rash, not of a characteristic nature, such as: infectious mononucleosis, dengue, bacteremia, typhoid fever, and tularemia.

Muscular Pains (or Generalized Pains). More or less marked muscular pains will be associated with variola, influenza, dengue, poliomyelitis, brucellosis, yellow fever, typhoid fever, and the leptospiroses.

Rachialgia. An intense rachialgia is characteristic of variola, but it may also occur in meningitis.

Enlargement of Lymph Nodes and/or Spleen. In rubella, there is an enlargement of lymph nodes, and also in plague, tularemia, lymphogranuloma venereum, and meningitis. The enlargement of lymph nodes is associated with splenomegaly in infectious mononucleosis, dengue, and brucellosis.

Flushing of the Skin. Flushing, particularly of the face, is found in dengue, scarlet fever, malaria, and yellow fever. In general, it is associated with any exceptionally elevated temperature, including heatstroke.

Stiffness of the Neck. This is a sign characteristic of meningitis, and may also occur in poliomyelitis.

Sweating. Sweating always occurs with fever, but profuse sweating could herald malaria, tularemia, brucellosis, and relapsing fever.

Neurological Symptoms, including paresis, paralysis, paresthesias, and the like, are found in: poliomyelitis, meningitis, and encephalitis.

Leukocytosis. Leukocytosis is a normal occurrence with fever, and is marked in bacteremia and scarlet fever.

Leukopenia. Leukopenia characterizes influenza, dengue, rubeola, rubella, exanthema subitum, variola (early stages), Colorado tick fever, and typhoid fever.

Other Laboratory Findings. Needless to remind the reader that, fortunately, there are a large number of laboratory procedures that will help to establish the diagnosis of many infectious diseases, such as is the case with salmonellosis, tuberculosis, viral infections, etc.

Systemic Infections

Variola (smallpox). A severe headache associated with rachialgia and muscle pains closely follows the sudden onset of fever, chills, and tachycardia. Nausea, vomiting, and prostration are frequently added distressing symptoms. The diagnosis ordinarily is made when the typical eruption appears, after the rise of fever: red macules which increase in size and turn into papules, then into umbilicated vesicles, and, finally, pustules. This occurs about the third or fourth day of fever, first noted on the face and head, thereafter spreading to trunk and limbs. The dermal lesions result in only one crop of eruptions (all elements appear as of the same age, and not in different stages as in the case with varicella).

No specific therapy is available. Symptomatic treatment is the only help to be offered. In the case of pain (head, spine, muscles, etc.), which may reach intolerable proportions, this kind of help will be welcomed. If pains, particularly cephalalgia, are not controlled by acetylsalicylic acid given alone (600 mg every 3 or 4 hours), a combination with codeine or any other similar drug may be tried.

> Acetylsalicylic acid, 300 mg, plus codeine, 30 mg, in a tablet, every 4 hours, or even more frequently if needed.

> Acetylsalicylic acid, 300 mg, plus acetophenetidin, 300 mg, in a tablet or capsule, one every 4 hours.

Narcotic drugs are not to be advised for these patients on a regular basis, but only in very exceptional conditions, such as intractable pain, and then under very strict control, to avoid excessive sedation, particularly to the point of depressing the respiratory centers.

> Morphine sulfate, 5 to 10 mg, by subcutaneous injection, repeated as tolerated and needed.

> Methadone, 10 mg, by subcutaneous injection, repeated as tolerated and needed.

> Meperidine, 100 mg, by subcutaneous injection or by mouth, repeated every 4 hours, as tolerated and needed.

Varicella (Chickenpox). The headache is mostly of a mild nature or may be absent. The diagnosis is made following the appearance of the eruption, which coincides with the rise in temperature; macules that turn into papules which vesicate, are not umbilicated, and finally fade in the form of pustules. The rash appears first on the trunk, and in several different crops (lesions of different age are present at the same time). The great majority of patients will show a mild disease (even without fever, in rare instances); but a severe case of varicella might cause confusion with a mild case of variola. In these very rare instances, a serologic diagnosis or detection of virus will be imperative.

There is no specific therapy for varicella; and regarding the treatment of headache due to this disease, most cases are so mild that the use of analgesia, even acetylsalicylic acid, is hardly justified.

> Acetylsalicylic acid, 300 mg, tablets, every 6 hours. This dosage will be enough in most instances; if needed, give 600 mg every 4 hours, preferably with meals.

Very rarely, stronger therapy will be required.

Herpes Zoster. Pain, at times a very severe neuralgia, may precede the skin lesions. These are similar to varicella, but are limited to only one side of the body, corresponding to the cutaneous distribution of one nerve. The disease may start as an ordinary infection, with fever, chills, and malaise; and pain in the head will be conspicuous in the cases of geniculate ganglion herpes (corresponding to the distribution of the ophthalmic branch of the fifth cranial nerve: head and forehead, around the eyes and the maxillary area).

No specific therapy is available, but pain can be relieved, and the disease shortened, by the adequate use of corticoids. It is extremely important to differentiate herpes zoster from herpes simplex, particularly when located in the ocular area, because corticoids are postively contraindicated in herpes simplex.

> Prednisone, start with 40 to 50 mg a day, in divided doses; decrease slowly to smaller amounts as soon as improvement is noted; and after 7 or 10 days of therapy, discontinuance will be started, also at a slow pace.
>
> Triamcinolone acetonide, 40-mg suspension for intramuscular injection in the gluteal area as the starting medication, to afford rapid relief; then, continue as above stated.

Other analgesics can be tried, as follows:

> Acetylsalicylic acid, 600 mg, in tablets, every 4 hours, preferably with meals.
>
> Codeine, 60 mg, by mouth, every 4 to 6 hours.
>
> Acetophenetidin, 300 mg, by mouth, every 4 hours.
>
> Propoxyphene hydrochloride, 65 mg, by mouth, every 4 hours.
>
> Meperidine, 100 mg, by mouth, every 4 or 6 hours.

Persisting neuralgia after disappearance of skin lesions might respond to infiltration of the affected area with triamcinolone acetonide (see above) and lidocaine solution.

> Lidocaine, 2% solution, 1 to 5 ml, for each specific painful area.
>
> Procaine, 0.5% solution; inject a total of 200 ml in some 50 to 100 different points; the procedure may be repeated once a week, for a few weeks.

Rubeola (Measles). Headache is a very minor symptom in this conglomerate of fever, upper respiratory infection complex, conjunctivitis, and maculae (first in the mouth, the Koplik's spots; then on the body, starting around the ears). A severe headache may be due to a complicating encephalitis. Serologic tests may confirm the diagnosis.

There is no specific therapy for rubeola. A number of patients, particularly of an older age, might request treatment of their headaches. Acetylsalicylic acid will be tried first.

> Acetylsalicylic acid, 600 mg, in tablets, every 4 or 6 hours as needed; preferably with meals. The dosage will be adjusted to age for smaller children.

If the headache is due to a complicating encephalitis (see corresponding paragraph), injections of hydrocortisone should be started immediately.

> Hydrocortisone, 50 mg per ml of solution; inject 50 to 100 mg every 8 or 12 hours, either subcutaneously, intramuscularly, or intravenously.

Rubella (German Measles). In the great majority of cases, the headache is of little importance. The infective syndrome, by itself, may be also a very minor one. Rhinitis and lympadenopathy (particularly postauricular and postoccipital) may be present. The diagnosis is made the second or third day, when fine macules of a pinkish color appear, first on the face, and become confluent at a later stage.

No treatment is known, but its common mildness rarely will require any intense therapy. The accompanying headache, which occurs only in a very few instances, will respond effectively to acetylsalicylic acid in small dosages.

> Acetylsalicylic acid, 300 mg, every 6 hours; increased to 600 mg, if needed. Give with meals.

Infectious Mononucleosis. A variable headache may be present; but a sore throat, lymphadenopathy, and splenomegaly are almost always present to establish the diagnosis. A rash similar to measles or scarlet fever may occur in a few cases. The Paul Bunnel test is positive, and typically enlarged lymphocytes are found in blood smears.

There is no specific therapy for infectious mononucleosis. Cephalalgia may be distressing, more for its duration than for its intensity. Since prolonged rest is essential for the treatment of the disease, it will also help in alleviating the headache. If needed, acetylsalicylic acid can be tried.

Acetylsalicylic acid, 600 mg, tablets, every 4 to 6 hours, preferably with meals.

Corticoids are also very effective for the general management of infectious mononucleosis, but their use is better reserved for selected cases with very serious symptomatology.

Prednisone, to start with 40 mg a day, in divided doses; decrease slowly to lower amounts when improvement is noted; then, after some 7 or 10 days of therapy, start discontinuance at a very slow rate.

Common Cold. Among the miseries of the common cold, headache is a frequent complaint. Rhinitis, coughing, and general malaise are the characteristic symptoms. Care should be taken not to mistake a common cold for other more serious diseases also accompanied by rhinitis, particularly if sore throat is present, or if other symptoms appear.

No specific therapy is available, and the frequently mentioned "miseries" of the common cold very rarely need any treatment. The repeated slogan "bed rest, plenty of liquids, and aspirin" is more of a commercial than medical advice, since all physicians know that rest is of paramount importance in many instances, liquids should be taken in strict balance with the liquids lost, and any drug is to be given only when needed. If needed, in the rare instances when headache becomes intolerable, acetylsalicylic acid may be tried, and also codeine if coughing increases the headache.

Codeine, 15, 30, or 60 mg, by mouth, every 4 to 6 hours.

Acetylsalicylic acid, 300 or 600 mg, in tablets, every 4 to 6 hours, preferably with meals.

In some instances a combination of codeine and acetylsalicylic acid will give better results than either drug alone.

Influenza (Grippe) and Similar Diseases. Sudden elevation of temperature, chills, headache, muscular pains, intense malaise, and weakness are characteristic. Respiratory involvement is almost the rule, while digestive symptoms occur less frequently. When these symptoms take place during an epidemic outburst, there are not diagnostic doubts. A common cold will show little or no severe constitutional symptoms. Bacterial diseases will present leukocytosis instead of the influenza leukopenia. A final diagnosis may be reached by isolation of the virus from garglings (early stage) or serum tests (acute phase and convalescence). The parainfluenza viruses provoke a disease identical with influenza on clinical grounds, the distinction being made only by laboratory tests (complement-fixation, hemagglutination-inhibition, etc.). The adenoviruses may also cause syndromes with a similar clinical picture (see below, "Other viral diseases"). Only appropriate laboratory tests will disclose the final diagnosis.

There is no specific therapy for these ailments, but the severity of most of their symptoms requires help from the physician, since they usually reach burdensome proportions. Because of the presence of fever and headache, acetylsalicylic acid should be tried first.

> Acetylsalicylic acid, 600 mg, in tablets, every 4 hours, preferably with meals. If needed, give the medication more frequently, to obtain effective analgesic and antithermic results.

Occasionally, when patients start to cough, codeine should be added to the above medication, but preferably at a low dosage.

> Codeine, 15 to 30 mg, by mouth, every 4 or 6 hours.

Because nasal obstruction may help to increase, or at least maintain the headache, it must be relieved with adequate therapy.

> Ephedrine, 1, 2, or 3% solution; instill a few drops (or use as a spray) into each nostril, repeating every 4 or 5 hours.

> Phenylephrine, 0.1 or 0.5% solution; instill a few drops (or use a spray) into each nostril, every 4 or 5 hours.

In the case of parainfluenza, same amounts of acetylsalicylic acid and codeine as stated above can be used. Essentially, the care is the same.

Other Viral Diseases. In addition to influenza, parainfluenza, and adenoviruses considered above [in "Influenza (grippe) and similar diseases"], several hundred other viruses are capable of inducing febrile illness accompanied with headache. Of all these viral diseases, AFRI, the *acute febrile respiratory illness* is one of the most frequent, with a symptomatology of a severe common cold, a mild influenza, or no symptoms at all (only an inflammatory reaction of the upper respiratory mucosae), mainly occurring during the cold months. A positive diagnosis is made only by laboratory tests. Another disease, ARD, or *acute respiratory disease*, has been noticed especially among recruits in the armed forces, showing headache, fever with chills, malaise and symptoms of upper respiratory tract infection (rhinitis, pharyngitis, cough), rarely with evidence of pneumonitis. *Herpangina*, as the name implies, is characterized by herpetic lesions (papulo-vesicular) on the tonsils accompanying a clinical picture of systemic infection (fever, headache, and other pains). In herpetic stomatitis the vesicles are large and spread in the mouth, and rarely there is a marked infectious syndrome. The virus can be isolated, and elevated antibody titer detected. *Aseptic meningitis* presents headache, stiff neck, pain in the muscles, fever, and other symptoms suggestive of bacterial meningitis, but the cerebrospinal fluid is not under increased pressure, is clear, and has a slightly increased cell count, sugar and protein closer to normal, no demonstrable pathogens.

In most viral diseases caused by adenoviruses (AFRI, ARD), the use of acetylsalicylic acid is recommended for the management of headache or generalized pains. Dosage should be adjusted for each patient.

> Acetylsalicylic acid, 600 mg, tablets, every 4 to 6 hours, as needed and tolerated, preferably at the same time that food is given.

If there is a disturbing cough, codeine may be given to ensure rest.

> Codeine, 15 or 30 mg, by mouth, every 4 or 6 hours.

Corticoids or antibiotics are not recommended in the virus diseases.

In herpangina, the treatment of pain is symptomatic as described above. Supportive treatment is indicated also in aseptic meningitis, and poliomyelitis of the nonparalytic type. Bed rest, adequate hydration, good electrolyte balance, sedatives, and acetylsalicylic acid, either alone or with codeine, should have major weight in the management of these diseases.

Colorado Tick Fever. Most patients will be found in, or coming from the western part of the United States, mainly from March to August. The onset is sudden, with fever, chills, and severe pain in the head and muscles. Accompanying symptoms are photophobia, nausea (with or without vomiting), anorexia, and a possible mild, nonspecific rash. When the diagnosis is not made from these symptoms, more confirmatory is their reappearance, following a remission of 2 or 3 days. There is leukopenia, a shift to the left, and the virus may be inoculated into laboratory animals and identified.

No specific therapy is known. Acetylsalicylic acid ordinarily controls pains, and perhaps other symptoms of the disease.

> Acetylsalicylic acid, 600 mg, in tablets, every 4 or 6
> hours, preferably with meals.

Other salicylates and coal-tar derivatives may also be effective.

Pleurodynia. Actually, this is a muscle neuralgia in the intercostal area, which may appear in an epidemic form (Borholm disease) due to coxsackie virus. Respiratory movements are decreased, and it might be confused with pleuritic pain. The infective syndrome ordinarily includes headache, fever, sore throat, and malaise; but the pain in the intercostal area (lower chest or epigastrium might be involved), frequently accompanied by local swelling and tenderness, gives the final diagnosis. In case of doubt (poliomyelitis, pneumothorax, pancreatitis, intra-abdominal perforation, etc.), isolation of the virus or the titer of antibodies can be performed in the laboratory.

No specific therapy is known for this disease, in which pain, including cephalalgia, may reach very severe proportions. The first trial should be given to acetylsalicylic acid.

> Acetylsalicylic acid, 600 mg, in tablets, every 4 hours,
> preferably with some food taken at the same time.

Together with acetylsalicylic acid, codeine should be given.

> Codeine, 30 to 60 mg, by mouth, every 4 hours, to
> be decreased to 15 or 30 mg every 6 hours as soon as the
> medication controls the situation.

If there is no relief with the above regimen, adequate alternates should be tried, as follows:

> Sodium salicylate, 600 mg, by mouth, every 4 or 6 hours.

> Anileridine, 25 to 50 mg, by mouth, every 4 to 6 hours.

> Meperidine, 50 to 100 mg, either by subcutaneous
> injection or by mouth, every 4 or 6 hours; but this
> medication should not be given for too long a time.

Dengue. This is not a frequent disease, but perhaps many cases are erroneously diagnosed as influenza, since its symptoms are almost of the same clinical category. In the case of dengue, they present a sudden onset, with severe pain in the joints and muscles ("breakbone fever"). If the diagnosis is not made in the first stage of the disease, when there is a transient flushing or frank eruption of a pale pink macular rash in the face, there is usually a remission of symptoms, lasting for 3 or 4 days, and then there is a second similar stage, when the eruption is more marked and similar to measles or scarlet fever. Superficial lymph nodes may be enlarged, and splenomegaly noted. Laboratory tests will detect leukopenia, and mouse antibody neutralization, hemagglutination, and virus isolation at times are needed because of confusion with yellow fever, typhus, malaria, or pappataci (sandfly) fever.

No specific therapy is available, and pain—excruciating, at times—is the main target of the treatment. For the headache, an ice cap is always a very good help. The most important drugs to be considered here are codeine and acetysalicylic acid; but in some instances other salicylates might also be effective.

Codeine, 30 to 60 mg, by mouth, every 4 or 6 hours, or even more frequently, if needed and tolerated.

Acetylsalicylic acid, 600 mg, in tablets, also every 4 or 6 hours, or more frequently if needed and tolerated. Give together with food.

Poliomyelitis (Infantile Paralysis). Patients with poliomyelitis may show a clinical picture ranging from mild (such as a light influenza or gastrointestinal discomfort) to extremely severe (headache, high fever, sore throat, vomiting, etc., such as in the case of meningitis). In the first instance, the disease will go unnoticed or will not give any clue until the appearance of paralysis; in the second, patients will have a very severe headache, muscle pain, stiff neck and back, hyperesthesia, paresthesia, weakness of muscles with loss of reflexes (both superficial and deep), at times rigidity instead of weakness, and finally paralysis. In rare instances, the severe form follows an initial mild one after a few days of apparent improvement. Paralysis of muscles with cranial innervation may result in difficult swallowing, with nasal regurgitation and nasal voice, indicating bulbar lesions. Spinal lesions will cause paraplegia. The flaccid paralyses that occur during a febrile disease as stated above, ordinarily indicate that poliomyelitis is the causative factor. Nonparalytic disease may show muscular disability, but spasm is substituted for paralysis. Polio virus and/or antibodies can be detected by special means.

There is no specific therapy for poliomyelitis. In mild cases, those of the nonparalytic type, bed rest is important, and adequate hydration, a good electrolyte balance, and the control of fever and pain are of great importance. For the relief of headache and other pain, and of fever acetylsalicylic acid will ordinarily suffice, either alone or with codeine or codeine substituting for it.

> Acetylsalicylic acid, 300 to 600 mg (dosage corrected for smaller patients) in tablets, every 4 to six hours, preferably with meals.

> Codeine, 30 to 60 mg (dosage corrected for smaller patients), every 4 to 6 hours.

At times, meperidine is advisable, to be given either by mouth or by subcutaneous or intramuscular injection.

> Meperidine, 50 to 100 mg (dosage corrected for smaller patients), every 4 to 6 hours. This drug should not be given for prolonged periods of time.

Septicemia (*Bacteremia*). Bacteria invading the circulating blood may provoke fever commonly of the hectic (septic) type, mostly with chills, at least at the onset, and headache, in many cases. Skin rashes are frequent (often purpuric or petechial). Bacteremia ordinarily spreads from a known infected area, and is suspected when from such an infection there is no improvement in due time, or if, instead, there is an exacerbation of septic symptoms. Of course, the site of origin may be unknown (cryptogenic bacteremia). Most commonly bacteremia follows: puerperal sepsis (after a delivery), erysipelas (following the characteristic well-delineated red area with swollen borders, located mainly around the mouth or the eyes, but also on limbs or trunk), tonsillitis, otitis, urinary sepsis, tooth abscess, etc. In turn, bacteremia may produce new focal sites of infection, particularly in the heart (check continuously for early detection of endocarditis), central nervous system (mainly meningitis), vascular system (thrombophlebitis), lungs (abscess, pneumonia, infarct), skeletal system (osteomyelitis), etc. Blood cultures will establish the diagnosis, in most instances.

The basic treatment depends on the offending infective organism and its sensitivity to antibiotics. These will be administered accordingly. It will not be forgotten that the control of the infection will result in the control of the headache, but the adjunctive use of analgesics and sedatives will give additional support. Codeine is the first choice.

> Codeine, 60 mg, by mouth or by subcutaneous injection every 4 hours.

Other analgesics, or combinations of analgesics, can be tried whenever needed, such as acetylsalicylic acid and codeine, acetylsalicylic acid plus codeine and acetophenetidin, etc., in recognition of the varying response of different individuals to medication.

Acetylsalicylic acid, 300 mg, codeine, 30 mg, tablets, one or two by mouth, every 4 to 6 hours.

Acetylsalicylic acid, 300 mg, codeine, 30 mg, acetophenetidin, 150 mg, tablets or capsules by mouth, one or two every 4 to 6 hours.

Scarlet Fever (Scarlatina). This formerly very frequent disease ordinarily starts with fever accompanied by headache and vomiting, sore throat, malaise, flushing of the face (with a pale area around the mouth), and the so-called strawberry tongue. The skin-red exanthem starts on the neck and the chest, and disappears under pressure (digital or with a glass slide); there are dark red lines, Pastia's lines, in the skin creases, and the rash covers the whole body in two or three days. It is to be remembered that the characteristic bright red rash (which gives the name to the disease) may be slight or even absent in some cases. Then the physician has to rely on the other symptoms of the disease to make the final diagnosis. Desquamation (even without detected exanthema) starts during convalescence, reaches its peak in three or four weeks, lasts up to ten weeks, and is more marked in the palms and the soles. The detection of a group A streptococcus with erythrogenic toxin will solve the diagnosis in dubious cases.

Antibiotic therapy, with penicillin, is specific for scarlet fever. Sore throat and headache are usually the chief complaints, for which acetylsalicylic acid and codeine are the drugs of choice, with copious water drinking to dilute the toxins.

Acetylsalicylic acid, 300 or 600 mg, in tablets, every 4 to 6 hours, preferably with meals.

If needed, codeine might be added, at a relatively low dosage of 30 mg for each 600 mg of acetylsalicylic acid.

Typhoid Fever. Let us not forget that nowadays all salmonelloses, including typhoid fever, may show such a mild symptomatology that they may run their course totally unrecognized or considered as a mild gastrointestinal upset. When fever is present, showing toxemia, headache becomes a part of the clinical picture accompanying the gradual increase in temperature. Either diarrhea or constipation may be present, as well as a relatively slow dicrotic pulse. When the severity of the symptoms steadily increases, the diagnosis will be suspected. The fever reaches a peak in about 1 week, is sustained for 1 or 2 weeks, and gradually decreases for about 1 week (but any type of fever may occur!); the typical typhoid roseola (rose spots), which disappears under pressure, is found on the abdomen and chest at about the second week. The diagnosis is confirmed by finding typhoid bacilli or positive laboratory tests.

Antibiotic treatment is specific, particularly with chloramphenicol or ampicillin. Corticoids may help to alleviate subjective symptoms, including headache, but they have to be given only at the very start of the disease and perhaps for no more than 5 days.

> Prednisone, 5 to 10 mg, every 6 hours, by mouth.

If the headache is severe enough to require especial attention, try first codeine injections.

> Codeine, 30 to 60 mg, by subcutaneous injection, every
> 4 or 6 hours, as needed and tolerated.

Acetylsalicylic acid and similar drugs should not be given because of gastrointestinal irritation. Analgesics with narcotic properties should be avoided or given guardedly because of the danger of increasing the stuporous condition of many of these patients.

Other salmonelloses will be detected only by laboratory procedures, since the clinical pictures are identical with typhoid fever.

The general trend for therapeutic advice will be similar to that for typhoid fever (q.v.), with less emphasis on antibiotic therapy, which may prolong the carrier state. Headache is burdensome only at times; and then it will require the use of codeine. Acetylsalicylic acid could be used, but with very special care because of its irritation of the gastrointestinal tract.

> Codeine, 60 mg, by mouth, every 4 or 6 hours, or by
> subcutaneous injection if not well tolerated.

Malaria. A severe headache accompanies the second stage (hot stage) of malaria, when flushing of the face and elevation of temperature take place. The sequence of chilling, heating, and sweating is almost pathognomonic of malaria. Other details and the detection of the parasite in blood smears will indicate the type of malaria parasite involved.

The headache present during the crisis of a malarial attack will subside with the treatment of such attack by means of antimalarial drugs, such as chloroquine and chlorguanide, which must be considered the first choice.

> Chloroquine, 1 g, to start, followed by 500 mg after
> 8 hours, and then 500 mg daily, for 4 days.

Amodiaquine, 600 mg, or even up to 1 g, to start,
followed by 400 mg daily, for 2 days.

Hydroxychloroquine, 800 mg, to start, followed by 400 mg
after 8 hours, and then 400 mg daily for 2 days.

Of course, quinine is still a drug of great therapeutic importance: it is not only an antimalarial, but also analgesic and antipyretic, per se. When the preferred antimalarials are not effective or available, quinine might be used.

Quinine, 1 g every 8 hours, during the first day of
treatment, followed by 600 mg every 8 hours for about 1
week.

Plague (*Bubonic Plague*). Headache may be present, but is not constantly found or characteristic of this serious disease, in which the diagnostic clue is given by the enlarged lymph nodes, or the syndromic complexes of pneumonia, pharyngitis, or meningitis, confirmed by the recovery of the infective germ.

Antibiotic therapy is specific and should be started immediately with streptomycin, the tetracyclines, or chloramphenicol. It will help to reduce the severe nervous symptoms, which include headache. The use of narcotic analgesics is to be discouraged; codeine, acetylsalicylic acid, or both are usually effective.

Codeine, 30 to 60 mg, by subcutaneous injection, every
4 to 6 hours, or as needed and tolerated.

Acetylsalicylic acid, 300 mg, plus codeine, 30 mg, capsules
or tablets, two every 4 to 6 hours.

Glanders (*Farcy*). Acute glanders, typically, has an abrupt and violent beginning with high fever, chills, and headache and prostration. Often a skin abrasion is the point of initial infection and forms a painful ulcer. The diagnosis is established by laboratory procedures when an acute disease appears following exposure to horses.

A chronic form is known with painful ulcers, and recurrent fulminating recurrences. Specific antibiotic therapy is to be prescribed whenever possible. For therapy, the soluble sulfonamides, especially sulfadiazine, continued for at least 20 days, and chlortetracycline and chloramphenicol are useful.

If the case is severe, associate two antibiotics or an antibiotic and a sulfa. The disease does not respond to penicillin or streptomycin.

90 DIAGNOSIS AND TREATMENT

A good therapeutic response will be accompanied by the control of the headache. Nevertheless, when cephalalgia is troublesome, use acetylsalicylic acid.

>Sulfadiazine, tablets, 0.5 g, four to twelve tablets daily.

>Chlortetracycline, tablets, 250 mg, four tablets daily, between meals.

>Chloramphenicol, tablets, 250 mg, four tablets daily between meals.

Continue antibiotic therapy for at least 2 weeks.

Tularemia. All forms of tularemia are characterized by a febrile attack, with headache and other symptoms of infection. The patient feels extremely weak; chills and sweating occur. At the site of innoculation, a papule appears and rapidly ulcerates, and lymphedema develops (which may suppurate and drain). An atypical pneumonia follows. Diagnosis is made after identification of the Pasteurella.

Streptomycin is the first choice for the specific treatment of tularemia, with a tetracycline or chloramphenicol as a second choice, these antibiotics being effective in the great majority of cases. Headache may become burdensome, at times, even to the point of requiring injections of codeine.

>Codeine, 30 or 60 mg, subcutaneously, every 3 or 4 hours, as needed and tolerated. Same dosage could be given by the oral route, either from the beginning of therapy, or after obtaining some relief from the use of injections.

Also, acetylsalicylic acid or equivalent analgesics could be tried in some patients for whom codeine might not be well advised.

>Acetylsalicylic acid, 600 mg, in tablets, every 4 hours, preferably with meals.

>Acetophenetidin, 300 mg, by mouth, every 4 hours.

>Propoxyphene hydrochloride, 65 mg, by mouth, every 4 hours.

Brucellosis (*Malta Fever, Undulant Fever*). Headache occurs in over 60% of patients during the acute stage of the disease, or during the phases of elevated temperature which are heralded by the onset of cephalalgia. The presence of sweating, generalized aches, weakness, anorexia, lymphadenopathy, splenomegaly, and chilly sensations might suggest the exact diagnosis. Orchitis, which seems to be relatively frequent in other countries, is not so prevalent in the United States.

Antibiotic therapy is advised for these patients. Usually, a tetracycline, either alone or, for seriously ill patients, in combination with streptomycin, is a wise choice. For the treatment of headache, codeine (to which many patients respond better than to other analgesics), acetylsalicylic acid, or a combination of both can be administered.

> Codeine, 30 or 60 mg, by subcutaneous injection to start, followed by the same dosage and timing after some effect is obtained. Give every 4 to 6 hours, according to results and tolerance.

> Acetylsalicylic acid, 300 to 600 mg, in tablets, every 4 to 6 hours, according to response, and better given with some food.

> Acetylsalicylic acid, 300 mg, plus codeine, 30 mg, in capsules or tablets, one or two every 4 to 6 hours, according to response.

In patients with severe toxemia, the adjunctive use of a corticoid might be of help, but never given for more than 3 or 4 days.

> Prednisone, 20 mg every 8 hours, by mouth.

> Hydrocortisone, 50 to 100 mg every 8 hours, by mouth.

Yellow Fever (Black Vomit). The essential features in yellow fever are: elevated temperature, albuminuria, jaundice, and hematemesis (black vomit). The disease begins abruptly with severe headache, generalized pains, flushed face, and a rise in pulse rate and temperature. A reliable diagnosis cannot be made, except by specialized laboratories. The disease will be found only in endemic areas, or in persons coming from these places.

No specific treatment is known, but the severe headache which accompanies most cases should be relieved. Because of the impairment of the gastric mucosa, salicylates should be avoided. Instead, codeine or meperidine can be given.

> Codeine, 60 mg, by subcutaneous injection, every 4 hours, as needed and tolerated. Subsequently, the oral route should be used, with the same amount of medication and same timing.

> Meperidine, 100 mg, by intramuscular injection, every 4
> hours, as needed and tolerated. As above, the oral route—
> same dosage and timing—may be used after obtaining
> some response.

Relapsing Fever (Recurrent Fever). An intense headache accompanies the disease after the first attack of fever and sweating. The clinical picture will subside by crisis, and after a period of remission, will reappear; additional relapses may occur, but at longer intervals. The diagnosis depends on the finding of Borrelia in peripheral blood.

Antibiotic drugs are usually effective for the treatment of relapsing fever. A tetracycline or chloramphenicol will be of use in most instances, but it has to be remembered that the antibiotic has to be given only during the attacks, *never* at the end of any relapsing attack or during the intervals, because of the possibility of provoking a serious Herxheimer reaction. The attacks are accompanied by a characteristic severe headache, which fortunately responds very well to the administration of codeine.

> Codeine, 30 or 60 mg, preferably to be given by mouth,
> every 4 to 6 hours. If needed, the subcutaneous route may be
> used, with the same amount of medication and timing.

The Leptospiroses (Weil's Disease and Others). The main symptoms are headache, photophobia, and fever. Generalized algias are also present, particularly in arms and calves. Conjunctival hemorrhage is almost characteristic.

Antibiotic therapy (penicillin or a tetracycline) is recommended, but not always effective. The headache usually responds to the administration of acetylsalicylic acid, codeine, or a similar analgesic.

> Acetylsalicylic acid, 300 or 600 mg, in tablets, every 4 to 6
> hours, preferably with meals.

> Codeine, 15 or 60 mg, according to response and tolerance,
> every 4 to 6 hours. An effective average dosage is 30 mg every
> 4 hours.

> Propoxyphene hydrochloride, 65 mg, by mouth, every 4
> hours.

> Acetaminophen, 600 mg, every 6 hours, by mouth.

The Rickettsial Diseases (Typhus, Rocky Mountain Spotted Fever, Q Fever, Trench Fever). In all rickettsial diseases, headache of a severe character is a paramount symptom. Elevated temperature and a rash are also common to most of them. A complete diagnosis relies on laboratory test. The rash of the typhus group begins on the back and chest; that of the Rocky Mountain spotted fever, on the flexor surfaces of wrists, ankles and back; that of trench fever, on chest and abdomen. In Q fever, a rash may be present or, possibly, respiratory symptoms.

Adequate antibiotics are extremely useful for the treatment of typhus, both epidemic and murine. Chloramphenicol and the tetracyclines are the first choice. For the treatment of cephalalgia do not give acetylsalicylic acid, since it increases the already profuse sweating of these patients, thus risking dehydration. Meperidine can be tried, but with caution, because in severe cases it may depress the respiratory centers. The first choice is codeine.

> Codeine, 30 to 60 mg, by subcutaneous injection or by mouth, every 4 to 6 hours, as needed and tolerated.

> Meperidine, 50 to 100 mg, by intramuscular injection or by mouth, every 4 or 6 hours, as needed and tolerated.

All other rickettsial diseases are to be treated in the same way as typhus (see above): antibiotic therapy may be carried out mainly with chloramphenicol or a tetracycline; codeine is the drug of choice for cephalalgia; meperidine has good effects, but may depress the respiratory centers; and acetylsalicylic acid is better avoided because of excessive sweating.

Syphilis. Headache may accompany all clinical forms of syphilis. In cerebral syphilis, pain may be excruciating. It may be present, also, as an intense pain in cases of gummata, osteitis, arteritis, meningitis, and particularly in tabes and general paresis. Some cases may suffer headache during eruption of the chancre. Consequently, a headache may not only be considered as part of the clinical picture, but also taken as a clue for the diagnosis of the disease. The clinical history and laboratory tests will give the final diagnosis.

Headache may be present during the secondary or the late stages of the disease; or may be a symptom heralding an otherwise ignored syphilitic infection. Antibiotic therapy is mandatory. Symptomatic treatment for cephalalgia will be carried out, whenever needed, with acetylsalicylic acid, codeine, for any other acceptable analgesic, for any one of them under regular schedule.

> Acetylsalicylic acid, 300 or 600 mg, in tablets, every 4 to 6 hours, preferably with meals.

> Codeine, 30 or 60 mg, by mouth, every 4 to 6 hours.

Propoxyphene hydrochloride, 65 mg, by mouth, every 4 hours.

Lymphogranuloma Venereum. This diagnosis is suggested by the presence of a shallow ulceration and the development of a well-marked regional lymphadonopathy, particularly in the inguinal area. The possibility of a complicating meningitis should be considered. In this rare complication cephalalgia is an indicative sign.

Chemotherapy, with a sulfa drug, alone, or with tetracycline is effective treatment. Headache is rarely severe, and should respond satisfactorily to acetylsalicylic acid.

Sulfadiazine, tablets, 0.5 g, two at once, then one four times a day.

Acetylsalicylic acid, 300 mg tablets, one every 4 to 6 hours, preferably with meals.

Local Infections

Meningitis. Inflammation of the meninges ordinarily follows an infection located elsewhere in the body, particularly otitis media, mastoiditis and sinusitis, ruptured brain abscess, infections in the orbit, or systemic infections. The disease is strongly suggested by a severe headache in a patient with fever and stiff neck. Positive Kernig's and Brudzinski's signs are characteristic. Laboratory tests are essential for the diagnosis.

Without specific treatment and before the inflammation of the meninges subsides, little effect is to be expected from the use of ordinary analgesics. Before using them, put on an ice cap and start a course with corticoids.

Cortisone, 25 mg, four or five times a day, by mouth.

Prednisone, 5 mg, also four or five times a day, by mouth.

Dexamethasone, 0.5 mg dosage for a total of 2 to 3 mg per day.

Then, either codeine, acetylsalicylic acid, or a similar analgesic could be used to some advantage.

Codeine, 60 mg, by subcutaneous injection or by mouth, every 4 hours.

Acetylsalicylic acid, 600 mg, in tablets, every 4 hours, preferably with meals.

> Propoxyphene hydrochloride, 65 mg, by mouth every 4 hours.
>
> Meperidine, 50 to 100 mg, by mouth, every 6 hours.

Encephalitis. Headache and neurologic symptoms accompany most forms of encephalitis, though the general clinical picture may be one so mild as to be unrecognized (as is found in most cases of St. Louis encephalitis) or be extremely severe (as in Eastern encephalitis, with hyperpyrexia, convulsions, and coma). Among the diagnostic possibilities are also the Japanese B, the Murray Valley, and the arthropod-borne encephalitides. Other intracranial complications to be looked for are due to systemic infections, such as brucellosis, measles, influenza, mumps, poliomyelitis, vaccinia, and varicella; or to parkinsonism, hemorrhage, drug therapy, or perhaps other causes. Generally speaking, the symptoms may begin suddenly or by steps, with cephalalgia, malaise, insomnia, chills, fever, and other symptoms, depending on the area most affected. Convulsions, myoclonus, hemiplegia, ocular paralysis, medullar or cerebellar symptoms, may occur when the cortex is affected; backache is common due to muscle spasm or irritation of the spine.

Etiological treatment can be carried out in many instances, when the infecting agent is known. Independently of this attack on the cause, relief of the burdensome headache is imperative. Corticoids may be of help, particularly when given early in the disease, and especially if it is of viral origin.

> Prednisone, 5 to 20 mg, every 6 hours, according to needs and results.

The first analgesic to be tried should be either acetylsalicylic acid or codeine, or a combination of the two.

> Acetylsalicylic acid, 600 mg, in tablets, every 4 hours, preferably with meals. Smaller doses are usually ineffective.
>
> Codeine, 60 mg, by mouth, every 4 hours.
>
> Acetylsalicylic acid, 300 mg, plus codeine, 30 mg, in capsules or tablets, two every 4 hours.

If insufficient relief is obtained by the above medication, meperidine could be tried, but not for too long a time.

> Meperidine, 50 to 100 mg, by intramuscular injection or by mouth, every 4 hours.

If excessive intracranial pressure is the cause of the headache, it should be lowered with infusions of mannitol or a urea-invert sugar preparation.

Sinusitis. Not only the sphenoid and ethmoid, but also the maxillary sinuses can cause, in addition to the local symptoms, a more or less marked cephalalgia. Frequently, the headache will be frontal, though it may be found at any other location in the head. The ache may be increased by coughing, by effort, or by percussion over the affected sinus. An X-ray plate will solve the diagnosis.

Both the acute and the chronic forms of sinusitis, particularly the latter, will be accompanied by headache. This will not be relieved until adequate drainage of the affected sinus is obtained. Vasoconstrictors and steam are the first steps to take in treating this form of cephalalgia. Thereafter, analgesics of the type of acetylsalicylic acid, codeine, etc. will be of help, either given alone or in combination.

> Codeine, 60 mg, by mouth, every 4 hours.
>
> Acetylsalicylic acid, 600 mg, in tablets, every 4 hours, preferably with meals.
>
> Acetylsalicylic acid, 300 mg, plus codeine, 30 mg, in tablets or capsules, two every 4 hours.

Oral Headache. Inflammation of the structures of the mouth, particularly in the teeth, even when the lesion is minor, may cause a headache. If the oral lesion is not obvious, the diagnosis might be established by exclusion.

Many of the disorders of the oral cavity are, or might be, accompanied by cephalalgia. In each case, an adequate therapy will be advised, with which the overall treatment can be started. Only thereafter, the help of ordinary analgesics will be advised.

> Acetylsalicylic acid, 600 mg, in tablets, every 4 hours, preferably with meals.
>
> Meperidine, 50 mg, by mouth, every 6 hours.

Aural Headache. It is well known how chronic otitis will provoke cephalalgia. The local symptoms will assist the diagnosis.

A goodly number of diseases of the middle ear are accompanied by headache, which will respond well in the majority of instances to the specific treatment, better carried out by an otologist. To comfort the patient, from the very beginning of trouble, codeine, acetylsalicylic acid, or both will be prescribed.

> Codeine, 60 mg, by mouth, every 4 hours.
>
> Acetylsalicylic acid, 600 mg, in tablets, every 4 hours, preferably with meals.
>
> Acetylsalicylic acid, 300 mg, plus codeine, 30 mg, in tablets or capsules, two every 4 hours.

Diseases of the Central Nervous System

Brain Tumors and Cysts. The main symptoms belong to the complexes of cranial hypertension and the localization of the new mass. An intense cephalalgia together with projectile vomiting and papilledema are characteristic of cranial hypertension. Also there may be found bradycardia, epileptic seizures, ophthalmoplegy, and behavioral disorders. The intense cephalalgia interferes with sleep, increases with effort, may be more severe at the site of the lesion, and is resistant to ordinary analgesics. It may mimic migraine. If the tumor localizes in the pituitary gland, the headache is mostly frontal and the patient may complain of extreme weakness.

Hydatid cyst of the brain is frequent in Europe and relatively rare in the United States, where children are more frequently affected than adults. Ordinarily, a previous cyst is found elsewhere in the body (liver). Headache may be the first manifestation of an expanding mass within the skull, even when it occurs in a patient in general good health. Diagnosis is made by X-ray examination and laboratory tests (eosiniphilia, Carson's test, complement fixation).

Surgery is the only logical approach to these problems, except for some tumors sensitive to radiation. For the relief of headache, prior to surgery, the best measure to be taken is the intravenous administration of a 50% glucose solution.

> Glucose, 50% solution; inject intravenously 25 ml—most cases will respond well to this amount—up to 50 ml.

Analgesics are of little value; and the most potent, the narcotic group, are not indicated for these patients. The risks of lumbar puncture (mobilization of the tumor to obstruct cerebrospinal pathways) make this procedure inadvisable.

Subdural Hematoma. A headache that appears immediately after an injury to the head, or after the first few days, particularly if accompanied with irritability and mental confusion, may be indicative of subdural hematoma. A spastic hemiplegia is a later confirmation of the intracranial bleeding. The cerebrospinal fluid will appear tinged with blood.

This condition requires surgery, particularly when progressing symptoms reveal the increasing pressure within the skull due to the increase in size of the lesion. Naturally, analgesics are of little help while the increasing pressure is still aggravating the pain. It is not to be forgotten that narcotic drugs should not be given whenever increased intracranial pressure is one of the causative factors of pain.

Subarachnoid Hemorrhage. The bleeding is most often heralded by a sudden and very intense cephalalgia, possibly following previous exertion of some kind. The headache may be frontal or occipital to start, then becoming generalized. Loss of consciousness may last for a few moments or hours in smaller hemorrhages, or until death in more severe ones. Neck stiffness is also constant; convulsions and fever are common. The spinal fluid pressure is elevated, as well as its content of red blood cells.

Even though analgesics are of little value in the treatment of cephalalgia caused by subarachnoid hemorrhage, codeine and acetylsalicylic acid should be tried for help.

> Acetylsalicylic acid, 300 to 600 mg, in tablets, every 3 to 6 hours, preferably with some food.

> Codeine, 30 to 60 mg, by mouth, every 3 to 6 hours.

As usual with these intracranial problems, narcotics are to be considered as contraindicated. If the diagnostic tapping is followed by alleviation of the headache and of other symptoms, lumbar puncture will be considered the best help for these patients, repeated until the bleeding stops.

Intracranial Abscess. Headache is variable, ranging from mild to severe pain; but convulsions are the first indication of an abscess, ordinarily, together with other signs of increased intracranial pressure, such as vomiting and papilledema. Sometimes a previous septic lesion developing neurological symptoms will suggest the formation of intracranial abscess.

Codeine may result in acceptable help in a few instances.

> Codeine, 60 mg, by mouth, every 4 hours.

Each case requires individualized therapy: surgery, antibiotics, analgesics, as indicated above.

Epilepsy. The diagnosis of epilepsy is obvious as soon as the first typical seizure occurs. Headache may be a part of the aura complex, and follows most attacks; but there are also headaches similar to migraine that appear between the principal epileptic seizures. It is to be noted that some relatives of epileptic patients, who show some of the epileptic stigmata, may suffer from typical migraine pains.

When epilepsy is due to a known cause (symptomatic epilepsy), the treatment should be addressed to this underlying cause, and measures against cephalalgia itself taken only whenever needed, since in the majority of instances there will be no need for analgesics. In all forms of epilepsy (either idiopathic or symptomatic) there is headache following the convulsive attacks. When this pain becomes bothersome, mild analgesics may be given, of the type of acetylsalicylic acid or codeine.

> Acetylsalicylic acid, 300 mg (rarely 600 mg will be needed), in tablets, repeating one or three tablets every 2 to 4 hours.

> Codeine, 30 mg every 6 to 8 hours; or repeated two or three times after the attack.

Neurosis and Emotions. Headache may be present among the characteristic symptoms of neurosis and emotions. It is often of a bizarre type and lacking in any features from which a diagnosis could be made. Care must be observed, however, not to take a neurotic or an emotional cephalalgia for an organic disease, or vice versa.

Any form of pain accompanying a neurosis, especially headache, is very likely to respond to sedatives and mild analgesics. Interestingly enough, it might yield just as well to the administration of a placebo. Needless to say, the neurosis, the basic problem, will respond better to psychotherapy, preferably by a specialist; however, under the skillful management of any understanding doctor the neurotic symptoms are likely to improve.

> Acetylsalicylic acid, 300 to 600 mg, in tablets, every 4 to 6 hours, preferably with meals.

> Codeine, 30 mg, by mouth, every 4 to 6 hours.

When the headache follows a more or less intense emotional shock (an accident, a distressing situation), the first attempt will be made to quiet the patient. Thereafter, if needed, codeine will be prescribed.

> Codeine, 30 to 60 mg, by mouth, every 4 hours, for only a few times.

If codeine fails, acetylsalicylic acid will be considered as an alternative.

> Acetylsalicylic acid, 600 mg, in tablets, every 4 hours, preferably with food; repeat if needed.

Circulatory Diseases

Hypertension. Many people know about their hypertensive bouts because of a revealing headache. Other symptoms also present are: dizziness, asthenia, palpitation, and insomnia. The diagnosis is made by taking the blood pressure with the sphygmomanometer. Frequently the headache occurs during the morning hours, is located in the occipital area, and increases with effort.

Most cases with headache due to elevated blood pressure will respond satisfactorily to mild analgesics, such as the following:

> Acetylsalicylic acid, 300 to 600 mg, in tablets, every 4 to 6 hours, preferably with meals.
>
> Propoxyphene hydrochloride, 65 mg, by mouth, every 4 to 6 hours.
>
> Acetophenetidin, 300 mg, every 3 or 4 hours, by mouth.
>
> Pentazocine, 50 mg, by mouth, every 4 hours.

Only in rare instances codeine will be needed.

> Codeine, 30 to 60 mg, by mouth, every 4 or 6 hours.

For the relief of nocturnal headache, to sleep with the head on a higher position than the rest of the body is helpful (blocks under the bed, extra pillows, elevation of the mattress, etc.).

Hypotension. In cases of hypotension, headache may also be an important symptom. It may be modified by the position of the body and by efforts. These patients ordinarily feel weak and faint easily (some, when getting up from bed). The headache is most frequently in the occipital area. All debilitating diseases may provoke hypotension.

Only a few patients will have headache, which may be relieved with mild analgesics, as in the case of hypertension discussed above. If syncope occurs, it will be treated according to the regular procedures.

Heart Failure. Congestion in the pulmonary and/or systemic circulation will interfere with oxygenation of tissues. Respiratory symptoms (dyspnea, coughing, and rales heard on auscultation) are conspicuous in left heart failure. Edema, epigastric distress due to enlargement of the liver, and congestion of abdominal viscerae causing anorexia and constipation are prominent in right heart failure. Headache of nonspecific nature may accompany either type of heart failure.

This condition is relatively prone to provoke headache, which sometimes requires drastic measures, such as the use of morphine, hydromorphone, meperidine, or anileridine; but on other occasions codeine may be good enough to control the situation.

> Morphine, 10 or 15 mg, by subcutaneous injection, every 4 hours.
>
> Hydromorphone, 2 mg, by subcutaneous injection, every 4 hours.
>
> Meperidine, 50 or 100 mg, by intramuscular injection or orally, every 4 hours.
>
> Anileridine, 25 mg, by intramuscular injection or by mouth, every 6 hours.
>
> Codeine, 60 mg, every 4 hours, by subcutaneous injection, or by mouth.

Also, there are patients who respond to milder analgesics, such as the salicylates and equivalents.

> Acetylsalicylic acid, 600 mg, by mouth, in tablets, every 4 hours, preferably with meals.
>
> Pentazocine, 50 or 100 mg, in tablets, every 3 or 4 hours.
>
> Propoxyphene hydrochloride, 65 mg, by mouth, every 4 hours.

Arteritis. Inflammation of the temporal arteries provokes headache, and local pain and tenderness. The pain exacerbates on pressure and during mastication. There is also fever and loss of weight.

When arteritis affects the temporal artery, it requires an immediate and active treatment for the prevention of blindness, as intracranial arteries might also be involved. Corticoids are mandatory in these cases.

> Cortisone acetate, 50 mg in each ml of the suspension; inject 100 mg, every 8 hours, intramuscularly, until symptoms begin to subside; immediately, start decreasing the injected amount, to 200 mg a day, and then to 100 mg a day (always in divided doses); and as soon as the situation is under control, discontinue gradually. Keep the reduced dosage at a level sufficient to ensure continuing action.
>
> Hydrocortisone, to start with 300 to 500 mg in 24 hours, the schedule being similar to the one above.

Prednisone, to start with 80 mg a day, in divided doses, the schedule being similar to the one developed for cortisone, above.

Dexamethasone, to start with 4 to 5 mg a day, in divided doses, the schedule as above.

With such elevated dosage, sodium retention is a possibility to be kept in mind; salt ingestion should be drastically reduced, additional potassium given, and frequent determination of electrolytes performed.

Metabolic and Toxic Conditions

All clinical syndromes in which the lack of an adequate oxygenation of cells is the main pathogenic mechanism may reveal dyspnea, cyanosis, asthenia, and, in some cases, nervous symptoms as well (convulsions, delirium), and almost constantly headache.

When hypoxia and anoxia are discussed, the effects of some toxic substances must be mentioned. In the following lines we will consider clinical syndromes accompanied by cephalalgia and due to toxic causes. Metabolic derangements may induce similar effects and symptoms.

High Altitude. Persons not accustomed to living in high altitudes may develop anoxic symptoms when they come to these places. If they are rapidly transported to a high altitude, the symptoms appear suddenly; dyspnea after light effort, dizziness, weakness, cyanosis, palpitation (tachycardia), possibly hemorrhage, and, almost always, headache. The chronic state of those who stay in high altitudes for long periods is revealed by dyspnea, dizziness, and headache, although the rule is no discomfort or disability after 2 to 4 weeks sojourn. Also, psychic aberrations may occur, particularly in the acute form.

In general, no analgesics should be used when headache is due to the poor oxygenation of high altitudes. Of course, narcotic analgesics are positively contraindicated in all instances, because of the possible depression of the respiratory center. The first approach is to decrease physical activity until the body accomodates to the new environment of an atmosphere poor in oxygen. When symptoms become annoying or dangerous, oxygen can be given by mask. As soon as the situation is under control, the headache will disappear.

Hypoventilation. Respiratory hypoventilation occurs in pneumonia, chronic emphysema, pneumothorax, or any other form of obstruction to the normal ventilation of the lungs, and incurs anoxemic symptoms, with disturbance of electrolyte balance, and, frequently, annoying headache. The particular symptoms of each of these disturbances will point out the diagnosis. Also, toxemias producing a depression of the respiratory centers (opium and related drugs) will induce hypoventilation. The inhalation of toxic gases will impair the oxygenation of blood and tissues. Carbon monoxide intoxication ordinarily begins with headache, and then other nervous symptoms (vertigo and loss of consciousness). The inert carbon monoxide–hemoglobin replacing the oxyhemoglobin gives the characteristic redness of the skin. Inert gases of all sorts may substitute for oxygen in some places, thus interfering with a good respiration. In acute poisoning by gases, particularly carbon monoxide, immediate 100% oxygen by inhalation is mandatory. Rest is required to decrease oxygen need, and will be maintained until respiration and oxygenation become normal. As in the case of symptoms brought on by high altitude, oxygen will be given by mask when they become bothersome or actually severe. Do not give narcotic analgesics, because they will depress the respiratory center, and use sparingly all other analgesics.

Do not forget that in cases of CO_2 retention, with hypoventilation and hypoxemia, oxygen may increase the inhibition of the respiratory center, thus making necessary the use of analeptics or respiratory stimulants.

> Ethamivan, by intravenous infusion, at a dosage of about 0.1 mg for each kg of body weight per minute as required.

> Caffeine sodium benzoate, USP, 500 mg to inject intramuscularly.

Cerebral Anoxia from Hematic Conditions. In acute posthemorrhagic anemia, there is some direct or indirect evidence or history of blood loss, and in addition there will be dizziness, faintness, more or less marked pallor, sweating and thirst, tachycardia, and progression into shock. In chronic blood loss, the evidence of some sort of bleeding is not always clear, but there are fatigability and weakness, and perhaps other symptoms of depleted vitality; but a blood count will give the final clue to diagnosis. The causative factor must be found. Arteriovenous shunts and anemia will also interfere with the adequate oxygenation of tissues. In some congenital heart diseases (patent ductus arteriosus or open foramen ovale), the mixing of venous with arterial blood will decrease the transported oxygen, causing cyanosis as an important symptom, together with other circulatory conditions; and headache is manifested by those patients old enough to tell about it. Among the symptoms of anemia—pallor, dyspnea, asthenia, and psychic changes—cephalalgia has an important place. Some toxic substances will interfere with respiration because of their power to transform hemoglobin into a different pigment. Toxic drugs are the nitrites, chlorates, and sulfas, among others. Headache will be a symptom in most of these intoxications.

In case of acute posthemorrhagic anemia, the treatment is that of shock; in chronic posthemorrhagic or iron deficiency anemia the treatment will be directed towards the blood deficiency. Regular analgesics will provide little and transient effect, such as acetylsalicylic acid and codeine.

> Acetylsalicylic acid, 300 to 600 mg, in tablets, every 6 hours, preferably with meals.
>
> Codeine, 30 mg, by mouth, every 6 hours.

Other anemias are to be treated following the same principles. In the case of headache due to cerebral anoxia caused by congenital heart disease or shunt, the symptomatic treatment, as stated above, might give some help; but the basic treatment is that applying to the underlying cause. If the cephalalgia is a consequence of a toxic reaction of a drug (sulfas, chlorates, etc.) first, discontinue that drug; secondly, try to eliminate it from the body; and last of all, try a mild analgesic, if it is really needed.

Toxic Headache. The following subjects will be included in this heading:

TOBACCO. Immoderately large amounts of tobacco will provoke headache together with other neurological symptoms (confusion, weakness, twitchings, convulsions), symptoms from the gastrointestinal tract (painful abdominal cramps, vomiting, diarrhea), and other symptoms, even collapse and coma if absorption has been excessive. Death may occur (respiratory paralysis). Intoxication by lobelia may cause similar symptoms.

COFFEE AND TEA. Caffeine intoxication may also begin with headache and other neurological symptoms. Pain of a burning nature is felt in the throat; ringing in the ears, tachycardia, and thirst may be dominant symptoms. As in the case of tobacco intoxication, anamnesis will reveal an inordinate use of these beverages.

CO AND OTHER VAPORS. These intoxicants must be considered professional poisonings. A patient with persistent headaches not due to other evident cause should be investigated from the industrial risk point of view: laborers who work in locales with an excess of carbon monoxide or any other toxic gas. Additional symptoms due to each particular toxic gas should be sought.

UREMIA. In chronic nephritis, headache is a very important symptom, but the usual clinical picture is that of a formerly known progressive renal insufficiency, with or without edema. An attack of a previous acute glomerulonephritis has occurred in the great majority of patients. In uremia, neurological, respiratory, gastrointestinal, and circulatory symptoms are involved, thus revealing the serious nature of the intoxication by nitrogen accumulating in the blood. It is a terminal phase of chronic kidney disease, and may also occur as a result of acute kidney diseases and regress when the basic condition improves. Laboratory tests will give an accurate diagnosis.

DIABETES. At the beginning of the disease, when hyperglycemia is not yet controlled, or whenever hyperglycemic bouts occur, headache is a common finding. Also, cephalalgia may occur whenever acidosis develops during the course of the disease. We should mention that headache may be present at the preclinical stage of the disease (prediabetes). Prediabetes is suspected when minimal changes in glucose tolerance occur in patients with relatives suffering from diabetes. When polydypsia, polyuria, polyphagia, and itching accompany the headache, there will probably be sugar in the urine, confirming the diagnosis of diabetes.

HYPOGLYCEMIA. This condition may result from an overdose of insulin or from going many hours without taking any food. There are headache, sweating, trembling, weakness, palpitations, psychological changes (similar to drunkenness, with which it has been confounded), and finally syncope, which may also occur early. The psychological symptoms may predominate when hypoglycemia develops slowly after use of long-acting insulins. Also, symptoms may appear at higher blood sugar levels when the hyperglycemia of a diabetic patient is lowered too rapidly.

TREATMENT. *Anoxic toxins* will induce anoxemia, which, as stated above (see "Cerebral anoxia from hematic conditions"), is to be treated with oxygen inhalation plus the basic therapy for each particular toxin. A severe *tobacco intoxication* may paralyze respiration; oxygen is also to be given in this instance, frequently together with artificial respiration. For the resulting headache, an ice cap is the best aid. In the case of headaches due to *coffee or tea intoxi-*

cation morphine is the drug of choice, because it will also help to decrease caffeine hyperexcitability.

>Morphine, 10 to 15 mg, by subcutaneous injection.

Also, *carbon dioxide and other gases* may also interfere with proper oxygen absorption, thus provoking a syndrome similar to any other hypoxic or anoxic condition. The administration of oxygen, frequently together with respiratory stimulants, is the correct therapeutic approach.

>Ethamivan, by intravenous infusion, at a dosage of about 0.1 mg for each kg and minute.

>Caffeine sodium benzoate, USP, 500 mg, to inject intramuscularly.

Headache due to *carbon monoxide intoxication* requires: immediate removal of the patient from the place of contamination; complete avoidance of any effort; artificial respiration (with oxygen inhalation); administration of mannitol or hypertonic urea, to combat cerebral edema whenever present.

>Mannitol solution; inject 2.5 g for each kg of body weight, by intravenous infusion.

>Hypertonic urea solution; inject 1 g for each kg of body weight, by intravenous infusion.

If needed, because of the severity of symptoms, an exchange transfusion can be given. Analgesics are of very little help in these cases. *Uremia, diabetes, and hypoglycemia,* as noted above, are frequently accompanied by headache. The basic treatment of each condition is paramount. In some instances, the use of a mild analgesic can be considered a good adjuvant therapy.

>Acetylsalicylic acid, 300 to 600 mg, in tablets, every 6 hours, preferably with meals.

>Codeine, 30 mg, by mouth, every 6 hours.

Ovaric Headache. Many headaches are intimately related to the ovarian function, such as menstruation, menopause, etc. On the other hand, headache (particularly migraine) is by far a disease of women, who suffer it much more frequently than men. Also, headaches are common symptoms in all forms of ovarian insufficiency. During pregnancy, headache may occur without any other known cause, but it must be suspected as a sign of toxemia gravidarum.

During the amenorrheic phase of ovarian insufficiency, during the premenstrual phase (for some women), and at the menopause or following removal of the ovaries, headache is a frequent and bothersome symptom. Hormones (estrogens, or a combination of estrogens and a progesterone) are the basic treatment. Any analgesic drug can be given as adjuvant, emergency treatment.

> Acetylsalicylic acid, 600 mg, in tablets, every 6 hours, preferably with meals.
>
> Acetaminophen, 300 to 600 mg, by mouth, every 6 to 8 hours, for one or two days.
>
> Pentazocine, 25 to 50 mg, by mouth, every 4 hours, for one or two days.
>
> Codeine, 30 mg, by mouth, every 4 to 6 hours.

It is to be noted that ovarian headache can be of cerebrovascular nature (migraine), and in these cases it should be treated accordingly, with analgesics as above or as stated in more detail below (see "Migraine").

Acidosis. Particularly in metabolic acidosis (which may follow excessive absorption of chloride, loss of bicarbonate, renal disease, diabetes), the clinical picture reveals headache, weakness, abdominal pain (do not mistake it for an acute abdomen!), hyperpnea, and nausea with or without vomiting. Signs of dehydration will be noted (inelastic skin, dry mouth, sunken eyes). The diagnosis is made by laboratory tests.

In the headache due to metabolic acidosis, the treatment has to be addressed to the cause (diabetes, renal failure, diarrhea, as the most frequent etiologic factors), and the metabolic imbalance corrected by intravenous infusions of bicarbonate whenever indicated. Once the acidotic state responds to adequate treatment, the headache disappears without the need of any analgesic drug.

In respiratory acidosis (depressed respiratory center, impaired mechanical respiration, carbon dioxide intoxication) the treatment is the same as for hypoventilation: rest, oxygen therapy, and avoidance of narcotic analgesics (see above, "Hypoventilation").

Alkalosis. Headache may be present, but the dominant symptoms are of neuromuscular irritability, particularly tetany. In the case of metabolic alkalosis, the deficit in water, sodium, chloride, and potassium has to be corrected by giving these either by mouth or by intravenous infusion, as the circumstances dictate.

Respiratory alkalosis, mostly due to neurotic hyperventilation but also to toxemia (lesions of the central nervous system, hepatic coma, salicylate poisoning, fever, etc.), will require the administration of oxygen, or simply (as in the case of neurotic hyperventilation) to breathe into a paper bag (do not use a plastic bag). Analgesics with a sedative, or the sedative alone, might be of some help.

> Acetylsalicylic acid, 300 mg, plus phenobarbital, 15 mg, capsule, one or two every 4 to 6 hours.

> Phenobarbital, 15 or 30 mg, by mouth, every 6 to 8 hours.

Headache in Allergy

Migraine. The cause of migraine is unknown, but we include the disease here because the allergic theory of its etiology has been one of the most favored. Headache is the dominant symptom, either affecting the whole head or, frequently, the right or the left side (hemicrania). During the attack, nausea and photophobia are also important symptoms. Often preceding the attack are photophobia, visual aura, scintillating scotoma, nervous irritability, and nausea. In many patients the recurrent pattern of these symptoms warns of the coming of the typical attack.

In cases thought to be due to allergic disease, if the causative allergen is found, desensitization or avoidance of the allergen will be a necessary treatment. Recently, there has been considerable question about allergy being the sole cause of migraine.

If the diagnosis is in doubt and the symptoms are slight, the chosen medication can be acetylsalicylic acid and codeine or a similar analgesic.

> Acetylsalicylic acid, 600 mg, in tablets, every 4 hours, while the attack lasts.

> Codeine, 30 to 60 mg, by mouth, every 4 hours while the attack lasts. In severe cases, codeine could be given in the same amounts, by subcutaneous injection.

> Acetaminophen, 600 mg, by mouth, every 6 hours, while the attack lasts.

> Pentazocine, 50 mg, by mouth, every 4 hours, while the attack lasts.

> Propoxyphene hydrochloride, 65 mg, by mouth, every 4 hours, while the attack lasts.

If no effect is noted following the first or second dosage, ergot derivatives will be used instead. In really severe cases, the ergot derivatives should be the first drug given by injection, particularly when vomiting does not allow oral medication.

> Ergotamine tartrate, 0.5 mg in solution, by subcutaneous injection; or, for more active and rapid effect, 0.25 mg in solution by intravenous injection. This will terminate the attack in most instances.

Do not forget that ergotamine, by the intravenous route, may increase vomiting, at times. Dihydroergotamine is a good, effective alternative.

> Dihydroergotamine, 1 mg in each ml solution, to be given by intramuscular or subcutaneous injection. Inject only 1 mg.
> In case of need, give it by vein.

The ergot derivatives mentioned above can be repeated after 1 or 2 hours, whenever necessary, and the therapy can be complemented with the same drugs given orally.

> Ergotamine tartrate, 1 mg, by mouth, every 4 hours the first day; every 8 hours, thereafter, as needed.

The addition of caffeine may be of help for some of these patients.

> Caffeine, 100 mg, by mouth, every 6 to 8 hours.

Histamine Headache. This headache shows some similarities to migraine. It affects one side of the head and the corresponding eye, temple, face, and neck. Other symptoms are localized vasodilation, edema, watery eyes, and running nose.

This headache seems to be very closely related to migraine (see above), and its treatment will follow the same rules; to start with a regular analgesic drug (acetylsalicylic acid, codeine, pentazocine, propoxyphene hydrochloride, etc.) or resort to ergot derivatives (ergotamine tartrate, dihydroergotamine) whenever the first trial fails or the attack is so severe that we may assume ergot treatment should be started from the very beginning, no matter that it is relatively frequent that ergotamine tartrate by intravenous injection can increase vomiting.

> Ergotamine tartrate, 0.25 mg, by intravenous injection; or 0.5 mg in solution, by the subcutaneous route.

> Dihydroergotamine, 1 mg in each ml of solution, to be given by intramuscular or subcutaneous injection. Also, in

emergent situations dihydroergotamine in the same amount of 1 mg can be injected intravenously.

Also, antihistaminic drugs can be tried, such as chlorpheniramine, cyproheptadine, etc.

Chlorpheniramine, 4 mg, by mouth, every 6 to 8 hours.

Cyproheptadine, 4 mg, by mouth, every 6 to 8 hours.

For analgesic medication please refer to the section on "Migraine."

Hay Fever. A frontal headache accompanies the classic symptoms of itching nose, eyes, and pharynx, watery nasal discharge, and sneezing.

Pollinosis requires complete and continuous treatment, which will be carried out according to the rules given by allergists. Additional treatment with antihistaminic drugs is a help, in most instances.

Chlorpheniramine, 4 mg, by mouth, every 8 hours.

Cyproheptadine, 4 mg, by mouth, every 8 hours.

The treatment of headache, per se, is of little importance, since it usually responds well to antihistamine therapy, either alone or together with sympathominetics of the type of ephedrine.

Ephedrine, 25 mg, by mouth, every 6 or 8 hours.

Pseudoephedrine hydrochloride, 60 mg, by mouth every 6 or 8 hours.

Anaphylactic Shock. A pounding headache with throbbing in the ears accompanies a sensation of extreme anxiety and uneasiness, and follows the injection of an offending allergen. Intense peripheral vascular collapse and other allergic symptoms may appear. Fatal cases are not rare.

Since the headache will subside when the anaphylactic shock is under control, no attempt to treat the pain will be made, but all efforts will be directed to save the patient from this threatening reaction by giving immediately epinephrine by intravenous infusion.

Epinephrine, 0.5 mg in 10 ml of saline solution, to inject slowly into the vein.

The rest of the treatment depends on the occurrence, or not, of respiratory difficulties and hypotension, which conditions will be treated accordingly, including resuscitation, if things go so far.

Headache and Diseases of the Digestive System

Gastrointestinal Diseases. Headache may accompany many gastrointestinal disorders, but rarely will be considered an important part of the symptom complex. Dyspepsia may provoke nausea, frequently with vomiting, weakness, sweating, vertigo, and headache. Food infection with gastroenteritis starts suddenly with headache, fever, chills, and abdominal symptoms including diarrhea. Staphylococcus toxin gastroenteritis shows similar symptoms, but fever and headache are inconstant. In cases of mucous colitis or irritable colon, the characteristic digestive symptoms (constipation and mucous depositions) may be accompanied by headache, anorexia, insomnia, etc. Cephalalgia is a part of the constipation complex.

As a frequent complication of constipation, dyspepsia, or gastroenteritis, headache may become annoying enough to need some sort of treatment by itself. In the case of dyspepsia and gastroenteritis, the administration of drugs that may irritate the gastrointestinal tract should be avoided, particularly acetylsalicylic acid. Give instead codeine, acetaminophen, pentazocine, etc.

Codeine, 30 to 60 mg, by mouth, every 6 hours.

Acetaminophen, 600 mg, by mouth, every 8 hours.

Pentazocine, 50 mg, by mouth, every 8 hours.

For constipation headache any analgesic can be given, including acetylsalicylic acid.

Acetylsalicylic acid, 600 mg, by mouth, every 6 or 8 hours, preferably with meals.

Of course, in all instances the treatment of the underlying cause of the digestive problem is imperative.

Hepatic Headache. An intense cephalalgia is a part of the acute yellow atrophy symptom complex which includes abdominal pain in the liver area, vomiting, very marked jaundice, and convulsions. Ordinarily, there is a preceding liver disease. In other chronic liver diseases, headache may be present, but it is never an important part of the symptomatology.

In severe or relatively severe hepatic conditions, such as in the case of acute yellow atrophy or fulminant hepatitis—most commonly of viral etiology, common viral hepatitis, some forms of cirrhosis, and alcoholic liver, the treatment of the frequently accompanying headache is only secondary. If hepatic functions are under great stress, it is better not to give analgesics. Nevertheless, the use of corticoids is advisable in many instances: some forms of hepatitis (fulminant, submassive, prolonged), some forms of cirrhosis (portal or postnecrotic), and alcoholic liver.

> Prednisone, 5 to 15 mg, by mouth, every 6 or 8 hours, for a few days, decreasing the dosage when improvement is noted, and starting discontinuance gradually after a few days of treatment.

> Triamcinolone acetonide, 40 mg, suspension, for intramuscular injection in the gluteal area, to start medication, and then continuing by the oral route.

> Dexamethasone, 4 or 5 g a day in divided doses; amount to be decreased as soon as improvement is noted; then start discontinuance after a few days of treatment.

Diseases of the Bones and Muscles of the Head

Paget's Diseases. Bone pain, including pain in the skull, is a common symptom of the disease, which is characteristically manifested by the early decalcification of bones. The decalcification produces bone softening and bowing; the changes occuring in the head lead to a triangular appearance of the face. The diagnosis is made by X ray.

Since no specific therapy for Paget's disease is yet known (in spite of the interesting attempts made in this regard, lately), most of its symptoms will have to be treated as they become apparent. Initial bouts of headache will respond well to common analgesics, such as acetylsalicylic acid, codeine, propoxyphene hydrochloride, etc.

> Acetylsalicylic acid, 600 mg, in tablets, every 4 or 6 hours, preferably with meals.

> Codeine, 60 mg, by mouth, every 4 or 6 hours.

> Propoxyphene hydrochloride, 65 mg, by mouth, every 4 hours.

> Acetaminophen, 600 mg, by mouth, every 4 or 6 hours.

In advanced cases, when pressure may be a contributing factor, X-ray therapy should be tried. Estrogens or androgens (according to sex) have been recommended also.

Endocranial Hyperostosis. In the Stewart-Morell syndrome (in Europe, Morgagni-Pende or Morgagni-Morell) there are symptoms of a very diversified nature, most of them of an individualized character. The only peculiar symptoms of the complex are the excrescences found in the inner layer of the skull.

The great majority of patients with this derangement will not complain of any symptom. Some may present more or less marked symptoms, among them headache. This pain is easily relieved with average treatment with analgesics, such as stated above.

Intracranial Calcifications. At X-ray examination, intracranial calcifications may be found in patients showing some neurological disturbances who also complain of headache. A syndrome of cranial hypertension may also be present in some instances. More rarely, epilepsy and vertigo will accompany the calcifications.

The basic treatment belongs to the neurologist and the neurosurgeon; but when pain is distressing, the patient might be helped by meperidine or codeine, and for less marked pain, with acetylsalicylic acid, propoxyphene hydrochloride, etc.

> Meperidine, 100 mg, by mouth, every 4 to 6 hours; but in very severe cases can be given by injection.
>
> Codeine, 60 mg, by mouth, every 4 to 6 hours; but in very severe cases can be given by injection.
>
> Acetylsalicylic acid, 600 mg, in tablets, every 4 to 6 hours, preferably with meals.
>
> Propoxyphene hydrochloride, 65 mg, by mouth, every 4 hours.

Other analgesics can also be considered for treatment.

Muscle Strain. The muscles of the back of the neck can be tense and tender in cases of anxiety, or of cervical spondyloarthrosis. In either instance, an occipital headache will be apparent. A characteristic gesture is pressing the neck muscles with one or both hands while moving the head backwards.

The headache due to muscle strain of the neck is relieved as soon as the neck strain subsides under treatment. An adjuvant dose of an analgesic is of additional help. Muscle relaxants should be considered for this purpose.

> Codeine, 60 mg, by mouth, every 4 or 6 hours.
>
> Acetaminophen, 300 to 600 mg, by mouth, every 6 hours.
>
> Propoxyphene hydrochloride, 65 mg, by mouth, every 4 hours.

Relaxation of muscles may be helped by medication of the type of meprobamate, carisoprodol, etc.

Headache and Physic Factors

Traumatic. It is obvious to expect the onset of a headache following any injury to the head. A very close surveillance, or an initial surgical approach, is the basic condition for a good treatment of head injuries. But because headache may reach intolerable proportions at times, the additional use of drugs for the relief of pain may also be mandatory: common analgesics if pain is not too severe, to include narcotics whenever needed. Nevertheless, for a safer attitude, all cases should be transferred to the hospital, particularly if the patient has been found unconscious, if a fracture is disclosed, if convulsions are present, or if shock develops.

> Codeine, 60 mg, by mouth or by injection, every 4 or 6 hours, as needed.

> Meperidine, 100 mg, by mouth or by injection, as needed and tolerated. Either meperidine, morphine, or any other narcotic, if given, will be observed very closely for its effect upon the respiratory centers, to avoid depression.

Heat and Heatstroke. Prolonged heat is a frequent cause of headache. It is well known how people sleeping in closed and overheated rooms awake with a headache. Excessive heating may provoke heat cramps or heat prostration. In the latter condition, circulatory collapse is manifested, heralded by headache, irritability, cramps, and weakness. In heatstroke (sunstroke) the symptoms are similar (headache, irritability, collapse), but an elevated body temperature over $40.5°C$ ($105°F$) is also present.

When excessive heat threatens collapse of the patient, headache is one of the premonitory symptoms, as is also the case in heatstroke. The administration of analgesics capable of inducing diaphoresis is contraindicated; and for the avoidance of depression of respiratory centers, narcotics also have to be avoided. In both instances, heat and heatstroke, the first attempt will be to decrease body temperature (particularly in the case of sunstroke) by using an ice cap and blankets cooled with water, or placing the patient into an ice-water bath. Rectal temperature will be checked frequently and not allowed to fall below $38°C$ (about $101°F$). These measures will alleviate the headache, without the need of any analgesic. The complete treatment will follow the well-established rules.

Ocular Causes of Headache

Most diseases of the eye will cause not only localized pain but also a headache. In the following lines we will consider the most important eye diseases that may provoke a secondary cephalalgia.

Glaucoma. The increased intraocular pressure in glaucoma is the cause of the principal symptoms of the disease. In the case of simple glaucoma (chronic open-angle, noncongestive), the course is slow with progressive loss of vision, frequent changes of glasses, and cephalalgia. It is characteristic to see halos around lights (electric or the like). In acute congestive glaucoma (narrow-angle) the symptoms are the same, but are manifested in the form of attacks of pressure and pain lasting for a few hours and recurring at variable intervals (weeks, months, or even years), until the typical fulminating attack occurs with its characteristic brutality.

Once the diagnosis of glaucoma is established, the patient must be sent to the ophthalmologist, since the essentials of treatment of this disease depend on whether it is primary or secondary, acute or chronic, congestive or noncongestive, open-angle or narrow-angle glaucoma, etc. The essential part of the treatment is to reduce intraocular tension, which when achieved will check the headache. In chronic noncongestive (simple) glaucoma, the drugs of the type of pilocarpine are first to be used.

> Pilocarpine, 1 or 2% solution; instill one or two drops, as needed, in the conjunctival sac.
>
> Physostigmine, 0.25% solution; instill one or two drops in the conjuctival sac, as needed. During sleep time, 0.25% ointment will be used instead.
>
> Carbachol, 1.5% solution; instill only one drop, and no more than three times a day.

The above drugs can be given alone, or one of them together with acetazolamide.

> Acetazolamide, 250 mg in tablets, once—but never more than four times—a day. In emergent situations, 500 mg solution is to be injected intravenously.

If the patient has aphakic eyes, the following medication is preferred.

> Isofluorophate, 0.1% solution; instill two drops every 8 hours, for three days; or 0.025% ointment, to be used during the sleep time.

In chronic angle closure glaucoma, pilocarpine (q.v.) is also the medication of choice. But in the case of acute angle closure glaucoma, either glycerin or acetazolamine may abort the attack.

> Glycerin, 1 or 2 g for each kg of body weight, mixed with an equal amount of water, by mouth.
>
> Acetazolamide, as above.

If these medications do not exert their expected action, and if the kidneys are in good conditions, use a solution of urea.

> Urea, 30% solution, inject intravenously from 1 to 1.5 g for each kg of body weight.

Secondary glaucoma finally could require treatment with corticoids and acetazolamide after diagnosis and removal of the primary cause (synechiae, hemorrhage, tumors, cicatrices, foreign bodies).

> Prednisone, 5 to 10 mg every 4 hours, to decrease as soon as improvement is noted, and to start discontinuance after a few days of treatment.
>
> Acetazolamide, see above.

The rest of the treatment, either medical or surgical, will be evaluated by the ophthalmologist.

For more details see the section "Ophthalmodynia," under the heading "Glaucoma."

Iritis and Iridocyclitis. In iritis there is pain in the eye (which pain radiates to the corresponding temple), photophobia, lacrimation, and edema of the upper eyelid. There are also blurring of vision and visible alterations of the iris (swelling, irregular pupil, posterior synechiae, hypopyon).

The symptoms of iridocyclitis are the same as in iritis; but the involvement of the ciliary body makes these symptoms more intense; a well-marked circumcorneal ciliary injection and more intense pains are noted.

Common analgesics can be given to these patients, such as:

> Acetylsalicylic acid, 600 mg, in tablets, every 4 hours, preferably with meals.
>
> Codeine, 60 mg (30 mg enough in some instances) by mouth, every 4 to 6 hours.
>
> Acetaminophen, 600 mg, by mouth, every 6 hours.

Pentazocine, 50 mg, by mouth, every 4 hours.

Propoxyphene hydrochloride, 65 mg, by mouth, every 4 hours.

Together with analgesics, the treatment is to be started by using corticoids and mydriatics.

Prednisone, 5 mg—more if needed—by mouth, every 8 hours; to decrease and discontinue administration as soon as possible.

Atropine, 1% solution, to instill one drop into the conjunctival sac, two or three times a day.

But the patient has to be referred to the ophthalmologist as soon as first aid has been given.

Strabismus and Faulty Accommodation. There are no problems for diagnosis. Headache is noted in all forms when an effort is made to accommodate for fusion of the image. In latent strabismus headache may be more conspicuous.

In all errors of refraction headache is present when efforts to overcome the error are made by the eyes. This is true in hyperopia (farsightedness), myopia (nearsightedness), and presbyopia (old age vision).

These conditions require corrective glasses (or surgery, in the case of strabismus). In the meantime, the frequent headaches presented by many patients can be relieved by common analgesics given either alone or together with muscle relaxants. Miotics are of help, but should be advised and prescribed by the ophthalmologist. Consequently, the physician will order the use of codeine or other analgesic, or meprobamate or other muscle relaxant.

Codeine, 30 mg, by mouth, every 6 hours.

Propoxyphene hydrochloride, 65 mg, by mouth, every 4 hours.

Meprobamate, 400 mg, by mouth, every 8 hours.

Carisoprodol, 350 mg, tablets, every 6 hours.

II. PAIN IN THE FACE

Less frequent than headache, pain in the face is not rare, and is always very bothersome. Furuncles, sinus infection, and trigeminal neuralgia are, perhaps, the prevalent forms of pain in the face. Fortunately, most of these cases will respond favorably to adequate therapy.

Trigeminal Neuralgia. A very severe pain presented in the form of relatively brief attacks involving one half of the face (in relation with the affected branch of the trigeminal nerve) is suggestive of the name "tic douloureux," or trigeminal neuralgia. There are frequently found trigger areas, which are hypersensitive and which may excite an attack of pain when irritated or merely touched. It will not be confounded with other forms of neuritis (tumoral, postherpetic, etc.). A good clue will be given by precipitation of attacks under the influence of washing the face, exposure to cold, eating, drinking, or even talking.

The first trial in treating this disease can be made with cyanocobalamine (vitamin B_{12}), in large amounts by the intramuscular route.

Cyanocobalamine, 1 mg (1000 μg) by intramuscular injection, daily for 10 days.

This treatment could be repeated, even without pain, after a 1- or 2-month interval, for a few times. The second trial can be with carbamazepine.

Carbamazepine, 200 mg, tablets; one to ten tablets daily, in divided doses according to results and tolerance.

Also, anticonvulsants of the type of diphenylhydantoin, may be used, and expected to be effective in many cases.

Diphenylhydantoin, 100 mg, tablets; one every 6 hours.

The final resource is surgical: first, the injection of alcohol into the ganglion or into the affected branches of the trigeminus, which may allay pain for months and even years; and secondly, neurosurgery.

Ophthalmic Herpes Zoster. Typical lesions of herpes zoster will be found over the cutaneous distribution of the nasociliary nerve or other branches of the ophthalmic, i.e., around the eye, from the forehead to the nose, on one side of the face. Other symptoms are: pain, edema, inflammation of tissues (conjunctiva ciliary body, and other locations). The final diagnosis usually is easy to establish.

Herpes zoster is usually accompanied by intense pain, and if localized in the ophthalmic branch of the trigeminus may also cause serious ocular lesions. An ophthalmologist should be consulted for all cases of ophthalmic herpes zoster. For this corticoids are advised (do not forget that corticoids are positively contraindicated in herpes simplex!).

Prednisone, to start with, at 40 mg a day, and rapidly decrease the dosage; but discontinuance has to be slow.

Triamcinolone acetonide, 40 mg in suspension; inject into gluteus muscle, in starting corticoid therapy, for rapid relief.

Other analgesics can be tried, as follows:

Acetylsalicylic acid, 600 mg, tablets, every 4 hours, preferably with meals.

Codeine, 60 mg, by mouth, every 4 to 6 hours.

Acetophenetidin, 300 mg, by mouth, every 4 hours.

Propoxyphene hydrochloride, 65 mg, by mouth every 4 hours.

Meperidine, 100 mg, by mouth, every 4 to 6 hours.

Persisting neuralgia after disappearance of skin lesion might respond to infiltration of the affected area with triamcinolone acetonide (see above) and lidocaine solution.

Lidocaine, 2% solution; use 1 to 3 ml.

Ocular lesions are to be treated by an ophthalmologist.

Sinus pain. Acute sinusitis will begin abruptly or gradually, with pain in the area corresponding to the affected sinus or sinuses, which increases or appears under pressure. Together with local pain, there are heterotopic pains radiating to the head, teeth, and ears. There can be fever, periorbital edema, photophobia, general malaise, and even vertigo.

Chronic sinusitis is less conspicuous in clinical appearance. Pain might be the only symptom, either headache, toothache, or simply local pain or tenderness over the sinuses.

Regarding both forms of sinusitis, note that local pain varies in accordance with the affected sinus: supraorbital in frontal sinusitis; teeth, cheek, and forehead in maxillary sinusitis; occipital, parietal, root of the nose, or in the neck in ethmoid or sphenoid sinusitis.

The final diagnosis is made by noting purulent discharge from the affected sinus and the use of transillumination or X rays, or direct irrigation by catheter or puncture.

In acute sinusitis, advise bed rest, light diet, moderate intake of fluids, local heating, local decongestants, adequate antibiotic therapy, and the use of analgesics.

> Papaverine hydrochloride, 150 mg, in slow-release capsules, one every twelve hours.
>
> Meperidine, 100 mg, start by subcutaneous injection and continue by mouth every 4 to 6 hours.
>
> Acetylsalicylic acid, 600 mg, in tablets, every 4 hours, preferably with meals.

Local decongestants also help to control pain, either when given by mouth or instilled into the nose.

> Pseudoephedrine hydrochloride, 60 mg, tablets, every 6 or 8 hours.
>
> Phenylephrine, 5% solution, three of four drops into the nostril of the affected side.

Broad-spectrum antibiotics are fundamental in the treatment of sinusitis, both acute or chronic, together with surgical procedures to be put into practice by the specialist.

Chronic sinusitis requires more specialized care, with irrigations, removal of polyps—if present—antrotomy, etc., and adequate antibiotic therapy. For pain, analgesics can be prescribed, as stated above.

Furuncle. The clinical appearance of furuncles located on the face is typical of those found elsewhere on the body: an inflammatory nodule located perifollicularly, which changes into a pustule. A central area of necrosis permits the final purulent drainage of the lesion. They are particularly painful when located on the ear, nose, or lip.

A large number of furuncles do appear on the face, but their treatment does not differ from furuncles located at other sites. Excepting for furuncles located in the area comprising the upper lip and the nasogenian ridge: here, there is a risk of meningeal spreading of the infection. For this reason, it is advisable not to touch these furuncles, and to use only systemic antibiotic therapy. Otherwise, warm compresses may help; and a little incision, when pus is well localized, will complete control of the infection. Local application of antibiotics is also helpful.

> Neomycin, 1%, ointment or cream, apply locally every 6 or 8 hours.
>
> Polymyxin B, 0.25% solution, ointment or cream, to be applied locally every 6 to 8 hours.

Erysipelas. This is, ordinarily, an acute disease beginning with pain, fever, and chills, and a localized red rash with a distinctly demarcated margin, which is firm to the touch and swollen (particularly at the periphery). Malaise, nausea, and vomiting are frequent occurrences; redness spreads peripherally, and in severe cases there are vesicles or bullae. A frequent starting point is the angle of the mouth. It is caused by a streptococcus.

Most cases of erysipelas will be found around the nose and mouth; but they may be present elsewhere on the body. The patient will keep bed rest, with the head elevated. Hot packs on the lesion help to control pain. Acetylsalicylic acid will serve for both pain and fever.

> Acetylsalicylic acid, 600 mg, in tablets, repeat every 4 hours, preferably with meals.
>
> Acetophenetidin, 300 mg, by mouth, every 4 or 6 hours.
>
> Acetaminophen, 600 mg, by mouth, every 6 hours.

Since beta-hemolytic streptococci strains causing erysipelas are mostly sensitive to penicillin, give this antibiotic.

> Procaine penicillin, 600,000 units solution by injection, every 8 or 12 hours.

Injuries to the Face. These may be of any kind: contusions, bruises, wounds, fractures, burns, etc. The diagnosis is easily made from clinical history and physical appearance. For fractures, particular symptoms and the evidence of the X ray will assure the diagnosis.

Except for contusions and bruises, all injuries to the face should be referred to a surgeon, either general or plastic. After a thorough cleansing of the lesion, some analgesic will be given, according to the intensity of the pain.

> Meperidine, 100 mg, by subcutaneous injection.
>
> Methadone, 10 mg, by subcutaneous injection.
>
> Morphine sulfate, 10 to 15 mg, by subcutaneous injection.

The pain of contusions will be treated with cool compresses and the aid of salicylates and similar drugs.

Acetylsalicylic acid, 600 mg, in tablets, every 4 hours, preferably with meals.

Codeine, 60 mg, by mouth, every 4 hours.

Acetophenetidin, 300 mg, by mouth, every 4 hours.

Propoxyphene hydrochloride, 65 mg, by mouth, every 4 hours.

Bruises may receive similar care, or will be treated with local anesthetic solutions; of course, after thorough cleansing and good protection with local antibiotics and covering.

Benzocaine, 5 or 20% ointment, apply locally, once or twice a day.

Bone pain. This pain may be due to an injury, an infection, arthritis, or a tumor; and treated accordingly. In all instances, if pain is severe enough, a narcotic analgesic will be used.

Codeine, 60 mg, by subcutaneous injection, every 4 hours.

Meperidine, 100 mg, by subcutaneous injection, every 4 to 6 hours.

Methadone, 10 mg, by subcutaneous injection, every 4 to 6 hours.

Morphine sulfate, 10 to 15 mg, by subcutaneous injection, as needed and tolerated.

Otherwise, a salicylate or similar drug will be given, much as follows:

Acetylsalicylic acid, 600 mg, in tablets, every 4 to 6 hours, preferably with meals.

Acetophenetidin, 300 mg, by mouth, every 4 to 6 hours.

Propoxyphene hydrochloride, 65 mg, by mouth, every hours.

Codeine, 60 mg, every 4 to 6 hours, by mouth.

The basic condition provoking pain will receive adequate care, be it arthritic, rheumatic, infective, or tumoral.

Tooth Pain. See below, section on "Stomatalgia."

Skin Diseases. See section on "Pain in the Skin," at the end of this volume, for other skin diseases that cause pain in the face.

III. STOMATALGIA

Pain arising from mouth structures is relatively frequent. Most of these pains belong to the domain of the dentist, because they are due to dental problems. The physician also deals with these pains, because they may arise, too, from other mouth structures.

For pain in the mouth (stomatalgia), the great majority of patients will have consulted the dentist. But in many cases the physician will have to decide what to do, either on an emergency basis, or because the disease is medical in the first place and not dental.

Teeth

Caries will not be painful unless pulpitis is present.

Pulpitis is revealed by a sharp and intermittent pain, not always well localized by the patient. But pulpitis may be secondary to causes other than caries, that is, physical or bacterial causes. The diagnosis is made by X-ray and electric examination.

Dental caries is painless until it reaches the dental pulp and causes pulpitis. At this stage, there is pain which may be relieved by cleansing the cavity very carefully, removing all food debris, and applying oil of cloves.

> Oil of cloves, soak a cotton applicator and put in the cavity.
>
> Clove oil plus zinc oxide powder, mix to make a semisolid mixture and apply to the cavity.

Further treatment is entirely in the dentist's domain; but in the meantime efforts will be made to avoid accumulation of food in the cavity.

Dento-Alveolar Abscess. The dento-alveolar abscess is secondary to suppurative pulpitis, and is characterized by local inflammation of the gingiva and extended edematous reaction to the nearby facial structures. This form of abscess usually follows an infected pulp. In other instances, it may appear without previous pulpitis. The use of analgesics is of help.

> Acetylsalicylic acid, 600 mg, in tablets, every 4 hours, preferably with meals.
>
> Acetaminophen, 600 mg, by mouth, every 6 hours.
>
> Codeine, 60 mg, by mouth, every 4 hours.

> Propoxyphene hydrochloride, 65 mg, every 4 to 6 hours, by mouth.

If needed, codeine may be given by injection, when the pain is very severe.

> Codeine, 30 mg, by intramuscular or subcutaneous injection.

If there is fever, an antibiotic should be added, and the antibiotic therapy maintained until some sort of surgery is performed. If there is a culture of the causative germ and a test of its sensitivity to antibiotics, the specific one should be used; otherwise, penicillin is to be advised.

> Penicillin (procaine), 600,000 units every 6 or 8 hours, by injection. Also, it could be given by mouth in appropriate dosage.

In the case of fluctuant swelling at the site of the root of the affected tooth, an incision should be made to drain the pus, and this collected and sent to the laboratory for culture and sensitivity to antibiotics. Also, hot saline mouth rinses may be of some help.

Other Mouth Pains

Gingivitis and Stomatitis. The inflammation of the gingivae provokes pain, swelling, redness, and bleeding of these structures. It is a syndromic complex that may reveal other diseases, particularly diabetes, leukemia, scurvy, pellagra, or intoxication by diphenylhydantoin (Dilantin) or heavy metals. In pregnant women gingivitis may occur during the first two months and will last until delivery. Pain is not rare, particularly in secondary forms or forms characterized by their severity.

Inflammation of the oral mucosae (stomatitis) may constitute a painful condition that occurs either independently or secondarily to other diseases. Symptoms may vary from a relatively mild inflammation with little pain, to extremely painful necrotizing or gangrenous lesions. Direct smears or cultures from the lesions will help to diagnosis the etiological factor; a general examination of the patient will help to disclose any underlying disease (scurvy, pellagra, agranulocytosis, leukemia, bacterial or fungal diseases, syphilis, scarlet fever, etc.). The more severe forms are discussed in the following paragraphs.

Gangrenous Stomatitis. Also known as noma, the condition presents a grayish slough of all the buccal mucosae, which swells and turns red and, finally, black. In spite of the extensive destruction, pain is not too severe. If the cause is known, treatment on that basis is of paramount importance (for instance, diabetes, pellagra, toxic agents—including drugs, pernicious anemia, leukemia, etc). Any irritating cause must be removed, such as calculus, local infection, redundant gingiva, etc. Local treatment will include mouthwashes with hydrogen peroxide, sodium borate or perborate, etc.

>Hydrogen peroxide, diluted in equal parts of water.

>Sodium borate, 1 teaspoonful in a glass of water.

>Sodium perborate, 1 teaspoonful in a glass of water.

The application of a local anesthetic on painful areas is a help also, in the form of mouthwashes or ointment.

>Lidocaine, 2% solution, a few drops in a tablespoonful of water.

>Benzocaine, 5% ointment, applied locally.

>Dibucaine, 1% ointment, to apply locally.

Vincent's Angina. Also known as necrotizing ulcerative gingivostomatitis. The condition presents a sudden onset with fever and painful bleeding of the gingival area, the oral mucosa, and the pharynx, including the tonsils.

In this condition, any analgesic can be given to relieve pain, but this will almost completely subside in the great majority of cases following the use of frequently repeated mouthwashes with hydrogen peroxide, followed by especially supervised mouthwash of diluted potassium arsenite solution.

>Hydrogen peroxide, mixed with equal parts of water, to be used as mouthwash, after each meal and at bedtime.

After using the peroxide mouthwash, follow with Fowler's solution dilution:

>Fowler's solution (potassium arsenite solution) 0.2 cc (three drops) diluted with one-fourth glass (60 cc) of water. Hold in mouth for 2 minutes and spit out. Do not swallow.

The analgesics to be used are the acetylsalicylic type.

Acetylsalicylic acid, 600 mg, in tablets, every 4 hours, preferably with meals.

Acetaminophen, 600 mg, by mouth, every 6 hours.

Propoxyphene hydrochloride, 65 mg, by mouth, every 4 hours.

These measures will help and should be followed: rest, a bland diet, a multivitamin preparation, and strict avoidance of smoking.

Aphthae. Aphthae are small, shallow ulcers, round or ovoid in shape. Most commonly, there is only one ulcer during each attack, and it may occur anywhere within the mouth. It is very painful, particularly to the touch. There is no specific treatment known for this very bothersome condition. Also, no local application will be of true help, except for anesthetic medication applied locally.

Lidocaine, 2% solution; apply one drop to the lesion before eating.

Mouthwashes are convenient, for the double action of cleansing and soothing the ulcerated site. Use hydrogen peroxide, sodium perborate, or sodium borate as suggested previously in "Gangrenous stomatitis." Some physicians advise the use of multivitamin preparations to prevent recurrences, but this has not been proved effective. The best measure is good oral hygiene.

Glossitis. The inflammation of the tongue may be either chronic or acute, primary or secondary, and may manifest itself under several different types:

GLOSSITIS IN SYSTEMIC INFECTIONS. It is not always painful, but on some occasions its intense inflammation may provoke discomfort. Pain may occur when fissures are formed.

TRAUMATIC GLOSSITIS. It is due to irritation from teeth or orthodontic devices in the mouth. Pain is the main manifestation. Heavy smokers and drinkers often show glossitis, not always painful.

PELLAGRA. In pellagra, glossitis may reach important proportions, but is not the principal symptom of the disease. Its manifestations vary from an inflammation occupying only the borders and tip of the tongue, to a massive ulcerative stomatitis.

ULCERS. Ulcers of the tongue are always painful, particularly when touched. They may be provoked by a neighboring irritating tooth, by coughing (if located on the frenum), by self-biting (epilepsy), or by a generalized stomatitis. Cancer of the tongue begins with a painful ulcer, which bleeds easily. Tuberculous ulcers are relatively large and very painful.

Whenever there is a known causative factor for glossitis, it should be treated accordingly. Locally, the pain will be relieved by the use of some anesthetic measure before eating.

> Lidocaine, 2% solution, a few drops in a tablespoonful of water, used as a mouth rinse.
>
> Benzocaine, 5% ointment, to be applied locally.
>
> Dibucaine, 1% ointment, to be applied locally.

A nutritive diet will be encouraged, multivitamins will be given, and a careful oral hygiene will be observed. All sort of toxins and irritants have to be avoided (spices, strong beverages, tobacco, etc.).

In the case of glossodynia, local anesthesia must be obtained by local injection, better if accompanied by corticoids orally. Also, antihistamines, sedatives, tranquilizers, and vitamins may be used with benefit; and estrogens in the menopausal woman. Glossodynia with xerostomia will force the use of pilocarpine.

> Pilocarpine, 20 mg a day, in divided doses.

Neoplasms. Ulcers or tumors located anywhere in the mouth, will suggest the possibility of cancer as soon as they are indolent, painful (burning sensation, most frequently), or bleed easily. Tumors do not become painful until their healing is delayed.

Malignancies in the mouth are treated by either radiation or surgery. For the treatment of pain, regular analgesics should be used first, and narcotics given whenever necessary.

> Propoxyphene hydrochloride, 65 mg, by mouth, every 4 hours.
>
> Codeine, 60 mg, by mouth or subcutaneous injection, every 4 hours.
>
> Meperidine, 100 mg, by mouth or subcutaneous injection, every 4 hours or as needed and tolerated.
>
> Morphine sulfate, 10 or 15 mg, by subcutaneous injection, as needed and tolerated.

Postextraction Pain. Pain follows most extractions of teeth, because of the traumatism and also because of the previous infection. Delayed pain indicates socket reinfection.

Irrigate the socket with warm saline, either saline alone or with a few drops of an anesthetic.

> Lidocaine, 2% solution.

> Cocaine, 5% solution.

Pack loosely with gauze strips soaked with a mixture of guaiacol and glycerine. Repack, every other day, after cleansing. Give also oral analgesics.

> Acetylsalicylic acid, 600 mg, in tablets, every 4 hours, preferably with meals.

> Codeine, 60 mg, by mouth, every 4 hours.

Arthritis. Arthritis of the temporomaxillar joint provokes severe arthralgia and limits the movement of the mandible. Ordinarily it affects only one side.

Rest of the mandibular joint will be helped by a soft diet, and the use of analgesics, relaxants, and, if needed, tranquilizers will complete the attempt to ameliorate suffering. When this treatment fails, it will be better to consult a specialist, particularly if the local injection of corticoids also fails.

> Acetylsalicylic acid, 600 mg, in tablets, every 4 hours, preferably with meals.

> Sodium salicylate, 600 mg, by mouth, every 4 hours, preferably with small amounts of thyroid extract (30 mg a day).

> Meprobamate, 400 mg, by mouth, every 6 hours.

Trauma to Mouth. A localized pain and perhaps abnormal mobilization of the affected parts may indicate a fracture of the bones of the mouth. These fractures are frequently compound. All severe injuries to the mouth are to be treated by an oral surgeon. In the meantime, efforts to alleviate pain will be welcomed.

> Meperidine, 100 mg, by mouth, every 4 hours.

> Codeine, 60 mg, by mouth, every 4 hours.

> Acetylsalicylic acid, 600 mg, in tablets, every 4 hours, preferably with meals.

> Propoxyphene hydrochloride, 65 mg, by mouth, every 4 hours.

If oral medication is not indicated, codeine, 30 mg, by subcutaneous injection, can be given every 3 hours if needed for pain. External application of an ice bag might impede excessive swelling.

Tonsillitis and Pharyngitis. Both chronic and acute tonsillitis provoke pain, which increases with the act of swallowing. The tonsils are swollen and red, with or without discharge or exudate. The diagnosis is easy. In all cases, an etiological factor should be searched for. Diffuse inflammation will pose the diagnosis of pharyngitis.

Both chronic and acute pharyngitis are characterized by pain, exacerbated on swallowing (dysphagia), and by redness of the pharynx. Fever may accompany the acute stage.

Adenoiditis occurs together with tonsillitis in most cases. Nasal obstruction is the main differential symptom.

Detection of the causative infective agent and its sensitivity to antibiotics will permit effective radical treatment. If the pain requires especial measures, it will help to swab the pharynx with an anesthetic solution.

Lidocaine, 2% solution, to soak a swab.

Cocaine 5% solution, to soak a swab.

Also, it will help to put an ice collar around the neck or to take analgesics by mouth.

Codeine, 60 mg, by mouth, every 4 hours.

Meperidine, 100 mg, by mouth, every 4 hours.

Acetylsalicylic acid, 600 mg, in tablets, every 4 hours, preferably with meals.

If an abscess develops, it should be opened for drainage, if necessary. A specialist will be consulted in many instances.

Peritonsillar and Retropharyngeal Abscesses. Severe pain at one side of the throat, with swelling and tenderness of the corresponding jaw and adjacent tissues, edema of the uvula, and symptoms of systemic infection are indicative of a peritonsillar abscess. The tonsil appears displaced on examination.

Most frequently in younger children, an accumulation of pus may collect between the posterior wall of the pharynx and the cervical vertebrae, thus constituting a retropharyngeal abscess. Symptoms are: pain exacerbated on swallowing, dyspnea, cough, and aphonia. The head stays extended; and the mouth, opened. Palpation of a soft, fluctuant tumor is diagnostic. The collection of pus extends in rare occasions to both sides of the neck.

For both peritonsillar and retropharyngeal abscess the effective treatment is surgical drainage when fluctuation is evident. The incision is made at the point of localized swelling or softening. Often these cases require the surgical skill and judgment of a specialist. Since this area is extremely sensitive, some sort of anesthesia can be given, but its effectiveness is impaired by the presence of violent inflammation.

> Cocaine, 10% solution; apply with applicator to the surface to be incised.

> Procaine, 2% solution; inject locally.

Wash the mouth with antiseptics after a thorough cleansing following evacuation of pus. Codeine is helpful after incision.

> Codeine, 60 mg, by subcutaneous injection, repeated two or three times, every 4 hours.

Laryngitis. Difficulty with talking (hoarseness) is the main symptom of laryngitis, either chronic or acute. Pain on swallowing may be more or less marked, as well as a constant ache located in the lower oropharynx. Diphtheric and tuberculous laryngitis must be ruled out in all instances. Also a thorough search must be made for neoplasm of the larynx and pharynx, particularly in chronic conditions. The causative factor may be primary or as a complication of respiratory or systemic infections and has to be basically treated and eliminated whenever possible.

For alleviation of pain: rest of the voice, a humid atmosphere, steam inhalations at frequent intervals (either water alone or with eucalyptol—1 teaspoonful added to each quart of water), and anesthetic lozenges (dibucaine, 1%) are advised. For cough, codeine and expectorants can be given if necessary.

> Codeine, 60 mg, by mouth, every 4 hours.

> Potassium iodide saturated solution (1 g for each ml of water), 300 to 600 mg (5 to 10 drops) in water every 2 hours.

> Glyceryl guaiacolate, 100 mg for each 5 ml of water or syrup; 5 to 10 ml every 2 to 4 hours.

A specialist should be consulted in most cases.

IV. OPHTHALMODYNIA

In most instances, in cases of ophthalmodynia a consultation with an ophthalmologist is imperative, since almost all the cases with pain in the eye do have a local disease to be treated by the specialist. That is to say, in a great number of diseases of the eye, there is accompanying pain.

Conjunctiva

Conjunctivitis. A painful sensation, as of a foreign body in the eye, is the first symptom noted. There is also lacrimation, and, in most instances, photophobia. A more or less marked discharge of pus is the rule. The characteristic redness of the conjunctiva makes the diagnosis. Care must be taken to differentiate the various types of conjunctivitis: chronic or acute catarrhal inflammation, gonococcal, and the different types of viral conjunctivitis and trachoma. In trichinosis, there are pain, subconjunctival hemorrhage, and an edema of the lids.

To treat the pain accompanying conjunctivitis, as is the case for most ophthalmopathies, it is necessary to treat the conjunctivitis itself. First, take material from the secretion for culture and sensitivity to antibiotics; immediately, remove foreign bodies, if any, whenever the procedure is within one's own capabilities. Rarely, pain will need local anesthesia, which can be achieved with holocaine or pontocaine, for example.

> Holocaine, 1% solution; instill one or two drops into the conjunctival sac.
>
> Pontocaine, 0.5% solution; instill one or two drops into the conjunctival sac.

Most frequently, as soon as the specific treatment with antibiotic suspensions or solutions is started, pain subsides. These antibiotics can be given alone or with corticoids. These are a must in the case of allergic conjunctivitis.

> Cortisone, 15 mg for each g of an ophthalmic ointment, to be applied every 6 to 8 hours.
>
> Dexamethasone, 0.5 mg for each g of ophthalmic ointment, to be applied every 6 to 8 hours.

132 DIAGNOSIS AND TREATMENT

Cornea

Keratoconjunctivitis. Pain is severe, and occurs with other symptoms of conjunctivitis (lacrimation, photophobia, purulent discharge), but on examination, small yellow-grey phlyctenulae are found on the conjunctiva or the limbus. In these cases a combination of antibiotics and corticoids should be given.

> Neomycin sulfate, 5 mg, plus hydrocortisone acetate, 10 mg, for each ml of ophthalmic suspension; instill two or three drops, every 4 to 6 hours.

> Neomycin sulfate, 5 mg, plus polymyxin B sulfate, 10,000 units and hydrocortisone acetate, 10 mg, for each ml of ophthalmic suspension; instill two or three drops into the conjunctival sac every 4 to 6 hours.

Again, the patient should be sent to the ophthalmologist for further treatment. Seldom will the pain be so annoying as to rquire the use of local anesthetics.

> Tetracaine, 0.5% solution; instill two or three drops into the conjunctival sac every 4 to 6 hours.

> Cocaine, 4% solution; instill two or three drops into the conjunctival sac, every 4 to 6 hours.

Interstitial Keratitis. Pain, lacrimation, photophobia, together with a grayish infiltration of the cornea (deep layers) and new growth of vessels around the limbus. A progressive loss of vision accompanies the disease.

Other forms of keratitis or inflammation of the cornea always cause pain, lacrimation, and photophobia, and, in some instances, loss of vision. Scattered punctate infiltrations of the superficial layers characterize superficial punctate keratitis; ulceration forming branched lesions which resemble the veins of a leaf (with knoblike ends) is called dendritic keratitis; a disc-shaped deep inflammation is disciform keratitis.

As indicated above, in the paragraph devoted to keratoconjunctivitis, a combination of antibiotics and corticoids will be advised, specially if syphilis is a factor; but the patient will be referred immediately to an ophthalmologist for further treatment.

> Cortisone, 15 mg for each g of ophthalmic ointment; apply to the conjunctival sac every 4 to 6 hours.

> Dexamethasone, 0.5 mg for each g of ophthalmic ointment; apply to the conjunctival sac every 4 to 6 hours.

> Neomycin sulfate, 5 mg, plus polymyxin B sulfate, 10,000 units and hydrocortisone acetate, 10 mg, for each ml of ophthalmic solution; instill two or three drops into the conjunctival sac every 4 to 6 hours.

Ulcers of the Cornea. Pain, lacrimation, and photophobia are present together with a localized point of necrosis in the cornea (grayish superficial lesion) that might perforate at a later stage.

The first step is to obtain material for germ culture and sensitivity and to give, immediately, adequate and specific local and general antibiotic therapy. If pain is very annoying, local anesthetics are to be prescribed.

> Pontocaine, 0.5% solution; instill two or three drops into the conjunctival sac every 4 to 6 hours.

> Cocaine, 4% solution; instill two or three drops into the conjunctival sac every 4 to 6 hours.

If the ulceration is deep, it will be almost mandatory to give atropine, and in all instances to refer the patient to the ophthalmologist.

> Atropine, 1% solution; instill one drop into the conjunctival sac, no more than three times a day (every 8 hours).

Uveal Tract

Iritis and Iridocyclitis. Pain (radiating to the temple), edema of the upper eyelid, lacrimation, and photophobia occur together with swelling and color changes of the iris and a miotic pupil, irregular from synechiae. There is marked congestion of the blood vessels around the cornea.

Iridocyclitis shows the same symptoms as above, but they are more severe, and the injection of the blood vessels of the conjunctiva is more marked.

Dilate the pupils with atropine.

> Atropine, 1% ophthalmic solution; instill one drop into the conjunctival sac every 8 hours.

Give local corticoids, of the type of cortisone, dexamethasone, etc.

> Cortisone, 15 mg for each g of the ophthalmic ointment; apply every 4 to 6 hours.

Dexamethasone, 0.5 mg for each g of the ophthalmic ointment; apply every 4 to 6 hours.

Prescribe analgesics to allay the pain, such as:

Codeine, 60 mg, by mouth, every 4 hours.

Acetylsalicylic acid, 600 mg, in tablets, every 4 hours, preferably with meals.

Propoxyphene hydrochloride, 65 mg, by mouth, every 4 hours.

The patient has to be treated by an ophthalmologist.

Endophthalmitis and Panophthalmitis. Intense pain in the eye, with marked congestion of the blood vessels and chemosis, rapid loss of vision, and production of pus, indicates the onset of an endophthalmitis (suppuration is limited to the retina and the uveal tract), or a panophthalmitis (suppuration involves the whole eye). An early diagnosis is imperative, and treatment requires an ophthalmologist.

The patient has to be treated by an ophthalmologist from the very beginning of the disease. But the severe pain which almost always accompanies it has to be relieved immediately, with codeine, meperidine, or even morphine.

Codeine, 60 mg, by subcutaneous injection or by mouth, every 4 hours.

Meperidine, 100 mg, by subcutaneous injection or by mouth, every 4 to 6 hours, as needed, but only for a short time.

Morphine, 10 to 15 mg, by subcutaneous injection every 4 hours, as needed and tolerated; also not for a prolonged period of time.

It is desirable if some secretion can be taken for culture and sensitivity to antibiotics, since antibiotic therapy is to be started as soon as possible, with the specific antibiotic or at least with a broad spectrum antibiotic. Antibiotic therapy, of course, has to be given systemically.

Optic Nerve

Optic Neuritis and Retrobulbar Neuritis. Optic neuritis provokes pain on eye motion accompanied by some sort of disturbance of vision (from enlargement of the blind spot to complete blindness of the affected eye).

Retrobulbar neuritis also presents pain, which is constant and aggravated by eye motion. Rapid loss of vision ensues, with only a little hyperemia of the retina.

The patient will be referred to an ophthalmologist, for the needed specialized treatment; but meanwhile analgesics can be given for the relief of pain, together with corticoids, which will serve a double mission: to allay pain and to avoid reactive irritation.

> Acetylsalicylic acid, 600 mg, in tablets, every 4 hours, preferably with meals.

> Codeine, 60 mg, by mouth, every 4 hours; or by subcutaneous injection, if needed, particularly at the start of treatment.

> Prednisone, 5 mg, one or two tablets every 6 hours; decrease the dose when pain subsides, and discontinue therapy very slowly after some 10 days of treatment.

Lacrimal Apparatus

Dacryocystitis. In the acute form, there is pain at the medial canthus of the eye, with redness and edema over the region of the lacrimal sac. Lacrimation and other symptoms may also be present. Pain may be relieved by the use of common analgesics.

> Acetylsalicylic acid, 600 mg, every 4 to 6 hours, preferably with meals.

> Codeine, 60 mg, by mouth, every 4 to 6 hours.

> Propoxyphene hydrochloride, 65 mg, by mouth every 4 hours.

Hot compresses, applied over the affected area for 10 minutes, three or four times a day, are also helpful. The rest of the treatment depends on an ophthalmologist for antibiotic therapy.

Eyelids

Hordeolum (Sty) and Blepharitis. In hordeolum, pain, redness, and swelling of the eyelid (the inflammation more localized at the site of the infection) are diagnostic features when restricted to the superficial layers of the eyelid.

Blepharitis does not cause actual pain but a sensation of discomfort (burning, itching) of the eyelid, which appears inflamed and secreting some pus.

Both are painful, but the use of analgesics cannot help very much. Local treatment can be given by the use of ophthalmic antibiotic ointments, either alone or with corticoids. This holds true for both diseases, but in the case of hordeolum the mixture of corticoids and antibiotics may abort the sty. Also, when needed, hordeolum may mature more rapidly by the use of hot compresses, applied for 10 minutes, three or four times a day. When pus is collected, an incision will drain it.

> Neomycin sulfate, 5 mg, plus hydrocortisone acetate, 10 mg, for each ml of ophthalmic suspension; instill two or three drops into the conjuctival sac every 4 to 6 hours.

> Neomycin sulfate, 5 mg, plus polymyxin B sulfate, 10,000 units and hydrocortisone acetate, 10 mg, for each ml of ophthalmic suspension; instill two or three drops into the conjunctival sac every 4 to 6 hours.

Orbit

Orbital Cellulitis. There is very severe pain in the orbit, exophthalmos, restricted mobility of the eye, edema of lids and conjunctiva, and frequently a history of infection elsewhere in the body (paranasal sinuses, mouth, etc.).

A help to the general treatment of orbital cellulitis (rest, hot applications, and antibiotics) will be to minimize pain with analgesics of the type of codeine, acetylsalicylic acid, etc.

> Codeine, 60 mg, by subcutaneous injection or by mouth, as needed, every 4 hours.

> Acetylsalicylic acid, 600 mg, in tablets, every 4 hours, preferably with meals.

> Propoxyphene hydrochloride, 65 mg, by mouth, every 4 hours.

Rarely, stronger analgesia will be needed, with morphine and similar drugs, but providing that emesis will not be a complication that might cause eye damage.

> Meperidine, 100 mg, by subcutaneous injection, every 4 hours, or as needed and tolerated. Do not continue this medication for long periods.

> Morphine, 10 to 15 mg, by subcutaneous injection, repeated every 4 hours, or as needed and tolerated.

Others

Glaucoma. In glaucoma there is always some sort of pain, ranging from mild to excruciating, related to the eye. When the cause of glaucoma is unknown, it is a primary glaucoma; if known, secondary glaucoma:

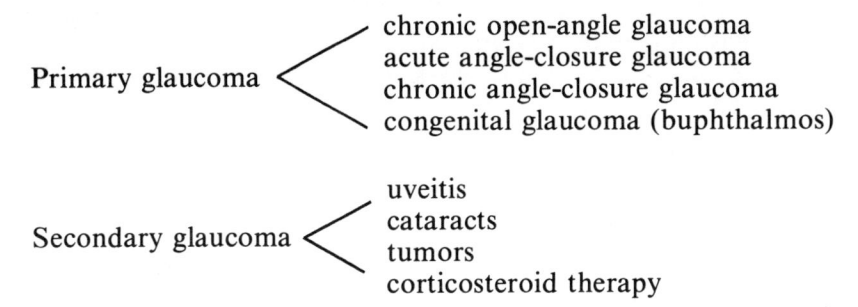

Primary glaucoma
- chronic open-angle glaucoma
- acute angle-closure glaucoma
- chronic angle-closure glaucoma
- congenital glaucoma (buphthalmos)

Secondary glaucoma
- uveitis
- cataracts
- tumors
- corticosteroid therapy

In chronic open-angle glaucoma there is a frequent need for change of glasses, and there are minor visual disturbances (halos around lights, mild pain, etc); the diagnosis depends on the finding of increased intraocular pressure, at times following provocative tests (water ingestion).

Acute angle-closure glaucoma is characterized by attacks of increased symptomatology of a relatively chronic situation (halos around lights, pain, etc), which last for a short time and recur frequently until the characteristic brutal attack takes place (severe pain, loss of vision, nausea and vomiting, chemosis, lacrimation, dilated pupil, turbid aqueous fluid, and highly increased ocular tension—even perceptible to touch).

In chronic angle-closure glaucoma repeated attacks are characteristic, similar to those in acute angle-closure glaucoma, but less marked. In congenital glaucoma there is a notable enlargement of the size of the eye.

Secondary glaucomas follow the clinical course of the causative factor, namely, the presence of uveitis, a space-occupying lesion (tumors) or cataracts, and the use of corticoids for the treatment of any disease. Under the circumstances, an attack of ophthalmodynia with increased ocular tension is diagnostic of secondary glaucoma.

The excruciating pain suffered by a great number of patients frequently requires emergency treatment to decrease intraocular tension, which, as is well known, causes the pain. But since the selection of therapies depends on whether it is a primary or secondary glaucoma, an open-angle glaucoma, etc., it will be better carried out by an experienced ophthalmologist.

Cases with chronic open-angle glaucoma will receive pilocarpine or physostigmine, or carbachol, or these drugs together with acetazolamide.

> Pilocarpine, 1% ophthalmic solution (or 20% if more convenient); instill one or two drops into the conjunctival sac, every 4 hours, or as needed and tolerated.
>
> Physostigmine, 0.25% ophthalmic solution; instill one or two drops into the conjunctival sac, every 4 to 6 hours, as needed and tolerated.
>
> Carbachol, 1.5% ophthalmic solution; instill only one drop each time, and no more than three times a day (every 8 hours).
>
> Acetazolamide, 250 mg, in tablets, better one a day, but never more than every 8 hours. In emergency situations, acetazolamide, 500 mg, can be given by intravenous injection.

When the patient has aphakic eyes, the lack of lens makes it preferable to use isoflurophate.

> Isoflurophate, 0.1% ophthalmic solution; instill two drops into the conjunctival sac every 8 hours, for three days; for night use more conveniently, isoflurophate, 0.025% ophthalmic ointment.

In chronic angle-closure glaucoma, pilocarpine is still the drug of choice.

In acute angle-closure glaucoma, the attack may be aborted by giving glycerin by mouth, acetazolamide by intravenous injection, or, in the case that both glycerin and acetazolamide fail, urea, also by vein.

> Glycerin, 1 or 2 g for each kg of body weight, in a mixture of equal parts with water.
>
> Acetazolamide, 500 mg, by intravenous injection; or 250 mg, in tablets, not more frequently than every 6 hours.
>
> Urea, 30% solution, give 1 to 1.5 g for each kg of body weight by the intravenous route, making sure that there is an adequate kidney function.

Secondary glaucoma can be treated initially with corticoids and acetazolamide.

> Prednisone, 5 to 10 mg, repeated every 4 hours, until symptoms subside; then decrease the dosage, and after 8 or 10 days of treatment reduce the dosage very slowly.
>
> Acetaxolamide; see treatment for chronic open-angle glaucoma.

Naturally, a patient with glaucoma has to be referred immediately to an experienced ophthalmologist.

For more details, look under the heading "Glaucoma" in the section on "Headache."

Errors of refraction cause cephalalgia, as discussed above, but also the sensation of strained eyes, which is not pain, actually, but only the uncomfortable feeling that something is going wrong. This will frequently cause headache (q.v.); but, at times, local pain may provoke discomfort. The patient will be referred to an ophthalmologist for corrective lenses which might prove the constant means of controlling pain. However, these pains will ordinarily respond to analgesics, though recurrence is to be expected.

> Acetylsalicylic acid, 300 to 600 mg, in tablets, every 4 to 6 hours, preferably with meals.
>
> Codeine, 30 to 60 mg, by mouth, every 4 to 6 hours.
>
> Propoxyphene hydrochloride, 65 mg, by mouth, every 4 hours.

Traumatic Lesions. The obvious nature of traumatic lesions, all of them accompanied by pain, makes unnecessary any discussion on this subject. Besides the surgical management urgently needed in most of these cases, the patient has to be relieved from the pain he is suffering. Because of its intensity, morphine will be the first thought, but it should not be used, because of the frequency with which it induces vomiting, endangering a damaged eye. In most instances, codeine will control the pain.

> Codeine, 30 to 60 mg, by intramuscular or subcutaneous injection, repeated as needed and tolerated.

V. OTALGIA

Otalgia, referred to as pain in the middle ear, can be extremely severe, so as to require direct treatment. This will not preclude the need to consult with a specialist. In other words, pain will be treated, according to its intensity, and first aid will be given, whenever needed, and the patient referred to an otologist.

External Ear

Furunculosis and External Otitis. The canal of the ear and the auricle itself are frequent sites for furunculosis. Pain is the dominant symptom. On examination, the presence of the furuncle is disclosed. In external otitis, severe pain, together with diffuse inflammation of the canal, are the main features. Pain has to be relieved with analgesics, and local heat applications started as soon as possible.

> Meperidine, 100 mg, by subcutaneous injection, every 4 hours; after two or three injections change to oral medication, 100 mg, every 4 hours.

> Codeine, 60 mg, by subcutaneous injection, followed by oral medication, as stated above for meperidine.

A thorough cleansing of the ear canal is imperative, and will be done immediately, gently using an irrigator or syringe with:

> Sodium bicarbonate, 3% solution; put 30 g (8 teaspoonfuls) in 1 liter of water.

After irrigation of the area, it will be dried with a cotton applicator. Thereafter, local treatment with antibiotic preparations will follow, either instilling the antibiotic solution or applying the solution to a loose cotton pledget in the canal, or, if preferred, applying an antibiotic ointment. To control the swelling of the canal, at times very annoying, particularly in the acute external otitis, but also in furunculosis, the use of aluminum acetate may be very helpful.

> Aluminum acetate, 5% solution (Burow's solution), 1 part in 10 (up to 40) parts of water.

Put a loose gauze strip or a piece of cotton into the canal, and keep it wet with the aluminum acetate solution by adding a few drops every 3 or 4 hours; but this is not to be done for more than 2 days. This will allow a better application of local antibiotics.

Furuncles are to be incised after pus is well localized; but the incision is not always advisable and should be left to the specialist.

Systemic antibiotic therapy must be started from the very beginning, and continued 2 days after the infection is cleared up. It is best to use the specific antibiotic, but, in any case, use a broad spectrum one.

Otomycosis. On rare occasion, otomycosis will cause pain in the canal. The infection will be easily noted. In the first place, as stated above for external otitis, the canal has to be well cleaned, better with the help of Burow's solution, but somewhat more diluted, in 20 to 40 parts of water.

>Aluminum acetate, 5% solution (Burow's solution).

As indicated above, put a loose piece of gauze in the ear canal and keep it wet by adding a few drops of diluted aluminum acetate solution, every 3 or 4 hours, but for no more than 2 days. Also, use the adequate antibiotic, either locally or systemically. If there is pain, use codeine or meperidine.

>Codeine, 60 mg, by subcutaneous injection, followed by oral administration, 60 mg, every 4 hours.

>Meperidine, 100 mg, by subcutaneous injection, followed by oral administration, 100 mg every 4 hours.

Other analgesics could also be used, when convenient.

>Acetylsalicylic acid, 600 mg, in tablets, every 4 to 6 hours, preferably with meals.

>Acetaminophen, 600 mg, by mouth, every 6 hours.

>Acetophenetidin, 300 mg, by mouth, every 4 hours.

>Propoxyphene hydrochloride, 65 mg, by mouth, every 4 hours.

Herpes zoster provokes a sudden onset of pain, a sensation of fullness in the ear, tinnitus, and slight deafness. Eventually, the characteristic vesicles appear, together with swelling of the area and a corresponding lymphadenopathy. Pain may reach an excruciating degree in cases of herpes zoster of the geniculate ganglion (7th and 8th cranial nerves may be involved). Analgesics should be given for relief: acetylsalicylic acid, codeine, a mixture of acetylsaliciclyc acid and codeine, meperidine, propoxyphene hydrochloride, and others.

>Acetylsalicyclic acid, 600 mg, in tablets, repeated every 4 hours, preferably with meals.

>Codeine, 60 mg, by mouth, every 4 hours; but if needed, might be given by subcutaneous injection.

>Meperidine, 100 mg, by subcutaneous injection, or oral administration, every 4 hours.

>Propoxyphene hydrochloride, 65 mg, by mouth, every 4 hours.

Corticoids may be useful both for pain and for the duration of the disease, which is lessened in many cases, particularly if they are given at an early date.

> Prednisone, 10 mg, by mouth, every 6 hours, at the start; to be decreased after 2 or 3 days, and after 7 to 10 days of therapy, to continue decreasing the dosage even more, but very gradually.

Also, cyanocobalamine (vitamin B_{12}) can be of some help.

> Cyanocobalamine, 1000 μg daily, by intramuscular injection, to continue for 1 or 2 weeks following disappearance of the lesions.

For more details, see other sections also dealing with herpes zoster.

Traumatic lesions are always obvious, and the diagnosis is easily made. Most injuries are due to foreign bodies inserted into the canal. These foreign bodies have to be removed at the earliest possible time; but since it is very easy to damage the eardrum during the removal, it is advised that the procedure should be done by a specialist or at least some one expert in the technic. Residual pain may be treated with local anesthetic solutions.

> Cocaine, 5 or 10% solution; instill in a few drops into the canal.

> Tetracaine, 2% solution; instill a few drops into the canal.

Contusions, wounds, frostbite, etc., will be treated as elsewhere in the body: cold compresses, local disinfection, stitches, etc. In the case of wounds, it is best to follow the advice of an expert on how to preserve the normal shape of the ear. In case of large hematomas, remove blood, apply pressure, and avoid infection by a sterile procedure. For residual pain use either local anesthetics, as stated above, or give analgesics.

> Acetylsalicylic acid, 600 mg, in tablets, every 4 hours, preferably with meals.

> Codeine, 60 mg, by mouth, every 4 hours.

> Propoxyphene hydrochloride, 65 mg, by mouth, every 4 hours.

Eardrum

Myringitis is often severely painful and produces more or less marked deafness and systemic symptoms (fever). On otoscopy, the eardrum is red and is often covered with vesicles. Give an analgesic to control pain: acetylsalicylic acid, meperidine, codeine, a mixture of acetylsalicylic acid and codeine, or other analgesics, as found more convenient.

> Acetylsalicylic acid, 600 mg, in tablets, every 4 hours, preferably with meals.

> Codeine, 60 mg, by subcutaneous injection, followed by oral administration every 4 hours.

> Meperidine, 100 mg, by subcutaneous injection, followed by oral administration every 4 hours.

In cases of local vesiculation, the use of local applications of warm aluminum acetate will undoubtedly help.

> Aluminum acetate, 5% solution (Burow's solution), 1 part in 10 or up to 40 parts of water.

A better control of the infection will be attained by the use of antibiotic therapy, both local and systemic, and using the specific antibiotic, if it is known, or at least a broad spectrum one. It will be imperative to continue antibiotic therapy for about 2 days after all symptoms of infection subside.

Also, the administration of corticoids will help for a better and perhaps more rapid disappearance of the infection.

> Prednisone or prednisolone, 5%, plus neomycin, 5% solution; instill a few drops, two or three times a day, into the ear canal.

It is to be stated that the treatment of myringitis stays within the domain of the otologist.

Injuries to the eardrum are the consequence of inserting objects (toothpicks, swabs, and the like) into the canal. A blow on the external meatus with sudden air compression might rupture the drum. Severe pain is the main symptom when the tissues are infected.

Foreign bodies inserted into the ear canal are the most frequent cause of injuries to the eardrum. Also, sudden changes in atmospheric pressure as in airplane flights or blows on the ear, may lacerate the membrane. Try not to use local manipulation under these circumstances. Keep the area dry, and give broad spectrum antibiotics, either by injection or by mouth, for at least 1 week, the time it usually takes for the spontaneous closure of the drum. But the best thing to do is to refer these patients to the otologist, after giving them some analgesics for the control of pain.

> Acetylsalicylic acid, 600 mg, in tablets, every 4 hours, preferably with meals.
>
> Codeine, 60 mg, by subcutaneous injection, followed by oral administration, every 4 hours.

Middle Ear

Otitis media is a common complication of infective diseases setting in the nasopharynx. Pain within the ear is common to all forms of otitis media. Other symptoms are: varying deafness, fullness inside the ear, tinnitus, and more or less marked constitutional symptoms (fever, malaise, etc.). Otoscopy will reveal an inflamed eardrum with, probably, bulging. In chronic otitis media there is also pain, but it may recede after a time.

Ordinarily, otitis media requires surgery, which will be better done by a specialist. Regarding pain, it may be relieved by means of analgesics when it is due to acute serous otitis, acute purulent otitis, chronic secretory otitis, and chronic purulent otitis.

> Acetylsalicylic acid, 600 mg, in tablets, every 4 hours, preferably with meals.
>
> Codeine, 60 mg, by mouth, every 4 hours.
>
> Propoxyphene hydrochloride, 65 mg, every 4 hours.
>
> Meperidine, 100 mg, every 4 hours; but this medication only for short periods of time.

In the case of complicating Eustachian tube inflammation, in acute serous otitis, in chronic secretory otitis, and in chronic congestive otitis, the use of a vasoconstrictor by the nasal route is advisable.

> Ephedrine, 1% solution, two or three drops, two or three times a day.
>
> Phenylephrine, 0.25% solution, three or four drops every 4 hours.

Inflation of the Eustachian tube is a procedure that should be left to the specialist. Needless to say, the use of antihistamines, systemic decongestants, and antibiotics can be a must in a great number of cases—if not all the cases.

Mastoiditis may provoke symptoms from the middle ear, but its main feature is pain felt over the mastoid, with or without edema at the same site. Vigorous treatment with antibiotics is the main procedure to follow, before mastoidectomy becomes necessary. If the specific antibiotic can be used, it is better. Otherwise, use a broad spectrum antibiotic. Since this is a problem to be solved by the specialist, the patient will be referred to him after receiving an injection of codeine to allay pain.

Codeine, 60 mg, by subcutaneous route.

Chronic cases should also be scheduled to receive specialized care because complications are manifold and prone to occur, including severe ones such as brain abscess, lateral sinus phlebitis, etc.

VI. DYSPHAGIA

As its name implies, dysphagia is only difficulty in the act of swallowing. But we include dysphagia in our review because most of its forms are also painful, either when it is a first stage dysphagia (pharyngeal dysphagia that occurs during the voluntary act of deglution) or when it is a second stage dysphagia (esophageal dysphagia that occurs during the involuntary act of food passing down the esophagus). The voluntary stage may be influenced by emotions, and the like; the involuntary stage is almost constantly due to organic causes.

The first paragraph in this section deals with difficulty in swallowing due to mouth lesions, which is not dysphagia, strictly speaking. But since it actually impairs the initial act of swallowing, it is included here.

Buccal Dysphagia

Buccal dysphagia occurs in all painful inflammatory diseases of the mouth, which were discussed under "Stomatalgia." Dysphagia due to parotiditis should be considered here, also. It is to be noted that in rare instances dysphagia precedes the pathognomonic swelling of the gland; there is pain on both sides of the mouth.

For more details, see the corresponding paragraphs in the above section on the treatment of stomatalgia. Only a brief summary will be given here about the treatment of pain in the mouth when it makes eating difficult.

For caries and pulpitis, cleanse the affected area and put a cotton plug with clove oil on the sensitive spot.

Dento-alveolar abscesses will be treated with analgesics of the salicylate type, and similar drugs; and if fever is also present, with antibiotics. As soon as pus is localized, the abscess must be incised.

In cases of buccal aphthae, local anesthetic medication will be given before each meal. Mouthwashes and vitamin therapy are also advisable.

Gingivitis and stomatitis will be treated according to the causative factor: diabetes, pernicious anemia, toxic agents (including drugs), leukemia, etc. Local irritants (calculus, infection, redundant gingiva, etc.) will be removed. Treat locally with cleansing solutions and use, if necessary, local anesthetics.

Start the treatment of Vincent's angina with analgesics of the type of salicylates and the like and wash the mouth with hydrogen peroxide (in equal amount of water). Clean the infected area and follow the mouthwash of hydrogen peroxide with a mouthwash of a dilution of Fowler's solution of arsenic, meticulously prepared and reliably supervised, as the systemic dose of undiluted Fowler's solution is 0.2 ml (three drops) a day.

Glossitis is better treated with anesthetic solutions and a very careful oral hygiene.

Injuries to the mouth should be referred to an oral surgeon, but pain has to be controlled with analgesics, mostly of the narcotic type, together with local application of cold (ice bags), starting at the first visit of the patient.

Postextraction pain will be treated with warm saline to cleanse the socket, a few drops of an anesthetic solution, repacking after cleansing every other day, and analgesics by mouth.

Pharyngeal Dysphagia

Again, dysphagia occurs in all painful inflammatory diseases of the pharynx, also discussed under "Stomatalgia." It is to be added now that a symptomatology similar to that of retropharyngeal abscess may be noted in cases with caries of the cervical vertebrae; but in this instance, pain may be absent. Diagnosis depends on the X-ray examination. There are also a few forms of dysphagia caused by spasms of the pharyngeal muscles, which may or may not be painful: rabies, tetanus, tetany, encephalitis, strychnine, intoxication, and perhaps others.

Pharyngitis and tonsillitis are, perhaps, the most frequent causes of pharyngeal dysphagia. The first step will be to identify the causative germ, determine its sensitivity to antibiotics, and give the indicated antibiotic. To treat the pain, swab the pharynx with anesthetic solutions and prescribe an anesthetic gargle containing phenol, 0.5%, particularly before meals.

Lidocaine, 2% solution, on a swab.

Cocaine, 5% solution, on a swab.

An ice collar around the neck is effective in many instances. Abscesses should be drained, whenever necessary; and a specialist consulted in selected cases. Analgesics of the type of salicylates and such may be given.

Acetylsalicylic acid, 600 mg, in tablets, every 4 hours, preferably with meals.

Acetaminophen, 600 mg, by mouth, every 6 hours.

Acetophenetidin, 300 mg, by mouth, every 4 hours.

Esophageal Dysphagia

This type of dysphagia is characterized by an obstacle to the normal progression of food from the pharynx to the stomach. In a few instances, pain or at least a feeling of thoracic oppression accompanies this type of dysphagia. Regurgitation also occurs (without the nauseating concomitant of vomiting).

Ulcers cause spasm and pain along with other symptoms of dysphagia. In the case of peptic ulcer, hemorrhage and epigastric pain may be present. Most esophageal ulcers are closely related to peptic ulcer and are to be treated as such, with bed rest (for at least a few days), avoidance of roughage and irritant food, frequent smaller feedings, and antacids. The administration of anticholinergics is very frequently a help.

Sodium bicarbonate, 1 or 2 g (less than a non-heaped half teaspoonful) every 1 to 3 hours, or at least before the administration of food or when pain is present.

Magnesium oxide (15 to 60 g, balancing the dosage individually, to avoid constipation) plus calcium carbonate (to complete a total of 120 g), to give a half or one non-heaped teaspoonful in half a glass of water, as stated above.

Belladonna tincture, 10, 20, or 30 drops, in water in accordance with effects and individual tolerance, half an hour before meals and at bedtime.

Propantheline bromide, 7.5 to 15 mg, in tablets, before meals and at bedtime.

If strictures are noted, dilation may be carried out after a careful study of the esophagus, better done by a specialist.

Diverticulosis. Pain occurs only at a later stage or when spasms occur. Regurgitation is the main symptom. A symptomatic treatment for pain or painful spasms rarely will be needed, and when these symptoms are present, surgery will be the best resource. Of course, codeine, papaverine, and the like might be given whenever required.

Codeine, 60 mg, by mouth, every 4 to 6 hours.

Papaverine hydrochloride, 150 mg, in slow-release capsules, one every 12 hours.

Cancer. In cancer, the initial dysphagia occurs without pain. Subsequently, epigastric or precordial pain is present, which is exaggerated by eructation. An early diagnosis requires further search for the cause of the pain.

Treatment is surgical, though chemotherapy and X-ray therapy may help. A specialist will take care of the patient. For pain, give narcotic analgesics.

Morphine sulfate, 10 or 15 mg, by subcutaneous injection, as needed and tolerated.

Methadone, 10 mg, by subcutaneous injection, as needed and tolerated.

Meperidine, 100 mg, by subcutaneous injection, as needed and tolerated.

Scars produced by corrosive liquids will induce dysphagia, painful mostly at the early stages. After a careful study of the esophagus, dilation will be carried out, preferably by a specialist. To avoid pain from spasms, give spasmolytic drugs.

Papaverine, 30 mg in 1 ml, for intramuscular administration, every 3, 4, or 6 hours (every individual dose ranging from 30 to 120 mg, as needed and tolerated).

Papaverine hydrochloride, 150 mg, in slow-release capsules, one every 12 hours.

Foreign bodies in the esophagus may cause discomfort and painful dysphagia. A sudden pressure, directed upwards, on the epigastric area may dislodge a number of these foreign bodies (there are reports of injuries to the stomach due to this maneuver; but in the case of a dreadful emergency, it is better to save the patient and then to operate on the injured stomach). Otherwise, extraction with the aid of an esophagoscope may be necessary, and a specialist will take care of the case.

Since the extraction has to be done usually as an emergency, there is no time for analgesics. This is to be left to the judgment of the attending physician.

Extrinsic Compression. Tumors in the neck (including goiter), mediastinal growths, lymphadenitis, and other causes of extrinsic compression of the esophagus may produce dysphagia. Only in a few instances (when inflammation is involved, or spasms are produced) does pain accompany this type of dysphagia.

The treatment, of course, has to be addressed to the causative factor; but when pain is the problem, it might respond to routine analgesics, though at times meperidine or even morphine is required.

> Acetylsalicylic acid, 300 to 600 mg, in tablets, every 4 to 6 hours, preferably with meals.
>
> Acetaminophen, 600 mg, by mouth, every 6 hours.
>
> Propoxyphene hydrochloride, 65 mg, by mouth, every 4 hours.
>
> Codeine, 30 to 60 mg, by mouth, every 4 to 6 hours, particularly effective if coughing is a factor.
>
> Meperidine, 50 to 100 mg, subcutaneously or, better, by mouth, every 6 hours.
>
> Morphine sulfate, 10 to 15 mg, by subcutaneous injection, repeated as needed and tolerated.

VII. PAIN IN THE NECK

Arthritis will be the causative factor in the greatest number of cases, but many instances of torticollis (wry neck) and a few instances of suboccipital neuralgia will also be encountered. To treat most of these patients will not be difficult.

Torticollis (Wry Neck). This is a spasm of the sternocleidomastoid muscle. There is pain on the side of the spasm, exaggerated when trying to move the head to a normal position from the forced torsion against the affected muscle. A spasm of the trapezius muscle can also be present. It will be kept in mind that torticollis might be an independent clinical entity (torticollis "a frigore"), but it is mostly secondary to other causes, usch as rheumatism, injuries, inflammatory lesions of the spine, neuritis, or even diseases of the central nervous system. The muscle appears tense and painful to the touch.

In torticollis, massage and heat applications are much more effective than analgesics, which only help a little, when they help at all. Anticholinergics may give more encouraging results.

> Belladonna tincture, five, ten, or more drops, in a little. water, every 4 to 8 hours, according to effects and tolerance

> Atropine sulfate, 0.5-mg tablet, half tablet or 1 tablet, by mouth, every 6 hours, or according to effects and tolerance.

Also, tranquilizers may help, as well as muscle relaxants, the latter preferred in most instances.

> Meprobamate, 400 mg, by mouth, every 6 hours.

> Carisoprodol, 350 mg, by mouth, every 6 or 8 hours.

More severe cases will need a head halter to apply traction to the head. Some will need a collar. These cases, of course, will be better under the care of the specialist, as well as cases of congenital torticollis which require very skillful care.

Rheumatism. In rheumatoid arthritis there are several painful and swollen joints involved. These joints are tender on palpation, the smaller joints more frequently in the adult type of the disease and the large ones in juveniles. Pain is worsened by inactivity; and the tense muscles induce the peculiar flexed position of affected parts.

Painful joints are also characteristic of degenerative arthritis, but there is no swelling or muscle involvement. Patients are over 40 years of age, are obese, and do not complain of systemic symptoms.

Patients with rheumatic fever are mostly young, and the rheumatic symptomatology—similar to that of rheumatoid arthritis (see above)—usually is accompanied by heart murmurs and follows a previous tonsillitis or pharyngitis. Other cardiovascular symptoms are present: precordial pain, arrythmias, and even heart failure. Skin rashes are not rare. The finding of a beta-hemolytic streptococcus is an important clue for diagnosis.

Rheumatoid or ankylosing spondylitis shows a tendency to induce the fusion of vertebrae, particularly in young patients. Ordinarily, the neck is affected later in the disease, after the involvement of lower parts of the spine. There are attacks of pain and stiffness lasting a few days or not too many weeks, and then subsiding for a time. X-ray and laboratory procedures will give the final diagnosis.

Hypertrophic spondylitis is a disease of older adults, appearing usually after 50 years of age.

For more detailed information on rheumatic pains, the reader is referred to the section on "Shoulders, Arms, and Hands" (see "Rheumatoid arthritis," "Degenerative arthritis," and "Rheumatic fever").

In rheumatoid arthritis, reasonable bed rest alternating with planned physical activity is advised, and the use of splints, or whatever is needed for articular rest, with moist or radiant heat to relax muscles and allay pain. As a last resort, chrysotherapy may be employed, but only after the failure of salicylates and corticoids.

In degenerative arthritis, avoid unnecessary stress on the affected joints; use supportive devices, whenever needed; apply heat locally; also, use orthopedic measures, if advisable; make the obese patients lose weight; and use medication as in the case of rheumatoid arthritis.

Rheumatic fever has an almost specific treatment in salicylates, which will be given as soon as possible in the disease, and at the proper dosage for each particular case. Penicillin and corticoids are also an important contribution to the overall treatment.

In spondylitis, each patient will receive the corresponding basic care, according to the type of infection; but all will benefit from analgesics for the relief of pain.

Hypertrophic spondylitis requires physical treatment in most instances: firm pillows and mattresses, neck collar or brace, traction. Analgesics are always of help, but strong narcotics should be avoided.

Deformities of the Cervical Spine

FUSION OF VERTEBRAE may be due to infectious diseases, injuries to the spine, or abnormal congenital development. A limitation of movements will be the natural consequences; and the diagnosis will depend on the clinical history and the X-ray findings.

THE KLIPPEL-FEIL SYNDROME is the fusion of all lower cervical vertebrae into one mass, showing a short and thick neck with poor movements in any direction. In this instance, other abnormalities are usually present.

CERVICAL RIBS cause pain in the shoulder and arm (scalenus anticus syndrome). the elongated rib may be felt on palpation (rarely on inspection). When pain, or at least discomfort, is present, it is mostly noted as paresthesias.

INCURVATIONS OF THE SPINE. All kinds of incurvations of the spine, namely, kyphosis, scoliosis, lordosis, or a combination of them, will cause pain in the neck and in the back. The diagnosis is made by simple inspection.

Fusion of vertebrae as a result of infective processes will introduce a situation entirely similar to that of the Klippel-Feil syndrome (q.v.), and will be treated the same way, but with special emphasis on the infection, if it is still present and amenable to therapy.

In the congenital Klippel-Feil syndrome, physical measures are to be preferred in almost all cases, even though pain is not too distressing and surgery is available. At times the advice of a specialist is desirable. Since the condition will last all life long, analgesics will be given with much care, and drug tolerance must be avoided.

> Acetylsalicylic acid, 300 to 600 mg, in tablets, every 6 hours, preferably with meals, to be discontinued as soon as possible.
>
> Codeine, 30 to 60 mg, by mouth, every 6 hours, to be discontinued as soon as possible.

Cervical ribs may cause pain spreading not only to the spine but also to the neck. Physical therapy is advised, with surgery as required and analgesics welcomed for the relief of pain. Either codeine, acetylsalicylic acid, or any similar drug may be prescribed as explained in the above paragraph.

Incurvations of the spine cause pain mostly because of muscle strain. The logical treatment, therefore, is to give cholinergics or muscle relaxants, but better if under the direction of a specialist.

> Tincture of belladonna, five to ten drops, in a little water, every 4, 6, or 8 hours, as needed and tolerated.
>
> Atropine, 0.25 mg, by mouth, no more than four times a day, according to tolerance.
>
> Meprobamate, 400 mg, by mouth, every 6 hours.
>
> Carisoprodol, 350 mg, by mouth, every 6 to 8 hours.

Suboccipital Neuralgia. It is characterized by pain in the back of the neck, at times more marked on one side, and by occasional muscle spasm. A sensitive point might be detected by pressing at the center of a line traced from the mastoid to the first cervical apophysis.

This form of neuritis (due to inflammation of the greater or lesser occipital nerve) responds very well to infiltration with an anesthetic solution into the tissues on the occipital area, at the level of the hairline.

> Procaine, 1% solution; inject up to 10 ml diffusely into the occipital area.

> Lidocaine, 1% solution; inject 5 to 10 ml diffusely into the occipital area.

Also, traction or a neck collar might result in help for many patients, particularly if analgesics are added.

> Acetylsalicylic acid, 600 mg, in tablets, every 4 hours, preferably with meals.

> Codeine, 60 mg, by mouth, every 4 or 6 hours.

> Propoxyphene hydrochloride, 65 mg, by mouth, every 4 hours.

> Acetaminophen, 600 mg, by mouth, every 6 hours.

When the above measures fail, surgery might be the best approach, if advised by a specialist.

VIII. PAIN ALONG THE SPINE AND LOWER BACK

A great number of medical and surgical conditions, either directly or indirectly related to the spine, are capable of causing pain in this area of the body. In most instances, this sort of pain may reach disabling proportions, thus making it imperative to relieve it as well as take measures to cure the causative factor. In other words, pain in the spine (rachialgia) may be a serious complication in the management of many a patient.

PAIN ALONG THE SPINE

Infectious Diseases

Smallpox (Variola). In smallpox the onset of the disease is characterized by fever together with a painful rachialgia and headache, myalgias, chills, and tachycardia. As has been stated before, the typical eruption establishes the diagnosis (macules, papules, umbilicated vesicles that turn into pustules, all of them appearing in only one crop of eruptions, first on the face).

The very few cases of variola that still can be found in some areas of the world will involve, in most instances, not only headache, but other pains, of which rachialgia is not the least. The first symptomatic remedy for the relief of this pain will be acetylsalicylic acid.

> Acetylsalicylic acid, 600 mg, in tablets, every 4 hours, or even more frequently (protect against hyperacidity).

If the results are not encouraging, also give codeine, as follows:

> Codeine, 30 to 60 mg, by subcutaneous injection or by mouth, every 4 hours, or even more frequently.

Other analgesics might substitute for the above-mentioned ones, in case of need, such as acetophenetidin, acetaminophen, or the like.

> Acetophenetidin, 300 mg, by mouth, every 4 hours.

> Acetaminophen, 600 mg, by mouth, every 6 hours.

Because of their effects upon the central nervous system, particularly the respiratory centers, do not give narcotic analgesics in these cases.

Meningitis and Meningism. Rachialgia is very frequent in most forms of meningitis, and accompanies the characteristic agonizing headache. There are fever, stiff neck, and positive Kernig's and Brudzinski's signs. Laboratory tests establish the diagnosis. Meningism will induce the same symptomatology but without evidence of meningeal infection.

In meningitis, or the milder reactions of meningism, the pain along the spine (like headache) will react better to efforts to decrease the inflammation of the meninges. Consequently, as soon as the diagnosis is completed, specific therapy will be started immediately, together with measures for dehydration and for electrolyte changes. Analgesics may be tried for relief of pain, but little is to be expected from them. Corticoids may help.

> Prednisone, 5 mg, three or four times a day; decrease dosage slowly as indicated and discontinue as soon as a good result is noted.

Influenza. In cases of grippe, a mild rachialgia, together with myalgias and other pains, accompanies the common and revealing respiratory symptoms. These discomforts ordinarily repsond well to the use of analgesics. The first to be used is acetylsalicylic acid; but also used are acetaminophen, acetophenetidin, etc.

> Acetylsalicylic acid, 300 to 600 mg, in tablets, every 4 to 6 hours, preferably with meals.

> Acetaminophen, 300 to 600 mg, by mouth, every 6 hours.
>
> Acetophenetidin, 300 mg, by mouth, every 4 hours.

A mixture of acetylsalicylic acid and codeine may also be used.

> Acetylsalicylic acid, 600 mg, plus codeine, 60 mg, by mouth, every 4 hours.

Pleuritis. If located at the central portion of the diaphragmatic pleura, pain is referred to the neck and shoulder. The hearing of a pleural friction rub is characteristic. Pain is mostly felt in the thorax, but rachialgia may be really burdensome. Nevertheless, common analgesics are usually effective in relieving these complaints.

> Acetylsalicylic acid, 600 mg, in tablets, every 6 hours, preferably with meals.
>
> Acetaminophen, 600 mg, in tablets, every 6 hours.
>
> Acetophenetidin, 300 mg, in tablets, every 4 hours.

Nevertheless, at times there is need of stronger drugs, either morphine or paravertebral procaine infiltration:

> Morphine sulfate, 10 to 15 mg, by subcutaneous injection, as needed and tolerated.
>
> Procaine, 1% solution, to inject 2 to 4 ml, or as required.

Codeine should be given a trial before resorting to stronger drugs since it helps mitigate the pain and allay cough reflexes.

> Codeine, 60 mg, by mouth or by subcutaneous injection, every 4 hours, or as needed and tolerated.

Spondylitis. A few infections may localize at the spine, thus giving the symptoms of rheumatic pains and limitation of motion, or even more important complaints. Tuberculosis is the most conspicuous one: severe pain may awake the patient from his sleep; X-ray plates will give a clue to the problem, but the diagnosis depends on demonstration of the bacilli by laboratory tests. Gonococcal spondylitis is frequent among patients infected with the gonococcus. In brucellosis there is a clinical picture similar to tuberculosis: pain occurs earlier, and suppuration is not so prevalent. And, of course, streptococcic infections may locate at the spine and provoke a spondylitic syndrome. In all these cases, the X-ray examination is very important.

Each individual case of spondylitis will require the corresponding basic care; but nearly all require also the help of analgesics for relief of pain.

> Acetylsalicylic acid, 300 to 600 mg, in tablets, every 4 to 6 hours, preferably with meals.

> Codeine, 30 to 60 mg, by mouth, every 4 to 6 hours.

> Propoxyphene hydrochloride, 65 mg, by mouth, every 4 hours.

> Meperidine, 100 mg, preferably by mouth, every 4 to 6 hours; subcutaneously if so needed.

Rheumatic Diseases

Rheumatoid Spondylitis. Also called ankylosing spondylitis because of its tendency to produce fusion of the vertebrae in younger people. Pain is the first symptom, starting at the lower portions of the spine and spreading upwards progressively. It is accompanied by stiffness of the column. The condition of the patient is worse when leaving his bed in the morning. Outbursts of pain and stiffness last only for days or weeks, and then subside for a time. The vertebrae are tender on pressure. X-ray examination and laboratory tests are essential for diagnosis.

In rheumatoid (ankylosing) spondylitis, in addition to physical care, the patient will receive analgesic and anti-inflammatory drugs.

> Acetylsalicylic acid, 600 mg, in tablets, every 4 hours.
> with meals or antacids.

> Sodium salicylate, 600 mg, by mouth, every 4 hours,
> with meals or antacids; the addition of small amounts
> of thyroid extract, 30 to 60 mg a day, may help for tolerance.

> Prednisone, 5 to 40 mg a day, to be decreased slowly and discontinued when effects are noted.

Indomethacin, phenylbutazone, or oxyphenbutazone are drugs to be tried, but always with due precautions, because of untoward effects, particularly hematologic (aplastic anemia, agranulocytosis, leukopenia, etc.).

> Indomethacin, 25 mg, by mouth, every 8 to 12 hours.

> Phenylbutazone, 100 to 200 mg, by mouth, every 8 hours.

> Oxyphenbutazone, 100 to 200 mg, by mouth, every 8 hours.

Hypertrophic Spondylitis. In opposition to rheumatoid arthritis, which is a disease of young people, osteoarthritis of the spine is a disease of elders. In fact, most people will show some osteoarthritic changes of their vertebrae after 50 years of age. Pain is of little interest, though aching and stiffness on motion can be detected in most cases.

Physical treatment is needed for most patients (firm pillow and mattress, neck collar or brace, traction). Analgesics are always of help for relief of pain.

> Acetylsalicylic acid, 600 mg, in tablets, every 4 to 6 hours, preferably with meals.

> Codeine, 60 mg, by mouth, every 4 to 6 hours.

Stronger narcotic analgesics are not recommended for these patients.

Metabolic

Climacteric Osteoporosis. The lack of estrogen may lead to a poor rate of bone matrix formation with subsequent decrease of bone mass. Pain is the main symptom of this condition; the diagnosis is made after an X-ray examination, and should be made before more severe symptoms arise (collapse of vertebrae).

This relatively frequent reaction of the climacterium is much improved with the administration of estrogens and progesterone (with due precautions because of recent warnings about induction of cancer), but requires some help with analgesics to alleviate the symptomatic pain. Salicylates and the like are desirable.

> Acetylsalicylic acid, 300 or 600 mg, in tablets, every 4 to 6 hours, preferably with meals.

> Acetophenetidin, 300 mg, by mouth every 4 to 6 hours.

> Acetaminophen, 600 mg, by mouth, every 6 hours.

> Propoxyphene hydrochloride, 65 mg, by mouth, every 4 hours.

Senile Osteoporosis. There is not a clear distinction between senile osteoporosis and climacterium osteoporosis, since senile osteoporosis may start after the climacterium. Pain is relieved by rest. Spontaneous fractures may occur when the disease is advanced.

In women, the treatment should be as for climacteric osteoporosis (see above). Androgens will be tried on men; and also other anabolic steroids. In general, analgesics will be of some help in relieving the pain of the disease.

Acetylsalicylic acid, 600 mg, in tablets, every 4 hours, preferably with meals.

Acetophenetidin, 300 mg, by mouth, every 4 to 6 hours.

Acetaminophen, 600 mg by mouth, every 6 hours.

Propoxyphene hydrochloride, 65, mg, by mouth, every 4 hours.

Codeine may be given together with acetylsalicylic acid, as follows:

Acetylsalicylic acid, 600 mg, plus codeine, 60 mg, by mouth, every 4 to 6 hours, preferably with meals.

Osteomalacia is a condition due to deficient calcification of bones. It is frequent during pregnancy and lactation. It may also occur in patients losing calcium in the urine or with other impairment of bone calcium deposition. Pain in the spine is a prominent symptom, and collapse of the vertebrae may occur later in the disease. Symptoms of tetany will be present when blood calcium is low.

Only a few patients will complain of bone pains, including rachialgia. Besides the specific treatment with vitamin D, a high calcium diet will be of positive help; but in many instances the physician will have to resort to analgesics, particularly acetylsalicylic acid, or any other similar drug.

Acetylsalicylic acid, 300 or 600 mg, in tablets, every 4 to 6 hours, preferably with meals.

Propoxyphene hydrochloride, 65 mg, by mouth, every 4 hours.

Acetaminophen, 600 mg, by mouth, every 6 hours.

Codeine, 60 mg, by mouth, every 4 to 6 hours.

Deformation of the Spine

Deformations of the spine are not painful per se in the great majority of the cases, but they may initiate pain on some occasions by pressure over neighboring roots or nerves, or by compensatory muscle stress. The pain localizes on the back in most cases; in other occasions, it radiates, according to the spread of the roots of nerves involved.

Cervical rib provokes pain to the shoulder and arm (scalenus anticus syndrome), although in a few cases pain may spread to the spine. Physical therapy is advised; at times, surgery is required; and the help of analgesics is frequently needed.

> Acetylsalicylic acid, 300 or 600 mg, in tablets every 4 to 6 hours, preferably with meals.
>
> Propoxyphene hydrochloride, 65 mg, by mouth every 4 hours.
>
> Codeine, 30 to 60 mg, preferably by mouth, every 4 or 6 hours.

Klippel-Feil syndrome or short neck, may give origin to torticollis. The diagnosis is obvious.

The approach to treat pain, not always a distressing symptom in this syndrome, is similar to the one scheduled for the cervical rib. Physical measures are required for practically all cases. Analgesics will help; but efforts will be made to use as little as possible, because the condition is a congenital, life-lasting one.

> Acetylsalicylic acid, 300 or 600 mg, in tablets, every 6 hours, preferably with meals, to be discontinued as soon as possible.
>
> Codeine, 30 to 60 mg, by mouth, every 6 hours, to be discontinued as soon as possible.
>
> Propoxyphene hydrochloride, 65 mg, by mouth, every 4 hours, to be discontinued as soon as possible.

Incurvations of the spine are lordosis, kyphosis, and scoliosis. Any of them may provoke pain in the back. Also, the diagnosis is obvious.

Since pain is mostly due to muscle strain, the logical approach is to use papaverine, belladonna, atropine, meprobamate, carisoprodol, etc. But the basic treatment should be directed by an orthopedist.

> Papaverine hydrochloride, 150 mg, in slow-release capsules, one every 12 hours.
>
> Tincture of belladonna, five to ten drops, three to six times a day, or more; according to needs and tolerance.
>
> Atropine, 0.25 mg, by mouth, up to four times a day, according to needs and tolerance.

Meprobamate, 400 mg, by mouth, every 6 hours.

Carisoprodol, 350 mg, by mouth, every 6 to 8 hours.

Diseases of the Spinal Cord

Spina Bifida. In spina bifida occulta pain is of little or no diagnostic interest; in cases with meningocele, some local pain may be present. Surgery is a must in most of these cases, but even after a good surgical repair of the congenital bifidism some pain may be felt. It will respond well, in the great majority of instances, to analgesics when these are given for a few days.

Acetylsalicylic acid, 300 to 600 mg, in tablets, every 6 hours, preferably by mouth.

Propoxyphene hydrochloride, 65 mg, by mouth, every 4 hours.

Codeine, 30 mg, by mouth, every 4 to 6 hours.

Acetaminophen, 600 mg, by mouth, every 4 hours.

Acetophenetidin, 300 mg, by mouth, every 4 hours.

Myelitis. Pain in the back may accompany some cases of myelitis; it is not an important symptom, since discomforts due to its nervous pathology are the dominant ones (paraplegias, paresthesias, and the like). The etiology of the myelitis should be found (syphilis, tuberculosis, bacterial, etc.).

Since most cases present serious complications, it is better to request the help of a neurologist. The general approach is: very good nursing care at all times; care of the bladder, including catheterization in most cases; care of the bowels, enemas, at least every other day; use of an air mattress, and turning the patient every 2 hours and at the same time giving thorough care to the skin. Also, since paraplegics are protein losers, this element in the blood must be kept at normal; and antibiotics will be given according to each individual infection. Alleviation of pain is a minor problem, because it will recede when the disease improves.

Spinal Epidural Abscess. Severe pain in the back is the first symptom; it is aggravated by motion of the spine. Other neurological symptoms are also present (paresis or paralysis, paresthesias, etc.). Of course, septic symptoms are present (fever syndrome).

Antibiotic therapy and surgery are the essentials of the treatment; the relief of pain is only secondary. Analgesics can be used, but little is to be expected from them.

> Codeine, 60 mg, by subcutaneous injection or by mouth, every 4 hours.
>
> Meperidine, 100 mg, by mouth, or 50 mg, by intramuscular injection, every 4 to 6 hours.
>
> Propoxyphene hydrochloride, 65 mg, by mouth, every 4 hours.
>
> Acetylsalicylic acid, 600 mg, in tablets, every 4 to 6 hours, preferably with meals.

Neuralgia

Suboccipital neuralgia includes pain in the back of the neck. If the pain is due to injury to the posterior branch of the second cervical nerve root, there is a sensitive point on pressure at the midpoint of a line from the mastoid to the first cervical apophysis. The pain is sometimes more marked on one side, and muscle spasms are occasionally present. This pain is due to neuritis of the occipital nerves (greater or lesser). Perhaps the simplest—and a very effective—treatment is local anesthesia, injecting the solution so as to diffuse it into the tissues of the occipital area at the level of the hairline.

> Procaine, 1% solution; inject up to 10 ml into the tissue of the occipital area.
>
> Lidocaine, 1% solution; inject up to 10 ml into the occipital area.

Also, the use of traction or a collar may be effective, particularly if helped with analgesics.

> Acetylsalicylic acid, 600 mg, in tablets, every 4 hours, preferably with meals.
>
> Codeine, 60 mg, by mouth, every 4 to 6 hours.

Surgery might be advisable when the above measures fail to give relief. The help of an orthopedist will be required.

Muscle Diseases and Reactions

As stated before, muscle strain is frequent whenever an abnormal position of the spine is maintained for a long time. Also, certain diseases of the muscles in the back may cause pain.

Strain. Excessive muscular effort will induce a reactive pain of the involved fibers. This occurs not only after violent and prolonged exercise, but also when an abnormal position is maintained for long periods of time: an example is pain of the occipital muscles in anxiety (the head is supposedly projected forward in an expectant attitude).

Muscle pain thus brought on is better treated by rest. Application of heat, and massage of the strained muscle, will help recovery by increasing blood circulation. The use of analgesics and muscle relaxants will also help.

> Acetylsalicylic acid, 300 or 600 mg, in tablets, every 4 to 6 hours, preferably with meals.
>
> Propoxyphene hydrochloride, 65 mg, by mouth, every 4 hours.
>
> Meprobamate, 400 mg, by mouth, every 6 hours.
>
> Carisoprodol, 350 mg, by mouth, every 6 to 8 hours.

For other details, see below, under the heading "Wry neck (torticollis)."

Fibrositis. The most frequent locations of symptoms of fibrositis are the neck and the low back. Also, the chest and shoulders may be affected. Pain and stiffness are the principal symptoms. Limitation of movement is not so important. The attacks are separated by periods of remission, and the symptoms worsen with bed rest. No lesions of the vertebrae are present in cases of fibrositis. A good point of differential diagnosis is that patients with fibrositis are better during periods of exercise, while those with organic bone lesions are not.

When this pain is felt in the spine, as well as in any other body area, the first measures to be taken are bed rest, heat, and massage. Of course, the help of analgesics is effective in most instances, either when taken alone or together with muscle relaxants.

> Acetylsalicylic acid, 600 mg, in tablets, every 4 hours, preferably with meals.
>
> Codeine, 60 mg, by mouth, every 4 hours.

Meprobamate, 400 mg, by mouth, every 6 hours.

Carisoprodol, 350 mg, by mouth, every 6 to 8 hours.

The small, painful nodules (trigger nodules) may be injected with either an anesthetic or a corticoid.

Procaine, 1% solution; inject 0.25 to 0.5 ml (even more) into the trigger nodules.

Hydrocortisone, 2.5% suspension; inject, as above, 0.25 ml or more into the affected nodules.

Trichinosis. Pain in the back of the neck is one of the early symptoms of trichinosis. A generalized symptomatology with diarrhea, and, later, pain over most of the muscles, fever, and intense eosinophilia, along with a history of previous ingestion of poorly cooked pork will be evidence for a diagnosis. Muscle pains, frequently located or extending into the spine, add to the symptomatology. Unfortunately, there is no specific therapy known. Pain will be relieved with corticoids and analgesics, given together.

Prednisone, 20 to 60 mg a day, by mouth, in divided doses, for 3 to 5 days; then decreased gradually and discontinued after 10 days.

Acetylsalicylic acid, 600 mg, in tablets, every 4 hours, preferably with meals.

Codeine, 60 mg, by mouth, every 4 hours.

Thiabendazole, by mouth, according to weight; 25 mg per kg of body weight, the dosage to be repeated every 12 hours during at least 5 days, but never for more than 10 days.

Wry Neck (*Torticollis*). This disorder was described above in the section on "Pain in the Neck."

The pain is mostly localized in the affected muscles, but aches may spread all over the spine or at least over the thoracic spine. Analgesics will provide only very modest relief. Better help is obtained by the use of tincture of belladonna, atropine, and muscle relaxants. Tranquilizers may help a little; and massage is to be encouraged.

Tincture of belladonna, five drops to ten drops—or more—three to six times a day, according to effects and tolerance.

Atropine, 0.25 mg, by mouth, up to four times a day, according to effects and tolerance.

Meprobamate, 400 mg, by mouth, every 6 hours.

Carisoprodol, 350 mg, by mouth, every 6 or 8 hours.

Diseases of the Mediastinum

Diseases of the posterior mediastinum occasionally account for pain in the spine—interscapular pain, not intense but very bothersome. Pain is exaggerated when the patient is in bed. Dysphagia may be present. The Horner syndrome may also be present.

Tumors are the main cause of mediastinal syndrome. They may be benign or malignant; radiography is the best diagnostic procedure. (Also, esophagoscopy or bronchoscopy can be used.)

The management is the same as for other tumors located elsewhere in the body: surgery whenever indicated for both benign or malignant growths and chemotherapy or radiotherapy as needed. Pain generally accompanies advanced malignancies, and in the great majority of instances it becomes intolerable; the pain is located either in the thorax or radiating to the spine, requiring the use of narcotics.

Morphine sulfate, 15 mg or more, by subcutaneous injection, repeated as needed and tolerated.

Meperidine, 50 to 100 mg, by subcutaneous injection, repeated as needed and tolerated.

Codeine, 60 mg, by subcutaneous injection, repeated as needed and tolerated.

Tuberculosis. Fibrotic types of pulmonary tuberculosis may simulate the mediastinal syndrome. Symptoms due to tuberculosis are also present. Perhaps, when pain along the spine is felt in cases of tuberculosis of the mediastinum, it is due to pleural reaction if not to direct infection of the surrounding structures. As in pleuritis, regular analgesics will be tried first—perhaps with some emphasis on codeine, because it may also alleviate coughing—and narcotics are the last resource.

Acetylsalicylic acid, 600 mg, in tablets, every 4 hours, preferably with meals.

Acetaminophen, 600 mg, by mouth, every 6 hours.

Acetophenetidin, 300 mg, by mouth, every 4 hours.

Propoxyphene hydrochloride, 65 mg, by mouth, every 4 hours.

Codeine, 60 mg, by mouth or subcutaneous injection, every 4 hours.

Morphine sulfate, 10 to 15 mg, by subcutaneous injection, repeated as needed and tolerated.

Aneurism of the Aorta. Circulatory or respiratory symptoms may appear first. Pain will be present, particularly when the aneurism injures the spine. Some relief might be afforded with analgesics, but the basic treatment depends on the judgment of specialists in cardiovascular conditions, who should be consulted.

Acetylsalicylic acid, 300 or 600 mg, in tablets, every 4 to 6 hours, preferably with meals.

Codeine, 30 to 60 mg, by mouth, every 4 to 6 hours.

Referred Pain (Heterotopic Pain)

Biliary lithiasis may provoke pain radiating to the spine and the right shoulder (in rare instances, the left shoulder). The treatment includes the care of an acute attack (colic), for which it is advised to give, first, an injection of papaverine; as the second choice, an injection of meperidine, or better, meperidine with papaverine; and only as a last resort, morphine. Bed rest, hydration, gastric suction for the relief of abdominal distention, and antibiotics are needed. In cholecystitis, antacids as well as antispasmodics and sedatives give good results.

Peptic Ulcer. Spinal pain may be present in a few patients. Peptic ulcers do not respond well to analgesics. Instead, give antacids and anticholinergics.

Pancreatitis. This disease also may cause pain in the spine in some patients. To control this continuous and boring type of pain, the best drug is codeine; meperidine will be the second (and cautious) choice.

In all three instances, the abdominal symptomatology is the focal point of the clinical picture.

LOW BACK PAIN

Low back pain can have its origin in the same causes discussed in "Pain along the Spine." Other more specific factors will be reviewed in the following topics.

Medical Conditions

Infective Diseases. Low back pain may be more prominent than the pain in the spine in smallpox, meningitis, influenza, and spondylitis.

Rheumatic Diseases. Except for the location of the pain, there is no difference in aches provoked by rheumatoid or hypertrophic spondylitis.

Metabolic Bone Diseases. Pain may be located low in the spine in climacteric osteoporosis, senile osteoporosis, and osteomalacia.

Deformities of the spine, such as scoliosis, kyphosis, and lordosis (particularly the latter) may initiate low back pain.

Diseases of the Spinal Cord. In diseases of the spinal cord, pain may be low when caused by spina bifida and myelitis.

Muscle diseases and reactions are as discussed above, except for those which refer to the cervical vertebrae.

Injuries

The mechanism of pain is similar for most types of injuries to the lumbar spine and the sacroiliac region. The main injury in this group is the strain of an unusual effort, particularly in lifting heavy objects; other efforts should be considered as well, such as violent movements of the trunk, jumping, or falling on the feet. In most instances, a protrusion of an intervertebral disk is the cause of pain.

Each individual case will require its own physical therapy or surgical procedure, but the adjuvant use of analgesics is to be advised to alleviate suffering.

> Codeine, 30 to 60 mg, by subcutaneous injection during the first 2 days, then by mouth; every 4 to 6 hours.
>
> Meperidine, 100 mg, by mouth, every 4 hours for 1 or 2 days; then resort to codeine or acetylsalicylic acid.
>
> Codeine, to follow after the use of meperidine, 30 mg, by mouth, every 4 hours.
>
> Acetylsalicylic acid, 600 mg, in tablets, every 4 to 6 hours, preferably with meals.

Acute Sprain. Ordinarily, the onset is sudden, with pain in the lumbar spine following either an unusually heavy effort or even a movement that is performed every day. The patient cannot straighten up or move, and the pain increases for the following 1 to 2 hours. Rarely, the symptoms develop later on. The muscles are tense and tender to pressure. In general, the symptomatology corresponds to that of fibrositis (q.v.).

Bed rest, local heat, and massage are almost the essentials of the treatment; but the use of analgesics and of muscle relaxants will provide a fairly effective relief of pain, particularly the analgesics.

> Acetylsalicylic acid, 600 mg, in tablets, every 4 hours, preferably after meals.
>
> Codeine, 60 mg, by mouth, every 4 hours.
>
> Meperidine, 100 mg, by mouth, every 4 hours.
>
> Meprobamate, 400 mg, by mouth, every 6 hours.
>
> Carisoprodol, 350 mg, by mouth, every 6 to 8 hours.

A mixture of acetylsalicylic acid and codeine can be given by using the same dosage as stated above for each drug alone.

Fractures. The symptoms of fracture are pain and muscle spasm. On examination there is local tenderness and perhaps a deformity. The diagnosis is made by X ray.

Absolute immobilization and surgical care are essential for these cases, but analgesics are needed, starting with codeine or meperidine, and thereafter salicylates or similar analgesics.

> Codeine, 30 to 60 mg, by subcutaneous injection during the first 2 days, thereafter by mouth; every 4 hours.
>
> Meperidine, 100 mg, by mouth, every 4 hours, for 1 or 2 days; then to be followed by any other analgesic.
>
> Acetylsalicylic acid, 600 mg, in tablets, every 4 hours, preferably with meals.
>
> Propoxyphene hydrochloride, 65 mg, by mouth, every 4 hours.

Disk Lesions

Disk lesions may be either traumatic or degenerative. Except for acute injuries (see above), forces acting constantly upon the last two vertebrae and their articulations will provoke low back pain. X-ray examination is imperative.

Protrusion of the Intervertebral Disk. This often produces low back pain, which frequently radiates to the thighs and is aggravated by effort. There are spasms, local tenderness, and limitation of motion. Neurological symptoms may develop (depression of reflexes, paresthesias, etc.). An X-ray picture ordinarily establishes the diagnosis.

In both the acute and the chronic stages of the disease, analgesics will be of help, as will muscle relaxants. Physical therapy is always needed, and surgical procedures are frequently a necessity.

> Acetylsalicylic acid, 600 mg, in tablets, every 4 hours, preferably with meals.
>
> Sodium salicylate, 600 mg, by mouth, every 4 or 6 hours.
>
> Codeine, 60 mg, by mouth, every 4 hours.
>
> Codeine with acetylsalicylic acid, same dosage as above stated for each drug.
>
> Meprobamate, 400 mg, by mouth, every 6 hours.
>
> Carisoprodol, 350 mg, by mouth, every 6 or 8 hours.

Chronic Low Back Pain

Chronic low back pain may be due to any one of the common causes of pain in this location. Lesions of the vertebrae or of the disks may be the causative factor; protrusion of disks (see above), sacralization of the 5th lumbar vertebra or lumbarization of the 1st sacral vertebra, spondylolysis, spondylolisthesis, etc. "Chronic low back" is continuous or intermittent low back pain, ordinarily aggravated by motion and mitigated by rest, heat, or massage. On examination, no abnormal signs or structures are found, except in cases mentioned in the foregoing paragraph. Patients do not complain of sharp pains, but of annoying dull aches that do not interfere too much with daily activities.

Besides the general measures necessary to handle these patients, the use of analgesics, particularly salicylates, is to be encouraged.

> Acetylsalicylic acid, 600 mg, in tablets, every 4 hours, to be decreased to 300 or 600 mg every 6 hours as soon as possible (take with meals, preferably).
>
> Sodium salicylate, 600 mg, by mouth, every 4 to 6 hours, preferably with small amounts of thyroid extract (30 mg a day).

At times, surgery is required for the total relief of some patients.

Psoitis may be due to an infection of the spine, and so will present rachialgia, but the main symptomatology belongs to the legs. The reader is referred to the corresponding paragraphs, below, for detailed information.

Heterotopic Pain

Some of the etiological factors for pain felt along other portions of the spine might be responsible as well for lumbar pain, particularly biliary lithiasis and chronic pancreatitis.

Kidney Diseases. In acute nephritis there is almost always low back pain present. In renal colic there is also pain referred to the lower portion of the spine. Similarly, low back pain may be provoked by pyelonephritis, hydronephrosis, and other kidney diseases; but in all instances, symptoms due to renal impairment are prevalent.

Genital Diseases. Diseases of othe uterus, either infective or tumoral, are well known causes of lumbar pain. Other signs and symptoms will be investigated whenever a woman complains of low back pain. Men will refer pain to the lumbar region when they suffer from prostatic diseases. A rectal examination will help in diagnosing these discomforts.

Hernia in Petit's triangle is a rare occurrence found among older people with habitual constipation or who do unusual strenuous exercise. The swelling in the lumbar region may be very small. Other symptoms of herniation may be found.

Pyelitis and pyelonephritis respond well to regular analgesics, when they are given together with antibiotics, fluids, and bed rest. In hydronephrosis papaverine or codeine should be given as a palliative before surgical repair of the obstruction. For a perirenal abscess or an abscess of the kidney, codeine, methylene blue, phenazopyridine, tincture of belladonna, or atropine is given; but the main thing to do is to treat the infection and to drain it, if that is indicated. Tuberculosis of the kidney has to be treated as such; to treat its pain (by codeine, meperidine, propoxyphene hydrochloride, etc.) is a minor problem. The pain from renal cancer requires morphine, meperidine, or codeine, but the basic treatment is the main concern. For the pain of polycystic kidney, papaverine, meperidine, codeine, etc., will be given. Renal lithiasis may require some sort of surgical intervention, but the pain may be relieved with codeine, papaverine, pentazocine hydrochloride, etc., morphine being the last choice.

Dysmenorrheic pains respond to an adequate hormonal treatment and to the usual analgesics. Primary dysmenorrhea is better treated

170 DIAGNOSIS AND TREATMENT

with papaverine, anticholinergics, or codeine. Salpingitic pains respond to regular analgesics, such as codeine, meperidine, etc.; but dysmenorrhea requires regulation of menstruation, and in case of infection antibiotics and surgery. For follicular cysts, give progesterone and regular analgesics; for luteal cysts, analgesics alone, if surgery is not needed. Surgery is the only treatment for ectopic pregnancy.

IX. THORACODYNIA

Pain in the thorax is a very common complaint of ailing people. Physicians may classify as thoracodynia any pain located between the neck and abdomen and beneath the skin, or as thoracalgia pain that originates in the thoracic walls. A distinction is frequently made relative to retrosternal pain, precordial pain, or pain in the side. A strict delimitation of each topographic location of pain is not so easy. Precordial pain (located at the area of the apex of the heart) and retrosternal pain (located somewhat to the right of the foregoing location, exactly behind the sternum) are ordinarily not distinguished from each other by the layman, and even physicians are not careful to separate the two since both may lead to the same diagnosis. For these reasons, we will divide this section into: (1) retrosternal and precordial pain, (2) chest pain, (3) mastalgia, (4) thoracalgia, and (5) referred pain.

Retrosternal and Precordial Pain

It is true that retrosternal and precordial pain refer in a great number of cases to heart diseases, particularly of the type of myocardial ischemia. But it must not be forgotten that many other diseases, either of the heart or of other organs, may also show this sort of pain, namely, retrosternal or precordial; and that the treatment might widely differ from one instance to another. The main situations are dealt with in the following paragraphs.

Angina Pectoris. The principal symptom, which gives its name (angor), is pain, substernally localized and possibly radiating to the left shoulder, the left arm, or the jaw. Discomfort may be felt on the right shoulder and right arm, and may also exist with little or no substernal pain. The pain lasts for only a few minutes; rarely as much as half an hour or one hour. There are no signs on auscultation or evidence of abnormal pulsations. A relation might be found to previous exertion, emotion, gastrointestinal upsets (overeating, indigestion, meteorism). Patients may or may not complain of palpitation, digestive symptoms, dyspnea, and weakness. Of course, a diagnosed anginal episode may be the first, or one in a series. The sequence of (a) provocation, (b) angina, (c) rest or nitroglycerin administration, and (d) relief is of diagnostic importance. During the anginal attack (not after it subsides!) there is a deflexion of the isoelectric line of the ECG at the RS-T junction, or an inversion of the T wave. Of course, signs of previous myocardial infarctions may help to establish the diagnosis of anginal pain. During the intervals between attacks, we repeat, there are no ECG abnormalities, in pure anginal crisis.

To treat anginal pain is to treat angina pectoris itself. The acute attack will be checked first by the patient's standing still or lying down from the beginning of the attack to its end, and by the classic use of nitroglycerin, which affords relief in less than a couple of minutes, at times accompanied by headache caused by the medication.

> Nitroglycerin, 0.5 mg, or less, sublingual tablet, to be repeated as needed.

It is to be recalled that the relief is of such a specificity that when it fails, suspicion of myocardial infarction will arise. Also, to be recalled: the abuse of repeated administration of nitroglycerin will lead to tolerance of the medication; and large doses can cause nitrite poisoning, with flushed face, intense headache, dizziness, initial violent heart action which diminishes shortly, faintness and muscle relaxation, irregular respiration, mydriasis, diarrhea, and final syncope and cardiorespiratory failure (see corresponding paragraph for nitrite poisoning).

Amyl nitrite pearls are a good substitute for nitroglycerin; the amount of the gas inhaled is varied according to tolerance and activity.

> Amyl nitrite, pearls, one pearl crushed and the gas inhaled.

General measures to be advised will be: engaging in physical activity, but at a good tolerance level; following a diet poor in fats, watching the cholesterol and lipid blood levels, and controlling body weight, to reach and stay at the right one; avoiding emotional or physical stress of any kind; observing bed rest whenever necessary; avoiding toxic habits (smoking, drinking, etc.), and any other individual error in hygiene. These general measures may help the patient to avoid, or at least decrease the frequency of anginal attacks.

For this purpose other vasodilators possessing slower and longer activity may be used:

>Pentaerythrityl tetranitrate, 10- or 20-mg tablets, one every 6 hours.

>Papaverine, 150-mg slow-release capsules, one every 12 hours.

>Mannitol hexanitrate, 15 or 30 mg by mouth, every 6 to 8 hours.

>Isosorbide dinitrate, 10-mg tablets, one every 6 hours.

>Erythrityl tetranitrate, 10 or 15 mg, sublingually, every 8 hours.

>Propanolol, 10 to 30 mg, by mouth, every 8 hours. Do not withdraw this drug at a rapid pace, since to do so may worsen angina.

The treatment of any coexisting disease should be pursued, particularly a cardiopathy, which should be at least supervised by a specialist.

Myocardial Infarction. The general pattern is the same as with angina pectoris, with a relatively slower start, no relation to exercise or emotion, but more severe pain, with accompanying fear of impending death; it is of more prolonged duration, and is not relieved by rest or nitroglycerin. A fall in blood pressure may occur. It is not exceptional in a case of myocardial infarction to encounter little pain and sparse symptomatology. A history of anginal attacks may be obtained in many cases, but some patients may not remember any previous coronary disability. Dyspnea is frequent in myocardial infarction, together with sweating and a feeling of extreme weakness (rarely, dyspnea, sweating, and weakness are the only symptoms). When acute left failure supervenes, the corresponding symptoms will appear (tachypnea, frothy sputum, lung congestion, and finally edema, hepatomegaly, etc.). Fever rises after the first day. Leukocytosis and increased serum glutamic oxalacetic transaminase (SGOT) are the rule. ECG findings (deflexion of ST segment and inversion of T wave) are characteristic.

As with angina pectoris, the treatment of pain induced by myocardial infarction is the treatment of the disease itself. The patient will be referred, immediately, to a cardiologist in a coronary care unit, under the most complete rest that is possible and under the influence of a narcotic analgesic.

Morphine, 10 to 15 mg by subcutaneous injection, or 5 to 10 mg by intranvenous injection, if so needed. Repeat after 30 minutes, if necessary.

Meperidine, 50 mg by intravenous injection, or 100 mg subcutaneously. Repeat after 30 minutes, if necessary.

At this time, the administration of anticoagulants might be started; but, if available, oxygen will be given during the trip to the hospital, since it may help to allay pain. The rest of the treatment, including the management of complications that might occur during that trip to the hospital, will be under the care of the specialist, and need not be outlined here.

Valvular Lesions. In younger patients, mitral stenosis may cause substernal pain, similar to angina, particularly after effort. The characteristic murmur is pre-systolic, increasing in intensity, until the first sound occurs. A thrill is felt in many patients. Pain due to cardiovascular diseases should receive the basic care given by the specialist. If the cause is a cardiovascular disturbance, some initial help will be offered by means of ordinary analgesics.

Acetylsalicylic acid, 300 mg tablets, one every 4 to 6 hours, preferably with meals.

Propoxyphene hydrochloride, 65-mg capsules, one every 6 hours.

In cases of acquired chronic valvular heart disease, rheumatic fever is to be considered the most frequent cause. Salicylates are almost specific, and will be given at average dosage in mild cases, and in large amounts in severe ones.

Acetylsalicylic acid, 300-mg tablets, two every 4 hours, preferably with meals.

Acetylsalicylic acid, larger doses: start with 60 mg for each kg of body weight in four or six doses given during 24 hours; increase to 90, 120, and even 180 mg per kg, also given in six doses in a day.

Sodium salicylate, 600 mg, by mouth, every 4 to 6 hours.

Sodium salicylate, larger doses: 1200 mg, by mouth, every 4 or 6 hours; increase to 2 g every 2 to 4 hours. It is to be noted that many patients do not tolerate salicylates well. The intravenous route has been advised for these patients, but it does not offer real advantages. It is better to use antacids to protect against local irritation; also, the use of small amounts of thyroid extract (30 to 60 mg a day) will increase tolerance in many cases.

Patients with rheumatic fever will also benefit from the administration of antibiotics (penicillin) and corticoids (prednisone). Such patients might accept a substitute of salicylates whenever salicylates do not show the desired effect after adequate use for 4 or 5 days. By this time, the patient should be under the care of the specialist; but if there is need of care, start immediately with the administration of corticoids.

Prednisone, 5 to 10 mg, by mouth, every 6 hours. After 3 weeks, the dosage should be decreased gradually, so that after a total treatment of 6 weeks, all is accomplished.
Higher dosages are needed, at times, up to 20 mg every 6 hours, or even 40 mg each time, for some special cases. In these instances, withdrawal will take a longer period of time.

The advice for additional treatment will be given by the specialist, particularly the one dealing with the general treatment of the disease itself, or of its complications, or the one dealing with the necessity for surgical procedures. This holds true particularly in those instances when rheumatic disease is not the problem.

Pericarditis. In acute fibrinous pericarditis, severe non-paroxymal pain may be present, accompanied by dyspnea and anxiety. Pain may be less severe in specific pericarditis, namely tuberculous, bacterial, rheumatic, etc. The characteristic to-and-fro friction rub is heard on auscultation (it does not stop when the patient holds his breath). The ECG may show changes that help to establish the diagnosis (initial elevation of RS-T waves principally). In acute benign pericarditis, pain is accompanied by fever, symptoms of respiratory involvement (cough, dyspnea, and in some cases continuation of a previous upper respiratory infection), and a course which can be mild or complicated by a mild pericardial effusion and/or other cardiac and respiratory symptoms (pleural effusion, shock, and very rarely, cardiac tamponade). Pain may be severe enough to require the initial use of morphine, or at least meperidine.

Morphine, 10 to 15 mg, by subcutaneous injection.

Meperidine, 100 mg, by intramuscular injection.

Thereafter, or if it seems advisable, starting with codeine, give such analgesics as acetylsalicylic acid, oral meperidine, or any other similar analgesic.

Codeine, 60 mg, by mouth, every 4 to 6 hours.

Acetylsalicylic acid, 600 mg, in tablets, every 4 hours.

Meperidine, 50 to 100 mg, by mouth, every 6 hours.

Corticoids are also of definite help.

Prednisone, 10 to 20 mg, every 8 hours during the first 3 or 4 days; thereafter, decrease gradually over about 2 weeks, and then discontinue.

According to each individual case, and in close communication with the cardiologist and the surgeon, evaluate the use of antibiotics, the necessity for surgical procedures, etc.

Cardiac tamponade only rarely causes pain. The diagnosis is based on the triad: increased venous blood pressure, increased diastolic pressure with narrowed pulse pressure, and distant heart sounds. Ordinarily, it follows a penetrating wound of the heart or is secondary to other heart disease. As soon as the diagnosis is made, the patient will receive an injection of morphine or meperidine:

Morphine, 10 to 15 mg, subcutaneously.

Meperidine, 100 mg, by intramuscular injection.

and a pericardiocentesis will be carried out for the slow removal of blood. The site for puncturing the pericardium (avoid touching the ventricle!) is at the level of the 5th or 6th left inter space, 1 cm inside the area of cardiac dullness or 7 to 8 cm to the left of the corresponding sternal line, the needle going inwards and slightly upwards, checking frequently for withdrawal of liquid. Also, access may be gained from between the xiphoid and the left sternal margin, inserting the needle directed upwards at a 30° angle, pointing to the midline. From either side, the pericardium is reached at a distance of about 3 to 5 cm. More rarely, at a distance of about 7 to 8 cm, when the first point of entrance is used. If things are done properly (which is not always possible, particularly in rural areas), the needle should be connected to a well-grounded electrocardiograph (for warning against entering the myocardium); the patient will be well-grounded, too (to avoid inducing fibrillation). A rubber tube between the needle and the syringe will facilitate the procedure.

Aortitis and Aortic Aneurism. Pain referred to the aorta, aortalgia, is very similar to anginal pain. It may also follow effort, emotion, or a heavy meal, but is less severe than the pure anginal attack. Some believe that aortalgia will occur only when there is an obstacle to the blood flow through the coronary arteries (true anginal pain). In the case of dissecting aortic aneurism, the clinical picture is very similar to that of myocardial infarction, with pain and shock; a lowered blood pressure in the legs, to levels equal or lower than that in the arms, occurs in this form of aneurysm, (also in coarctation of the aorta, aortic embolism, etc.). X-ray examinations will support the diagnosis in many cases.

Most cases of aortitis will not show pain, unless the coronary arteries are affected. In this instance, treatment will be that of angina pectoris (q.v.). On the contrary, most cases with aortic aneurism will have pain, even very severe as with dissecting aneurysm. The final treatment is surgical, no matter that the results of the procedure are in doubt. In the meantime, efforts will be directed to decrease the hypertension which is present in many instances. If there is hypertension propanolol must be given.

> Propanolol, 20 mg, by mouth, every 6 hours; or 1 to 2 mg by the intramuscular route, every 6 hours.

Emphysema. Pain is of little value in the diagnosis of emphysema. A few patients will complain of precordial pain, exaggerated following effort, that may cause anxiety. The main symptomatology consists of cough, dyspnea, hyperinflation of the chest, and some radiolucency in the X-ray plate.

The treatment of emphysema will be indirect and follows the overall treatment of the condition. Anyhow the use of codeine is advisable, under the circumstances:

> Codeine, 60 mg, by mouth, every four to six hours,

but not to the point of complete control of coughing, since cough is needed to cleanse the airways. Bronchodilators and corticoids (these in severe cases) may be additional help in alleviating pain, when present.

> Aminophylline, 100 or 200 mg, in tablets, three or four times a day.

> Prednisone, 5 or 10 mg, once or twice a day; discontinue gradually as soon as possible

Diseases of the Mediastinum. Any disease of the mediastinum may bring on precordial or substernal pain. Tumors, particularly malignant, are to be considered first; X-ray examination is the best diagnostic procedure, together with bronchoscopy and/or esophagoscopy.

Each disease must receive adequate therapy, but in case of pain the great majority will respond to common analgesics, such as:

Acetylsalicylic acid, 300 or 600 mg, in tablets, every 4 to 6 hours.

Acetaminophen, 600 mg, in tablets, every 6 hours.

Propoxyphene hydrochloride, 65-mg tablets, every 4 hours.

Codeine—particularly if there is coughing—30 to 60 mg, by mouth, every 4 to 6 hours.

Very rarely meperidine will be needed, and less frequently, morphine.

Meperidine, 50 or 100 mg, by mouth, every 6 hours.

Morphine, 10 or 15 mg by subcutaneous injection, as needed.

Referred Pain from the Digestive System. Diseases of the liver may provoke heterotopic pain in the retrosternal area. Biliary colic may radiate in such a way as to mimic an anginal attack. No other cardiovascular symptoms will be present; symptoms are, mainly, of digestive nature. Pain or pressure over the biliary area may reach severe proportions. In peptic ulcer, also, pain is occasionally referred to the precordial area. The rest of the symptomatology will be that of peptic ulcer: pain following digestive disturbances and alleviated by antispasmotics and antacids.

Referred Pain from the Urinary System. Very rarely, renal colic will encourage an erroneous diagnosis of angina pectoris, because of its retrosternal location.

Pulmonary infarction, pleuritis, pleurodynia, and pneumothorax may cause retrosternal or precordial pain, but they mainly give rise to a very characteristic chest pain, which is evaluated in the following categories:

	page no.
Biliary colic	189
Peptic ulcer	188
Renal colic	201
Pulmonary infarction	179
Pleurodynia and pleuritis	180
Pneumothorax	181

Chest Pain

The importance of chest pain, particularly in pneumonia, has been stressed by European physicians, who speak of a *point de côte*, *punto de costado*, or the like, in their semipopular jargon. Pulmonary diseases, in fact, frequently begin with a more or less severe chest pain.

Pneumonia. The sudden onset of pneumonia is ordinarily characterized by a sharp pain in the same side of the thorax, accompanied by elevation of temperature, chills, headache, and cough, with or without expectoration. Anyhow, the production of a pinkish sputum rapidly turning into a rusty one is one of the characteristic features of pneumonia. Dyspnea with tachypnea and a special expiratory grunt are very frequently found. Children may have convulsions at the onset of the disease. Soon, fine rales are heard on auscultation, and finally all the well-known signs and symptoms of the disease are well developed. Nevertheless, there are forms of pneumonia which present very little symptomatology. In all cases, the roentgenological examination is fundamental to the diagnosis. Once the presence of pneumonia is established, it is imperative to know the etiological factor in order to plan adequate treatment. The acute disease with marked symptomatology will most probably be a pneumococcal infection. In hemolytic streptococcal pneumonia the pharynx is almost always swollen and inflamed, the tonsils are covered with exudate, and not rarely there is a large pleural effusion. Staphylococcal pneumonia ordinarily occurs as a complication of other staphylococcal infections, either postoperatively, following attacks of influenza, or as a form of hospital (or any other concentration of people) infection by resistant strains. Klebsiella pneumonia is suspected when consolidation rapidly spreads from lobe to lobe. In tularemia pneumonia there is a history of some contact with wild animals, particularly rabbits. The onset of viral or mycoplasma pneumoniae infection is slow and shows few symptoms. Aspiration pneumonia follows the introduction of foreign matter (food) into the respiratory system.

Bronchopneumonia. Bronchopneumonia is an infection of the lung, restricted to the alveoli contiguous to the bronchi. Consequently, it can merely be considered a variety of pneumonia. A typical bronchopneumonia starts at several different foci at the same time. The onset is gradual, insidious, either in primary cases or even when it is secondary to an infection, particularly influenza. Very rarely, if at all, the staphylococcus will be responsible for the disease. Bronchopneumonia is not as typically developed as lobar pneumonia; the symptoms and signs are less marked, less organized in a sequence, and ordinarily the final crisis is lacking. Some patients will not show symptoms or signs; the disease is merely a radiologic finding; in other cases, symptomatology may be severe or extended for long periods of time. Bronchopneumonia will be suspected when pneumonia signs intermix with symptoms of a previous infective disease: influenza, measles, whooping cough, typhus, scarlet fever, smallpox, plague, typhoid fever (pneumotyphus), ornithosis, and perhaps others.

Depending on the nature of the infective germ, the etiologic treatment will be carried out with the specific antibiotic starting as soon as possible. The control of pain is merely a palliative measure, with little effect upon the disease. To obtain this symptomatic action, the physician will advise bed rest, oxygen administration, good hydration, and analgesics.

> Codeine, 60 mg, by mouth, every 4 to 6 hours.

> Acetylsalicylic acid, 600 mg, in tablets, every 4 hours, preferably with meals. This schedule is particularly useful with elevated temperature; but dosage will be decreased as indicated.

> Acetaminophen, 600 mg, by mouth, every 6 hours.

Pulmonary infarction is characterized by sudden onset of side pain, followed by dyspnea and cough (with bloody sputum). The symptoms resemble those of pneumonia, and may mimic also those of myocardial infarction, pleurisy, or pericarditis. The diagnosis is suggested very strongly when venous thrombosis is present elsewhere in the body (more frequently in the legs). Small infarcted areas will show few symptoms; large infarctions cause much trouble: acute pain and dyspnea, cyanosis, and finally symptoms of shock. If an ECG is made (myocardial damage suspected), only signs of right ventricular strain will be found (cor pulmonale); but other signs are not uncommon (S-T depression, T inversion, etc.). It is to be noted that the location of pain may vary with the location of the pulmonary infarction: at the left lower lobe, the pain is precordial or retrosternal; pain may be referred to the shoulder, the abdomen, etc.

The first choice in the treatment of pulmonary infarction has to be given, in most cases, to morphine, or meperidine as an alternate.

> Morphine, 5 mg by intravenous injection; or 10 or 15 mg by the subcutaneous route, to repeat as needed.

Meperidine, 50 mg by intramuscular injection, to repeat as needed.

If cough is severe, also give:

Codeine, 30 mg by the intramuscular route, up to six times a day; or 60 mg, by mouth, every 4 to 6 hours, when no heroic doses are needed.

Rest and oxygen therapy are important.

Atelectasis. In the case of a sudden obstruction of the lower air passages with a foreign body or thick secretion, side pain will be the first symptom, rapidly followed by dyspnea, cyanosis, fever, and shock. Objective findings will be reduced expansion of respiratory movements, and diminution of respiratory sounds. In slowly developing atelectasis due to tumors, symptoms are minimal except for coughing; once the obstruction is completely established, the symptoms are the same as for acute atelectasis. X-ray and bronchoscopic examination are essential for diagnosis: retraction of ribs and diaphragm, airless shadow, visualization of the obstruction.

Only when the collapse is sudden, massive, or infected is there pain; and whenever there is pain, its treatment should be added to the basic one. In general, narcotic analgesics should not be used. Use instead:

Acetylsalicylic acid, 600 mg, in tablets, every 4 to 6 hours.

Acetaminophen, 600 mg, by mouth, every 6 hours.

Acetophenetidin, 300 mg, by mouth, every 4 to 6 hours.

Nevertheless, better results are obtained by relieving obstruction and infection.

Pleurodynia and Pleuritis. In pleurodynia the pain is a chest pain and extends over the entire lower anterior chest, even to the epigastrium. Its onset is sudden, accompanied by fever and symptoms of upper respiratory infection (sore throat, headache, and malaise), and pains spread over other muscles of the body. Painful muscles may appear swollen, and they are tender on palpation.

In fibrinous pleurisy there is a sudden side pain with fever and malaise. The pain may be mild; more frequently it is very intense and related to respiration and coughing. It may radiate to the neck, shoulder, or abdomen, according to the location of the pleurisy. A shallow tachypnea is almost a rule, as well as a friction rub heard on auscultation (do not take for pleuritic friction rub, the one heard on auscultation of dehydrated patients). In pleurisy secondary to tuberculosis, pneumonia, pleurodynia, pericarditis, mediastinal diseases, rheumatic fever, uremia, polyarteritis, systemic lupus erythematosus, and perhaps others, the symptoms of the underlying disease will enrich the clinical picture. When pleural effusion is present (serofibrinous pleurisy), the clinical picture may be either abrupt or develop gradually with pleuritic pain, after a period of time. Depending on the amount of fluid, the symptoms will be less or more severe (from mild to severe dyspnea and circulatory embarrassment) and the physical findings less or more marked (interfering with the normal sounds heard on auscultation). The best aids to diagnosis are X-ray examination, and collection of pleural fluid for examination when it is present.

Pain itself will respond in most instances to:

> Codeine, 60 mg by mouth, every 4 hours, or 30 mg by intramuscular injection, every 4 hours; shift to the oral route as soon as possible.

Whenever needed, either meperidine, morphine, or any similar drug can be given.

> Meperidine, 50 to 100 mg by intramuscular injection, 4 to 6 times a day.

> Morphine, 10 to 15 mg, by subcutaneous injection, repeated as needed.

If all these measures fail to control pain, use:

> Procaine, 10% solution, up to 5 ml, by injection,

for paravertebral infiltration to block intercostal nerves.

Pneumothorax. In traumatic or secondary pneumothorax, the diagnosis is relatively obvious. Not so with a spontaneous pneumothorax occurring in an apparently healthy person. Most frequently, the onset is dramatic, as in myocardial infarction or acute abdomen, with sharp side pain, severe dyspnea, and dry cough. X-ray examination and the physical signs (diminished or absent respiratory sounds, hyperresonance, hyperinflation) confirm the diagnosis.

No matter that the pain may be considerable, its treatment is of little consequence while the intrapleural tension is present. The simplest measure to be taken is to give oxygen therapy; also a tracheal tube with suction will help clear the bronchi and expand the lung. As a last resort, surgery may be needed.

Cancer. Pain of a pleuritic type is a late symptom; cough is of paramount importance. Dyspnea may appear either early or late in the course of the disease. Other symptoms belong to the common symptomatology of cancer.

As in all forms of advanced malignancies, morphine is the drug of choice.

> Morphine, 10 to 15 mg, by subcutaneous administration, repeated as needed.

Alternatives might be meperidine or codeine as follows:

> Meperidine, 50 to 100 mg, by intramuscular injection, repeated as needed.

> Codeine, 30 mg, by subcutaneous injection, repeated as needed.

Surgery or chemotherapy will be considered as the possible basic treatment, whenever indicated. Other measures will be taken, according to circumstances.

Mastodynia

Pain in the breast is a true mastalgia, or pain in the mammary gland, in the great majority of instances. It may be related to normal incidents of life, due to diseases of the gland itself, or referred from diseases located on other parts of the body.

Incidences of the normal sexual life are frequent cause of what we could call physiologic (?) pains. At puberty, both males and females may complain of mastalgia, which is accompanied by swelling of the gland. In the male, this mild form of gynecomastia is transitory; in the female, the first stage of the normal development of the gland. One of the symptoms of premenstrual tension is mastalgia. In these cases, pain is ordinarily mild, but some women may exaggerate its significance psychologically; also the pain and swelling migiht be more intense and prolonged. Or, repeated bouts of mastalgia may occur during the days preceding menstruation, suggesting the possibility of a true mastopathy, particularly fibrocystic mastitis. Mild pain during pregnancy and lactation are almost the rule, while more severe pain will suggest the presence of a true mastopathy.

Mild analgesics will be adequate.

> Codeine, 30 or 60 mg, by mouth, every 4 to 6 hours.

Propoxyphene hydrochloride, 65 mg, by mouth, every 4 hours.

Acetylsalicylic acid, 600 mg, in tablets, every 4 hours.

Acetaminophen, 600 mg, by mouth, every 6 hours.

Acetophenetidin, 300 mg, by mouth, every 4 to 6 hours.

Diseases of the Mammary Gland. In acute mastitis there are severe pain, redness of the affected gland, and elevated temperature. The condition is more frequent during lactation, and affects the primipara more frequently. The physiologic initiation of lactation may provoke an elevation of temperature, with pain and swelling of the gland, but it is of short duration and does not present the true characteristic of bacterial inflammation. In fibrocystic or sclerocystic mastitis, also called cystic mastitis, there is mastalgia during the days preceding menstruation, more severe than in pure premenstrual tension. The differential diagnosis is based upon the finding of round or elongated masses within the gland. It is to be noted that pain is felt in both breasts, but only one may show nodules (one or none). The nodule is tender and is easily mobilized. At the onset of the disease, the nodule may be found only during the days with pain, and disappears after the menstruation is over. When the disease is well established, the nodules may become confluent, and a true cystic condition develops. The diagnosis is favored when the patient complains of discomfort in both breasts, no matter that nodules are found only in one (of course, the bilateral incidence is almost the rule). The final distinction between cystic mastitis and tumors in the gland is given by adequate X-ray exploration and/or biopsy. In tuberculosis of the mammary gland, ordinarily secondary to tuberculosis elsewhere in the body, a nodular, tender inflammation occurs, frequently following pregnancy, lactation, or trauma. No objective symptoms (retraction of skin and nipple) are similar to those found in cancer, but an important differential feature is that cancer rarely will provoke pain or be tender.

Analgesics may be used as stated in the above paragraph. In cases of infection with abscess formation, the abscess has to be excised or incised and drained. In cases of trauma, cold (or hot) compresses will be of help. In chronic cystic mastitis, besides the use of analgesics, surgery is indicated in many cases (from the excision of the affected area to mastectomy). At times, relief is obtained by simple aspiration of larger cysts, a procedure to be preferred in older women close to the menopause.

Referred Pain. Only in rare instances, no pathologic changes are found in the mammary gland; the pain may be only referred from lesions within the thorax, particularly pleurisy, heart lesions, and pulmonary tuberculosis. Also, with no local lesions of the pain and no diseases that may accompany heterotopic pain, mastalgia is likely suggested to be of psychogenic origin: most frequently among women fearful of cancer. For treatment, see corresponding entries.

Thoracalgia

Pain in the walls of the thorax, thoracalgia, may be due to lesions in the ribs or sternum, the muscles, or the nerves.

Diseases of the Ribs or the Sternum. Traumatic lesions, particularly fractures, are of relatively easy diagnosis, easier if clarified by an X-ray examination. Localized pain is always present. The symptoms of osteitis, osteomyelitis, syphilis and tuberculosis of the bones, osteosis, and similar diseases are not different (except for the location) from the same diseases in larger bones (see below, in the sections on "Chronic Abdominal Pain" and "Limbs"). It is to be remembered that the sternum is tender to percussion in most cases with diffuse lesions in the skeleton, such as patients with Recklinghausen's disease or patients with leukemia.

In each individual case, the basic treatment will be carried out, and only mild analgesics should be used; pain is usually moderate or even mild, and in many cases its intensity will be a good measure of the results of specific therapy.

> Acetylsalicylic acid, 300 mg, tablets, two every 4 to 6 hours, preferably with food.
>
> Codeine, 30 or 60 mg, by mouth or by intramuscular injection, every 4 to 6 hours (either alone or in combination with acetylsalicylic acid).

In the case of tumors, except for small nonmalignant growths, all should be removed surgically. If there is pain, it should be treated with either regular analgesics or even narcotic drugs, whenever indicated.

> Acetylsalicylic acid, 300-mg tablets as above, two every 4 hours with meals.
>
> Propoxyphene hydrochloride, 65-mg tablets, one every 4 hours.
>
> Codeine, 30 or 60 mg, either by mouth or intramuscularly.

> Meperidine, 100 mg, by subcutaneous injection, every 4 hours, or as needed and tolerated.
>
> Morphine sulfate, 10 or 15 mg, by subcutaneous injection, repeated as needed and tolerated.

Intercostal Neuralgia. In most instances, the diagnosis is obvious: pain along one of the intercostal spaces, ranging from moderate to excruciating. It may be due to lesions of the vertebrae (rheumatism, vertebral cancer or tuberculosis, traumatism), syphilis (tabes dorsalis), diseases of the mediastinum, or, more frequently, herpes zoster. An intense intercostal neuralgia, with burning sensation, will suggest herpes zoster.

Infiltration of the affected nerve, close to its emergent paravertebral site, will be attempted with anesthetic solutions.

> Procaine, 1 or 2% solution, up to 4 or 5 ml into each point; more if required

Bed rest will be advised, and analgesics given, if needed.

> Codeine, 60 mg, by subcutaneous injection, repeated as needed.
>
> Methadone, 10 mg, by subcutaneous injection, repeated as needed.

Causative agents, if known, will be eliminated (poisons, infections, metabolic and nutritional defects, cancer, and particularly herpes zoster and herniated disk).

Multiple Myeloma. An unexplained thoracalgia in a person over 40 years of age might make one think of multiple myeloma. Palliative treatment with analgesics will be carried out, together with other measures that are to be taken (splints, dietetic supplements, and particularly the use of alkylating drugs). The analgesics may be started with:

> Acetylsalicylic acid, 600 mg, in tablets, every 4 hours,

and similar agents; or resort to stronger ones, like morphine, whenever needed.

> Morphine sulfate, 10 or 15 mg, by subcutaneous injection, every 8 hours or as needed.

Heterotopic Pain

Heterotopic pain has been discussed under "Retrosternal and Precordial Pain" and "Mastodynia." Any of the diseases considered there may radiate pain elsewhere in the thorax. But we will give special emphasis to diseases due to the abdominal organs, such as biliary or renal colic, peptic ulcer, and most of the clinical incidences known as acute abdomen.

Subdiaphragmatic Abscess. There is discomfort in the lower part of the chest. Pain (radiating to the shoulder) and tenderness elicited by pressure applied beneath the lower ribs and directed inward may reveal a subphrenic abscess if other signs of infection are also present, particularly following a surgical procedure or a perforation of the gastrointestinal tract or the gall bladder. Other cases may relate to infection of other abdominal organs, including spleen, pancreas, and liver. The symptoms of the primary disease are always present. On X-ray examination, elevation and immobility of the diaphragm are of great importance. Gas might be found on some occasions. The great majority of subphrenic abscesses are found on the right side.

Subdiaphragmatic abscess requires the advice and participation of a surgeon. To treat infection and pain will help, and antibiotics will be given—specific, if the germ and its sensitivity are known, or those specific for the intestinal flora, like gentamycin and kanamycin. Analgesics will be of the type of codeine, papaverine, meperidine, or even morphine.

Hepatic Abscess. It is amebic in nature, and other symptoms of amebiasis can be found. Pain, or only discomfort, in the area of the liver may appear gradually or suddenly. It is exaggerated by motion and radiates to the lower chest or right shoulder.

Hepatic abscesses are usually responsive to emetine and chloroquine given together, or metronidazole. If drainage is needed, it is better to aspirate than to open.

Biliary Lithiasis and Colic. Almost always the initial symptom of biliary lithiasis is biliary colic; a sharp, cramplike pain in the epigastrium and lower right side of the chest, radiating to the right shoulder, together with nausea and vomiting.

Surgery is almost always the final goal, but meanwhile antacids, anticholinergics, and sedatives may be of help. For the chronic pain and/or colic, narcotic analgesics (morphine, methadone, meperidine, etc.) are needed.

Acute and Chronic Cholecystitis. Ordinarily, acute cholecystitis begins with a biliary colic, moderate elevation of temperature, and history or signs of previous biliary lithiasis. In chronic cholecystitis there is pain and tenderness in the liver area. In instances both of acute and of chronic cholecystitis, pain may radiate to the right lower part of the chest.

In acute and chronic cholecystitis the procedure is the same as that discussed above for biliary lithiasis. Surgery is the final solution, and meanwhile antacids, anticholinergics, and sedatives can be given. More acute pain might require narcotic analgesics.

Renal Colic. The characteristic extremely violent pain radiates from the corresponding flank down to the scrotum or labia; but in more than one case referred thoracic pain is present also.

Renal colic requires the immediate injection of morphine, meperidine, or similar narcotic analgesics.

X. ACUTE ABDOMEN

An acute, severe pain in the abdomen is one of the very frequent reasons why patients call the physician, and one of the most difficult situations faced in medical practice, since the symptoms will not always give a good clue to the diagnosis. In most instances, the physician will be aware of the seriousness of the clinical picture. By "acute abdomen" is commonly meant a severe abdominal condition demanding a surgical procedure. Actually, "acute abdomen" includes all diseases causing a sharp, violent pain in the abdomen; and the needs, in the way of treatment, whether surgical or non-surgical, are finally decided on after critically searching out and analyzing the acute gastrointestinal aggregate of symptoms.

For these reasons, we will discuss here the medical and surgical conditions giving an imposing symptomatology centering around acute abdominal pain. The clinical picture will show a patient immobilized by suffering even when the pain has subsided after the adminisration of a potent analgesic. It is almost constant to find rigidity of the abdominal muscles, the presence of nausea with or without vomiting, a soft and rapid pulse with hyper- or hypothermia. The facies abdominalis, or hippocratic facies, is pale, the nose and upper lip drawn up in an anxious expression. The basic diagnosis of "acute abdomen" is relatively easy; more difficult is the fundamental diagnosis of the causative factor.

It is to be noted that a great number of conditions provoking acute abdominal pain are strictly operative processes requiring surgery as the main resource; but in most instances the alleviation of suffering will be, if not considered a mere human act of charity, a beneficial medical approach welcomed by the patient. In other words, even as a secondary step in the overall treatment, to treat pain is to help recovery.

Diseases of the Digestive System

Peptic Ulcer (Gastric or Duodenal). In peptic ulcer, either gastric or duodenal, pain is mostly of moderate degree, and only occasionally may appear acute. This acuteness, together with a more intense tenderness on palpation, might be suggestive of peritoneal irritation, mainly due to a penetrating lesion. The diagnosis has to be based on the exacerbation of symptoms from a chronic lesion; plus heartburn, abdominal distention, salivation, anorexia, nausea, etc. In all instances, the diagnosis depends mainly on X-ray examination, and other laboratory procedures (gastric acid concentration, etc.).

During the acute stage of the disease, patients will request help for the abdominal pain. Analgesics are not, of course, the best help to be offered under the circumstances, but a judicious use is made of antacids and anticholinergics (parasympatholytic drugs). For years, sodium bicarbonate has been the one favored, particularly by patients.

> Sodium bicarbonate, 1 or 2 g (less than half a level teaspoonful) every 1 to 3 hours, day and night during the acute stage; thereafter, 1 or 2 hours following meals.

This medication is not to be advised for long-term use, as it increases acidity by compensatory oversecretion and always by the acid-producing glands of the stomach. It is better to prescribe a mixture of magnesium oxide and calcium carbonate.

> Magnesium oxide (15 to 60 grams, balancing the dosage individually, to avoid constipation) plus calcium carbonate (to complete a total of 120 g), to give a half or one level teaspoonful in half a glass of water, every 1 or 2 hours until resolution of the ulcer.

Since the use of calcium may induce hypercalcemia, the blood calcium should be checked regularly, every 2 to 4 weeks, particularly at the beginning of therapy. Several of the pharmaceutical specialties, and even OTC preparations, may be of help to these patients.

The number one anticholinergic drug is belladonna, which may be used alternatively with its active principle, atropine.

> Belladonna tincture, 10, 20, or 30 drops in water, half an hour before meals and at bedtime. The dosage will be scheduled according to effect and individual tolerance.

> Atropine, 0.5 mg, tablets; half or one tablet 30 minutes before meals and at bedtime, according to results and tolerance.

Other parasympatholytic (anticholinergic agents) can also be used, as follows:

> Dicyclomine hydrochloride, 20 mg in tablets, before meals and at bedtime.

> Propantheline bromide, 7.5 to 15 mg in tablets, before meals and at bedtime.

During the acute stage, bed rest is imperative (even for 1 to 3 weeks), and a special diet should be followed, avoiding all sort of irritants to the gastric mucosa (alcohol, spices, etc.), those which stimulate the secretion of acid (meats, coffee, tea, etc.), or those which the patient usually does not tolerate well. The diet has to be semibland, poor in fats (including milk and cream), not too bulky, and given on a rigid, regular schedule. It is best to add preparations of vitamins and minerals to this diet. At the beginning, the diet should be almost liquid (or with little amounts of milk).

Biliary Colic. In most instances, particularly when previous attacks have occurred, the diagnosis is made by the patient himself because of the location of a sudden, acute sharp pain at the right side of the upper abdomen. Very frequently, it radiates to the back or the right shoulder; more times to the right arm, very rarely, to the left shoulder. The pain is intermittent and is accompanied by more or less marked nausea, with or without vomiting, sweating, and extreme hyperactivity. Ordinarily the attacks follow a heavy meal. A pure biliary colic runs its course with or without moderate fever; a notable elevation of temperature, with chills, occurs only when there is some sort of infection (cholecystitis). On palpation, there is tenderness, and not too frequently the sensation of an enlarged tender mass in the region of the gallbladder. This tenderness is found even with a typical location of pain (heterotopic or diffuse pain, without radiation). Reflex spasm of the abdominal muscle may occur. Following the attack, jaundice and dark urine may appear. There are no urinary symptoms (dysuria and hematuria), as in renal colic; no red urine, as in porphyria; no cardiovascular symptoms, as in myocardial infarction; no increased abdominal borborygmi, as in intestinal obstruction.

The very severe pain of biliary colic has to be controlled as soon as possible, because it is really excruciating. Papaverine should be given initially, since it may suppress, in many cases, the spasmodic contractions of the biliary duct muscles, and thus the colic.

> Papaverine hydrochloride, 60 to 100 mg, by intramuscular injection; repeat if needed.

Because morphine may increase biliary spasm, it should be avoided as much as possible; and in case of papaverine failure the second choice will be meperidine (which might also be the first drug to use in these cases).

> Meperidine, 100 mg, by intramuscular injection.

But, also, meperidine may increase biliary spasm. Only after the failure of both papaverine and meperidine, or if the pain is intolerable, we can use morphine (with caution because of possible increase of spasm).

> Morphine sulfate, 10 to 15 mg, by subcutaneous injection, or by intramuscular route, if preferred; repeat if needed.

Adjunct therapy will be the use of a nasogastric tube for suction when there is abdominal distention, bed rest, and re-hydration by the venous route in all cases when it seems necessary. After the colic is over, the advisability of surgery will be discussed with the specialist. Because in most instances of biliary colic the disease of the ducts has an infective component, or for the prevention of later septic complications, the use of antibiotics seems advisable. If the specific one can be found and used, that is best. Otherwise, a broad spectrum drug will be used.

> Ampicillin, 250 mg, every 8 hours, by mouth or intravenously.

> Tetracycline, up to 500 mg every 6 hours, by mouth, or 250 mg every 6 hours, intravenously.

Pancreatic Colic and Acute Pancreatitis. In both acute and chronic pancreatitis, pain is not exactly of a colicky nature, since it is constant and widespread, with a principal left epigastric location. It is a very severe, agonizing pain, constantly accompanied by shock in acute hemorrhagic pancreatitis, and without shock but with the appearance of a very ill patient in acute and chronic pancreatitis. The sudden, severe pain is exaggerated in certain positions, such as lying supine, and it may radiate to the chest (substernal), the flanks, or the back. Tenderness is elicited on pressure on the epigastrium, where some muscular rigidity is also found. Consequences of pancreatic juice spreading into the chest cavities are: pneumonia, pleural effusion, and pulmonary atelectasis, the symptoms of which diseases may play an outstanding role in the overall clinical picture. Laboratory findings may help to diagnose a pancreatic condition: elevated serum amylase (over 300 Somogyi units), roentgenographic examination, leukocytosis, etc. In pancreatic colic there is no hard rigidity of abdominal musculature as in peritonitis from viscus perforation (peptic ulcer, gallbladder, etc.); there is no radiation to the shoulder, but there is relatively good general condition as in biliary colic; there is no early elevation of serum glutamic oxalacetic transaminase, as in myocardial infarction; there are no urinary symptoms (hematuria, dysuria), as in renal colic of the left kidney; there is no fecal vomiting and visible peristalsis, as in intestinal obstruction; nor is there bloody diarrhea, as in mesenteric thrombosis.

Since severe pain is the principal symptom, to treat it should be the first aim. Start treatment with papaverine hydrochloride, which may suppress the spasm of the duct and allay pain. Meperidine will be given next, if papaverine cannot control it. If both fail, atropine will be given; and only as a last resort morphine will be used, but very cautiously since the risk of increasing the muscle spasm is greater with morphine than with meperidine.

Papaverine hydrochloride, 60 to 100 mg, by intramuscular injection. To be repeated if needed.

Meperidine, 100 mg, by intramuscular injection.

Atropine, 0.4 to 0.6 mg, by subcutaneous injection.

Morphine sulfate, 10 to 15 mg, by subcutaneous injection.

These drugs may be repeated judiciously. A nasogastric tube to counteract gastrointestinal distention will be a good help. Bed rest is mandatory and since nothing should be given by mouth, intravenous fluids (and even blood in cases of hemorrhagic pancreatitis) are a must. Peritoneal dialysis will be considered for selected cases. As complications arise, they should be treated adequately. Check for hypocalcemia, and, if it is present, monitor it; treat with calcium salts if they are needed.

> Calcium gluconate, 10% solution, inject 10 ml, every 4 hours.

In case of infection, use antibiotics: the specific one, if known; or at least a broad spectrum antibiotic or those against fecal flora.

> Tetracycline, up to 500 mg, every 6 hours, by mouth; or 250 mg, every 6 hours, by intramuscular injection.

> Ampicillin, 250 mg, every 8 hours, by mouth or intravenously.

> Kanamycin, 50 mg for each kg of body weight for 24 hours, in four installments, taking care to note any toxic reactions.

> Gentamycin, 1 to 3 mg for each kg of body weight, each 24 hours, in three or four installments.

Intestinal Colic. Intestinal colic is the main manifestation of acute gastroenteritis (food poisoning). Commonly, it follows the ingestion of a noxious substance (food, alcohol, drugs, poisons), extensive burns, uremia, and even infective diseases, of which dysentery and typhoid fever are the principal examples. Pain is intermittent, of a colicky type, accompanied by nausea and/or vomiting, and other gastrointestinal symptoms such as borborygmi, flatus, and diarrhea. Malaise, prostration, distended abdomen, and even muscular rigidity are usual findings. Tenderness is elicited on palpation, particularly in the lower abdomen. There is no fever, except in cases of infective origin. The patient will adopt and continuously change bizarre positions to alleviate his suffering. Persistent vomiting may lead to alkalosis; persistent diarrhea, to acidosis. Hypokalemia may also occur (muscular weakness, leading to muscular paralysis). All symptoms should subside in less than 2 days in pure intestinal colic; otherwise, efforts should be made to establish a correct and complete etiologic diagnosis. Of course, there will be no leukocytosis and constipation as in the surgical abdomen and infective diseases; no signs elicited on sigmoidoscopy, like dysentery and ulcerative colitis; nor the accompanying symptoms of intestinal obstruction, pancreatitis, appendicitis, and others.

This extremely frequent reaction may occur due to several different entities, some of them covered in the corresponding paragraphs elsewhere, and treated in accordance with the etiology. But a common approach could be delineated at this time. Paregoric, elixir or tincture, is a classic. Adults may take full doses; smaller patients, according to age and weight; but infants should not be given paregoric.

> Paregoric elixir, 4 ml or up to 10 ml, if needed, in water; may be repeated every 4 hours.

A combination of opium and belladonna may even give much better results, as in the following prescriptions.

> Paregoric elixir and belladonna tincture, equal parts or double amount of paregoric (perhaps better), 1 to 1.5 ml, every 4 to 6 hours.

> Opium, 65 mg and belladonna, 8 mg, for one suppository; insert one every 4 hours.

Also, as a symptomatic antalgic treatment, anticholinergic drugs (parasympatholytics) can be useful, particularly if there is diarrhea.

> Belladonna tincture, 10 to 30 drops, every 8 hours, according to tolerance.

> Atropine, 0.5 mg, tablets; half a tablet, every 8 hours, according to need.

> Dicyclomine hydrochloride, 20 mg, tablets every 6 to 8 hours.

> Isopropamide iodide, 5 mg, tablets, every 12 hours.

> Propantheline bromide, 7.5 to 15 mg, tablets, every 6 or 8 hours.

Ulcerative Colitis. A history of a young adult, 20 to 40 years of age, complaining of attacks of bloody diarrhea accompanied by abdominal cramps of increasing severity which become intolerable with no pause at all, including the possibility of a serious toxemia—all the above coming together with evidence obtained from proctosigmoidoscopic and X-ray examination—will be a good base for the diagnosis of ulcerative colitis.

In ulcerative colitis bloody diarrhea is the main complaint, while mild abdominal cramps might be the only complaint of pain. Nevertheless, at times, this pain is very disturbing, and it should be treated, following the lines mentioned above for intestinal colic. It is to be added that in these cases bed rest is imperative, and intravenous infusions are needed in almost all instances. Anemia should be treated if there is severe loss of blood. Tranquilizers or sedatives are good for these patients. Also, corticoids are to be prescribed for all patients, to be gradually decreased when symptoms subside.

Prednisone, 5 to 10 mg, every 6 hours.

Salicylazosulfapyridine, 500 mg, tablets; two to four tablets every 6 hours, in individualized dosage that has been advised for these patients.

Peritonitis. Peritonitis is always secondary to an infection, either acute or chronic, located elsewhere in the body, but mainly in the adjacent organs. In a way, the symptomatology will depend on the causative factor; but in most instances the patient will appear acutely ill, and complain of an agonizing, constant pain in the abdomen. Because pain is exaggerated with motion, patients stay motionless and their respiration is very shallow, to avoid moving the diaphragm (during intestinal colic the patient freely moves his abdomen—diaphragm—when breathing). To obtain diaphragmatic immobilization the patient adopts a peculiar position with flexed legs, so as to use only thoracic respiration. Muscle rigidity (guarding) of the abdominal wall also helps to immobilize this part of the body: a continuous rigidity in peritonitis, in contrast with relaxation in other colicky pains. Pain and tenderness elicited on palpation may be somewhat diffuse at the beginning; sooner or later, they are localized at the area of the underlying infective focus (appendix, stomach, etc.). Tenderness may be obtained by rebound (pressing and suddenly relieving presure over a distant abdominal point). Rectal and vaginal examinations may also reveal painful spots, and even painful masses. Unless the patient goes into shock, elevated temperature is the rule, tachycardia with weak pulse is present, and chills are frequent. To check the pulse every 10 minutes is a good practice, since it progressively increases in rate, so helping the diagnosis.

The hippocratic facies referred to in the introductory lines is a characteristic of this diagnosis. The general condition seems very poor. Of course, it is less severe in localized peritonitis; but the less acute or even absent pain of peritonitis with large effusion does not exclude the extreme severity of the condition. Also, very young or elder patients may show little complaint of their symptoms, regardless of the seriousness of the disease. The reach for the underlying causative factor is fundamental to an adequate treatment; but it is at the same time a good clue to the estimate of the extent and character of the peritonitis. All pain and related symptomatology may subside if paralytic ileus ensues as a complication.

Because peritonitis is almost always secondary to a previous disease, symptoms of the original sickness precede and accompany the peritonitis: diseases of the gastrointestinal tract are of primary importance, particularly perforations from peptic ulcers, appendicitis, cancer, and diverticulitis; diseases of the female pelvic organs are important among women, particularly infections following salpingitis, abortions, or the puerperal state.

Polymorphonuclear leukocytosis is an important laboratory sign; it may be less consipicuous in the elder and in cases with severe infections, thus indicating a poorer prognosis.

A patient with peritonitis should be transferred immediately to a hospital, under the care of a surgeon, generally requiring repair of a perforated viscus. For the treatment of pain, most patients will benefit from the use of:

Meperidine, 100 mg, by intramuscular injection.

A nasogastric tube, for suction, intravenous fluids, and antibiotic therapy will also be required.

Gentamycin, 1 to 3 mg per kg of body weight daily, in divided doses.

Kanamycin, 50 mg per kg of body weight daily, in four installments.

When using the above-mentioned antibiotics, one must take care to watch for the relatively frequent toxic reactions they are prone to provoke.

Perforation of a Viscus. A patient with a known, more rarely with an unknown, *peptic ulcer* suddenly suffers an extremely violent pain in the abdomen, exactly of the type described in the foregoing lines on peritonitis. Almost always, it happens spontaneously without any preceding effort, trauma, or any other condition suggestive of causing the perforation. The pain is accompanied by profuse sweating, immobility, rigidity of the abdominal wall, and a change of the initial relatively slow and full pulse into a rapid, weak one which introduces other symptoms of shock, such as low blood pressure, collapse of veins, increased thirst, and decreased renal output. Bloody vomit is a good diagnostic clue. If the ulcer is not on the anterior wall of the duodenum or in the pyloric region of the stomach, symptoms may be somewhat different: ulcers of the posterior wall may give origin to a localized peritonitis. If there is no history of a previous ulcer, the diagnosis becomes extremely difficult. A roentgenographic exploration will be needed; the finding of air within the abdominal cavity is almost pathognomonic.

Surgical repair must follow this diagnosis immediately. Since the pain is extremely severe, meperidine should be given, a nasogastric tube placed for continuous suction, and shock watched for and prevented or treated if needed.

> Meperidine, 100 mg, by intramuscular injection.

It is good to remind the reader that an *acute erosive gastritis* will give the same clinical picture as a perforation, after the total erosion of the stomach wall.

All efforts will be directed towards the finding of an offending cause, mainly toxins, or alcohol, or drugs, or acetylsalicylic acid. If there is such a causative factor, it should be totally eliminated. If pain is intense enough, give meperidine; otherwise, give antacids by mouth. The disease should be terminated in less than 2 days.

> Meperidine, 100 mg, by intramuscular injection; repeat every 6 hours, or as needed and tolerated.

> Sodium bicarbonate, powder, half a level teaspoonful or less, with water.

> Any of the OTC preparations—without aspirin!

Intestinal Perforation. This condition may result from any intestinal erosive disease, but most cases are due to typhoid fever or appendicitis. In the course of the disease a sudden clinical picture resembling an acute peritonitis will take place, with a drop in temperature and the onset of pain, especially marked on the lower right abdomen. In cases of intestinal diverticulosis, cancer, and tuberculosis a perforation can also occur. A roentgenological examination will disclose the presence of air in the abdominal cavity.

Once the diagnosis is made, and there is no doubt as to the need for an urgent operation, a surgeon will be immediately consulted. There is little time to think of palliative measures; but they will help the patient to allay pain and apprehension, and it is imperative to prevent the almost inevitable infection of the peritoneum with the intestinal flora. Pass a tube to protect against distention, and start the administration of intravenous fluids to avoid shock.

Meperidine, 100 mg, by subcutaneous or intramuscular injection. There is no need to repeat.

Gentamycin, 1 to 3 mg for each kg of body weight and period of 24 hours, in divided doses. Watch for toxic reactions.

Kanamycin, 50 mg for each kg of body weight and period of 24 hours, in four installments. Watch for toxic reactions.

Perforation of the Gallbladder. The sudden onset of the peritonitic syndrome (q.v.) in a patient with acute cholecystitis (biliary colic), particularly if symptoms of obstruction are present (jaundice), will point to the diagnosis of perforation of the gallbladder. If the perforation occurs toward a neighboring organ (liver, diaphragm, stomach), the clinical picture will be that of localized peritonitis, pancreatitis, subphrenic abscess, etc.

In general, the procedures to follow are similar to those outlined for "Intestinal perforation," "Peritonitis," and "Perforation of a viscus," q.v. As in these cases, the help of a surgeon will be required immediately.

Mesenteric Vascular Occlusion. This condition provokes a sudden, very severe pain of the abdomen, frequently accompanied by bloody stools and vomiting. Most cases are due to arteriosclerosis, fibrillation, or polyarteritis.

For mesenteric vascular diseases (ischemia or occlusion), the only logical approach is surgery. To help with analgesia, give:

Morphine sulfate, 15 mg, by subcutaneous injection.

It does not mean that surgery has to be delayed in any way. Small frequent feedings may help in cases of ischemia. Intravenous infusions will be given when shock develops, particularly in mesenteric vascular occlusion.

For more details, see below.

Gastric and Intestinal Obstruction. The clinical syndrome of acute intestinal obstruction is centered around severe abdominal pain and vomiting. The syndrome varies depending on the location and the nature of the obstruction: it is more severe with obstruction of higher portions. Pain is of an agonizing colicky type; but if the obstruction is in the colon, pain will be intermittent, of a crampy character. vomiting of food is rapidly followed by biliary emesis; to wait for fecaloid vomiting to establish the diagnosis is an error, because of the late occurrence of this symptom. Small amounts of feces can be passed out in very low colonic obstructions; but a total suppression is the rule. Unfortunately, the suppression of feces is not an early symptom, and not reliable as a basis for diagnosis. It occurs later in the case of high obstruction, and is not complete in the case of lower colonic obstruction. Initially, there is abdominal rigidity, which changes soon, little by little, to the distended abdomen of meteorism. A pronounced epigastric distension corresponds to gastric dilatation; a distention of the middle part of the abdomen points to a small intestine obstruction; an obstruction of the colon produces a peripheric, horseshoe-like distension. Later in the course of the disease, the dilatation becomes generalized. Visible peristaltic contractions may occasionally occur, corresponding to the intestinal portion struggling against the obstruction.

We are not interested here in the late events occurring in the course of the disease, leading to dehydration and an abnormal electrolytic balance. The diagnosis of the course of the obstruction is the second step: stricture, intussusception, volvulus, compression, impaction, etc. An early laparotomy is both diagnostic and therapeutic.

In many cases of gastric obstruction there is severe pain (and vomiting). The first measure will be to give antacid:

> Sodium bicarbonate, half a level teaspoonful of powder, or less.

> Any of the OTC preparations; before feedings.

A bland diet (not to be given while pain persists) is advisable, together with vitamins and mineral capsules. If this fails, as frequently it does, a nasogastric tube for continuous suction will be placed (watch the electrolyte concentration, and correct deficits, when present). Note that the tube should be used as soon as the formal diagnosis of gastric obstruction is made. Surgery will be considered when the obstruction is due to an underlying peptic ulcer.

In cases of intestinal obstruction the patient will be confined to bed, and surgery will be considered from the beginning, and performed as soon as the patient is ready, particularly in cases of strangulation or infarction. Pain has to be controlled immediately, since it may reach intolerable proportions. In these instances, give:

> Meperidine, 100 mg, by intramuscular injection.

> Codeine, 60 mg, by intramusuclar injection.

> Papaverine hydrochloride, 60 to 100 mg, by intramuscular injection.

A Levin tube has to be used for continuous suction, and parenteral fluids will be given, according to the electrolyte profile, particularly following vomiting. Sedatives and tranquilizers may help for tension and restlessness. Shock will be watched for, and treated at the start.

Acute Dilation of the Stomach. After a more or less prolonged period of time in which the patient complains of discomfort and fullness of the stomach, epigastric pain appears at the same time that vomiting of huge amounts of liquid begins. The triad of abdominal distension, pain and vomiting will suggest acute gastric dilation. When it occurs in a bedridden patient following surgery, or with pneumonia or heart insufficiency, or with one who is a drug addict, the condition leads to dehydration, loss of electrolytic balance, and shock.

To pass a Levin tube will be the first measure to take, which will serve to empty the stomach by continuous (mild) suction. In most cases this will solve the problem within 1 or 2 days. Electrolyte balance and hydration will be checked and restored in case of need by means of intravenous fluids. Nevertheless, since nothing should be given by mouth until dilation is controlled, the intravenous catheter is needed to pass at least glucose in saline solution. When dilatation seems to be under control, suction will be stopped, and fluids given by mouth; and if the fluid passes into the duodenum, the tube will be removed.

Acute appendicitis begins with an acute, continuous pain, which may vary in intensity in a colicky manner, principally located at the epigastrium, but aggravated by pressure over the right iliac fossa, particularly the appendicular points (McBurney, etc.), where the skin may seen hyperesthesic, and the muscles are somewhat rigid. Rebound pain following release of pressure over a distant point (the left iliac fossa) is also elicited. There are anorexia and nausea; vomiting may or may not occur; there is moderate fever with increasing tachycardia and leucocytosis. The intensity of the clinical picture varies with the severity of the attack, and also with the anatomical location of the appendix. An appendix located retrocecally or retroperitoneally will provoke little muscle rigidity; a lower location in the vicinity of the pelvis will be tender on rectal or vaginal examination only. Congenital abnormal situations may also occur, and the local symptoms will depend on the anatomical location of the appendix (at the left side, closer to the liver, etc.). Good diagnostic points are: pain localized to the appendicular region and increasing leukocytosis.

Surgery is recommended at the earliest possible stage. If pain is severe, a previous intramuscular injection of meperidine should be given, provided that surgery is not postponed because of the transient, apparent improvement. When the patient cannot be operated on, meperidine or codeine should be given.

> Meperidine, 100 mg, by intramuscular injection, repeated every 4 to 6 hours.

> Codeine, 60 mg, by subcutaneous injection, every 4 to 6 hours.

Bed rest will be imposed, a nasogastric tube for continuous suction passed, intravenous fluids given, and antibiotic therapy started (it is best to use high dosages).

Familial Mediterranean fever or familial paroxysmal polyserositis is a puzzling cause of severe painful attacks in the chest, abdomen and joints. Although this disease is found only in those with a heritage from the Mediterranean area, it has become more widespread due to the ease of travel. Incidence can occur in infancy and most cases have their onset before the age of twenty. The attacks last usually a few hours, but often occur once a week with varying periods of remission. The symptoms are often similar to infections of the serous membranes such as appendicitis, gall bladder disease or gynecological infections.

The cause of the disease is not known and no evidence exists that it is due to an infection. Symptoms include moderate elevation of temperature, at times severe abdominal pain with rigidity, constipation or diarrhea, nausea, chest pain and symptoms of pleuritis, swelling and redness of joints, anorexia, malaise and occasionally, jaundice. Blood findings vary; sedimentation rates and white cells are elevated but no laboratory findings are consistent in this disease. The long duration of the disease and frequency of the painful attacks are likely to subject the patient to harmful amounts of analgesics.

In relieving the symptoms of these patients it is well to take full advantage of the simpler substances such as

> Acetylsalicylic acid, 600 mg., by mouth, every three hours.

> Propoxyphene, 65 mg, by mouth, every three hours.

> Codeine sulfate 30 mg., by mouth, every three hours if needed.

If sedatives are needed give

> Chlordiazepoxide, 20 or 25 mg, by mouth, three or four times a day.

The diagnosis is largely dependent on the history of familial incidence and recurrence of the typical attacks; therapy can be planned on a short term basis, since the attacks are self-limiting.

Typhoid Fever. During typhoid fever some patients show symptoms suggesting peritonitis, which are actually due to acidosis. Before diagnosing the relatively frequent complication of typhoid fever, namely, intestinal perforation, think of the possibility of acidotic pain (relieved by the treatment of acidosis).

Not all cases of typhoid fever will present abdominal pain, but when present, it might be really severe. Irritant or narcotic analgesics should not be given to these patients. Use instead:

Codeine, 30 to 60 mg, every 4 to 6 hours.

Propoxyphene hydrochloride, 65 mg, in tablets, every 4 to 6 hours.

If diarrhea becomes a troublesome complication, it will be better to give:

Paregoric elixir, up to 4 ml, in water, every 6 hours.

Tincture of belladonna, 10 to 20 drops, in water, every 4 to 6 hours.

The rest of the routine is well established: bed rest, hydration, electrolytic balance to be maintained, adequate nutrition, and antibiotic therapy (chloramphenicol to be first choice, ampicillin possible alternative).

Diseases of the Urinary System

Renal Colic (Ureteral Colic). The attack frequently begins with vague low back pain that soon turns into an excruciating pain felt from the corresponding costovertebral area and flank down to the corresponding side of the external genitourinary organs (penis and teste, in the male; labia majora, in the female) or even the thigh. Precordial pain is not a rarity. Sweating, vomiting, and syncopal symptoms may accompany the intense pain that appears intermittently, in a colicky fashion, and remains as a less severe discomfort between attacks of colic. If the physician does not examine the patient at the beginning of the crisis, it will be prudent to determine the exact nature of the pain, because further on the course it becomes more generalized, suggesting an abdominal crisis, particularly intestinal obstruction. Typical signs and symptoms are: dysuria or anuria; hematuria, with or without small clots; chills and fever; and the expulsion of solid sediment (sand, calculus). Unfortunately, not all patients present the mentioned typical features. Pain is elicited on pressure over the renal area or over the ureter. Ordinarily, the clinical picture will suggest the diagnosis, which is confirmed by laboratory tests: the urinalysis shows micro- or macrohematuria and plenty of urates or other salts; a radiologic examination might reveal a calculus, either directly or using contrast media.

The diagnosis of renal colic must be completed by identifying the cause of the obstruction: lithiasis provoked by an excess of uric acid, phosphates, calcium, alkaptonuria, hypovitaminosis A, oxalates, cystine, etc.; or pyelitis, hydronephrosis, kinks or strictures of the ureter, cancer, and renal tuberculosis.

Pain is the main symptom; it is among the worst pains man can suffer, and must be controlled as soon as possible.

> Morphine sulfate, 10 mg, by intravenous or intramusuclar injection; to be repeated in 10 to 15 minutes; and then every 3 to 4 hours, as needed, by subcutaneous injection.

> Meperidine, 100 mg, by intramuscular injection, repeated in 1 or 2 hours; and then every 3 or 4 hours, as needed.

The patient will be referred to the urologist for further evaluation and treatment.

Pyelonephritis. The common clinical picture shows sudden fever, with chills and aching pain in one of the costovertebral areas; on palpation, tenderness is felt at that point. Pain and tenderness may vary: they may be felt on both costovertebral areas, or may be milder, so as to be merely a low backache with no pain elicited by palpation. Signs of discomfort in the bladder, with dysuria, may or may not be present. A positive diagnosis is made by a urinalysis presenting numerous leukocytes and bacteria. An obstruction found in the X-ray is highly suggestive of pyelonephritis, when it accompanies the foregoing clinical picture.

For the relief of pain, analgesics of the type of salicylates are preferred. Acetylsalicylic acid will be the first choice.

> Acetylsalicylic acid, 300 or 600 mg, in tablets, every 4 to 6 hours.

> Acetaminophen, 300 or 600 mg, in tablets, every 6 hours.

> Acetophenetidin, 300 mg, in tablets, every 4 hours.

A good hydration is necessary, so that urinary output may reach at least 2 or 3 liters a day; hydration is achieved even by intravenous infusion when there is vomiting. The basic treatment will be antibiotic therapy, in accordance with the findings after the urine is checked for culture and sensitivity of germs. A combination of trimethoprim and sulfamethoxazole has been praised as effective, recently.

Hydronephrosis. Frequently, hydronephrosis does not present any evident symptomatology until the disease is well advanced. In other cases, it causes colicky pain of the same type as renal colic. There are colicky pains accompanied by a tumor, which is either a permanent or a transitory tumor (Dietl's crises). There is tenderness on the area of the renal pelvis. In most instances there will be found fever, pus in the urine, and less frequently hematuria; but the exact diagnosis is seldom made without intravenous or retrograde pyelograms.

In acute hydronephrosis the treatment of pain is only secondary. Perhaps codeine should be the first choice, but other analgesics may also be tried.

> Codeine, 30 or 60 mg, by mouth, every 4 to 6 hours, or by intramuscular injection if so required.

> Propoxyphene hydrochloride, 65 mg, by mouth, every 4 hours.

The patient will be referred immediately to the urologist, since some surgical procedures are needed in almost all cases.

Perirenal Abscess and Carbuncle. In occasional cases pain in the corresponding costovertebral area will be severe enough to justify the diagnosis of "acute abdomen," only suggested because of the sudden onset of fever, chills, and prostration which accompany pain, nausea and vomiting. Tenderness on palpation is elicited, thus suggesting an inflammation in the region of the kidney, confirmed by roentgenographic examination.

The symptoms and diagnostic procedures for renal carbuncle are the same as above.

The relief of pain is only a small part of the treatment, totally depending on antimicrobial therapy: antibiotics, sulfa drugs, and other chemotherapeutic agents. Surgery may be of great importance for many patients, so that the urologist should take care of the situation at the earliest possible moment. Palliative treatment of pain will be carried out with general analgesics.

Codeine, 60 mg, by mouth, every 4 hours.

Other similar analgesics can be used; but internal urinary antiseptics are perhaps of better use in these cases, such as the classic methylene blue or phenazopyridine.

Methylene blue, 65 to 130 mg, by mouth, every 8 hours, warning about discoloration of the urine and staining of clothes.

Phenazopyridine hydrochloride, 200 mg, by mouth, every 8 hours, warning about discoloration of the urine and staining of clothes.

Parasympatheticomimetic drugs may also be of help.

Belladonna tincture, 10 to 30 drops, in water, every 4 to 8 hours, according to tolerance.

Atropine, 0.5 mg, tablets; half a tablet or one tablet, every 8 hours, according to effects and tolerance.

Diseases of the Genital Organs

Ovulation Pain (Mittelschmerz). A great number of women complain of pain corresponding to the day of ovulation. Pain may be intense in many instances, but only rarely will it reach the dramatic intensity of "acute abdomen." If this pain occurs, the diagnosis may be made by the lack of objective symptoms in the pelvis, except for polycystic or sclerocystic ovaries, which in many instances are the causative factor.

In most instances, common analgesics will control ovular pain.

Acetylsalicylic acid, 600 mg, in tablets, every 4 hours, preferably with meals, for 1 or 2 days.

Codeine, 60 mg, by mouth, every 4 hours, for 1 or 2 days.

Very rarely, because of the severity of the pain, it will be advisable to suppress ovulation with anticonceptional pills.

Dysmenorrhea. Like ovulation pain, only exceptionally will dysmenorrhea reach catastrophic extent. Its close relationship with menstruation and the lack of objective findings will clear up the diagnosis. It must be realized, however, that dysmenorrhea may be the symptom of an endocrine or gynecologic disorder (endocrine imbalance, diseases of the uterus and the adnexae, pelvic tumors, etc.) Appendicitis heralded by menstrual pain is not exceptional.

In premenstrual tension, common analgesics, as stated above, will easily control pain. Acetylsalicylic acid, codeine, propoxyphene hydrochloride, acetaminophen, acetophenetidin, etc., will be prescribed for these dysmenorrheic women. When the analgesics do not control pain, diuretics—together with them, or given alone—can be used, starting a few days before menstruation.

>Chlorothiazide, 500 mg, by mouth, every 8 to 12 hours.

>Hydrochlorothiazide, 50 or 100 mg, by mouth, every 12 hours.

>Acetazolamide, 250 mg a day, by mouth, in divided doses.

In primary dysmenorrhea, it is best to use codeine, belladonna, atropine, or papaverine; and in most instances, particularly when dysmenorrhea persists for long periods, advise hormonotherapy.

Acute Adnexitis. This painful disease also will only rarely reach the dramatic proportions of "acute abdomen." But it may start with severe pain in either of the iliac fossae (more frequently the right), with fever and even peritonitic symptoms. The diagnosis is made by gynecologic examination, though it will not always differentiate readily among the several other gynecologic problems. In abruptio placentae, intense abdominal pain, vaginal bleeding, and shock might be the first symptoms.

These patients will be referred to the gynecologist, since surgery and antibiotic therapy are the essentials of their treatment. First help will be to delay menstruation with contraceptive pills, allay pain with analgesics like codeine or meperidine, and start antibiotic therapy after recovering material for evaluation of the causative germ (nature and sensitivity to antibiotics).

>Norethindrone plus mestranol tablets, one a day.

>Codeine, 60 mg, by subcutaneous injection, every 6 hours.

>Meperidine, 100 mg, by subcutaneous injection, every 6 hours.

Rupture of an Ectopic Pregnancy. In tubal rupture (from ectopic pregnancy), pain and shock in a woman with symptoms of pregnancy and an adnexal tumor are the outstanding symptoms. Ordinarily, there is a previous diagnosis of pregnancy. When a pregnant woman presents an acute abdomen, the situation is presumably a rupture of an ectopic pregnancy, unless a different disease is the proven cause. If there is no known pregnancy, a pregnancy test is mandatory. There are intense abdominal pain, not always localized; vomiting; shock (with symptoms of internal hemorrhage, namely, tachycardia and gradually increasing anemia); and the possibility of detecting the adnexial mass by bimanual palpation. The gradually increasing anemia favors the diagnosis even when other symptoms are less conspicuous.

The patient will be referred immediately to the gynecologist, since surgery is the only treatment. Whenever it is needed, replace lost blood and give some sedation. There is usually no need for analgesics; or if they are required, use the common ones, such as acetylsalicylic acid, codeine, etc.

Diseases of the Respiratory System

The clinical picture of the diseases of the respiratory system, of course, is characterized by symptoms in the air passages, lungs, and pleura; that is to say, mainly in the thorax. But heterotopic pain is very frequently felt in the abdomen, and symptoms of "acute abdomen" are not exceptional in respiratory diseases.

Pneumonia. When the infection centers in the right inferior lobe, abdominal pain, particularly in the right iliac fossa, is more frequent than pain in the thorax. An erroneous diagnosis of appendicitis can be made, more easily among young people and children. Ordinarily, there is no pain on pressure over the corresponding iliac fossa, but it may occur in some rare instances. Naturally, the bulk of symptomatology is respiratory; however, severe appendicitis may provoke a secondary pleuritis, on the right side.

It is not rare that pneumonia provokes abdominal pain, but the essentials of its treatment will not vary at all: etiologic antibiotherapy, oxygen administration, bed rest, and analgesics only if really needed, starting with papaverine or codeine.

> Papaverine hydrochloride, 30 or 60 mg, (or even 120 mg, if needed), by subcutaneous injection, every 4 to 6 hours.
>
> Codeine, 60 mg, by subcutaneous injection, every 4 to 6 hours.

Other analgesics could also be used.

Pleurisy and Pleurodynia. By the same token, in these two conditions a referred abdominal pain in the right abdominal fossa is frequently found, although no pain on pressure over the fossa is felt; and, on the other hand, pleural symptoms are evident. But, as we said before, care should be taken for a possible pleuritis secondary to a severe suppurative appendicitis.

First, treat the causative infection, if any. Pain will usually respond to codeine or meperidine. Only if these fail, morphine can be given, or paravertebral infiltration performed with procaine, to block intercostal nerves.

> Codeine, 60 mg, by mouth, or 30 mg, by intramuscular injection; repeat every 4 hours, and shift to the oral route as soon as possible.
>
> Meperidine, 50 or 100 mg, by intramuscular injection, every 4 to 6 hours, as needed.
>
> Morphine, 10 to 15 mg, by subcutaneous injection, repeated as needed and tolerated.
>
> Procaine, 2% solution; use up to 5 ml, by injection to block intercostal nerves.

Pneumothorax. Spontaneous pneumothorax may also give pain in the right iliac fossa, as in the foregoing discussed diseases.

Even with severe pain, the use of analgesics is not well indicated while intrapleural tension is elevated. Give oxygen therapy and use a chest tube for suction, trying to expand the lung. If these measures fail, surgery is to be considered.

Pulmonary Infarction. A pulmonary infarction of the inferior right lobe may provoke pain of the type of "acute abdomen," with more resemblance to biliary colic or occlusion of the mesenteric vessels; but there will be extreme dyspnea, hypotension, bloody sputum, and profound anguish.

Since in most instances cough is present, codeine is well indicated.

> Codeine, 30 mg, by intramuscular injection, every 4 hours; or 60 mg, by mouth, every 4 hours, when no heroic doses are needed.

But morphine is frequently required, or meperidine, as an alternative.

> Morphine, 5 mg, by intravenous injection; or 10 to 15 mg, by the subcutaneous route, to repeat as needed.
>
> Meperidine, 50 mg, by intramuscular injection, repeated as needed and tolerated.

These patients will rest in bed and receive oxygen therapy.

Diseases of the Circulatory System

Myocardial Infarction. The habitual pain of myocardial infarction is located in such a way that sometimes it seems to be abdominal rather than epigastric or thoracic. In such cases the clinical picture reminds one of an "acute abdomen," including vomiting and even some sort of muscular rigidity. It may resemble a biliary colic in a cholecystitic patient (with vomiting, elevated temperature, and leucocytosis). An infarction may be diagnosed because of a previous history of anginal attacks; the special crushing, agonizing characteristic of the pain, and its peculiar radiation to the left shoulder and jaw; the fall of blood pressure (particularly in hypertensive patients); and fever with leucocytosis. The electrocardiogram will give typical records, the erythrosedimentation rate will increase, and the serum glutamic oxalacetic transaminase (SGOT) will rise for 2 or 3 days and then fall.

For details, see the corresponding paragraph in the section devoted to treatment of thoracodynia. The essentials are: give morphine or meperidine, repeating as needed; immediately afterward, send the patient to a cardiologist in a coronary care unit; use oxygen therapy during the trip; and keep the patient under absolute bed rest.

Aortitis and Aortic Aneurism. An aortitic attack may begin during exercise or after a meal. Inflammatory or sclerotic lesions of the abdominal aorta may give origin, in some instances, to an abdominal colicky pain, located at the epigastrium and radiating bilaterally; some authors call it abdominal angina. A few patients discover that pain is released in the genupectoral position. A roentgenographic examination will reveal the abnormal condition of the abdominal aorta.

In most instances, the aneurism is arteriosclerotic. Pain is located in the epigastric region, also radiating bilaterally, and occasionally radiating to the back. Pain is more sharp and severe after the aneurism erodes the vertebrae. Palpation and radiologic examination may establish the final diagnosis.

In most instances of aortitis the care required will be as for angina pectoris, q.v.; in cases of aneurism, reduce hypertension (if there is none, give propanolol), and resort to surgery.

> Nitroglycerin, 0.5 mg, or less, sublingual tablet, repeated as needed.
>
> Amyl nitrite pearls: crush one and inhale the gas.
>
> Propanolol, 1 or 2 mg, by intramuscular injection, every 6 hours; or 20 mg, by mouth, every 6 hours.

Carotid Syncope. As indicated by the name, syncope is the main feature of the disturbance, and the only diagnostic clue in the close relationship of the syncope with irritation of the region of the carotid sinus (motion, pressure). In rare instances, an "acute abdomen" with pain and diarrhea may occur.

In these cases, the emergency care will be to give, with no delay, an intravenous (or intramuscular, if veins are difficult to find) injection of atropine.

> Atropine, 0.6 to 0.8 mg, solution; inject in the vein or intramuscularly.

Heart failure. Ordinarily there is no diagnostic problem in these cases, since the heart failure is obvious before it can be associated with abdominal symptoms. When pain occurs, it is paroxysmal and centers over the gallbladder region. Of course, other symptoms of heart failure are also present: dyspnea, hepatomegaly, edema, cyanosis, oliguria, and enlargement of the heart area.

Pains provoked by heart failure ordinarily respond well to codeine or other analgesics.

> Codeine, 60 mg, by mouth, every 4 hours.

> Acetylsalicylic acid, 600 mg, in tablets, every 4 hours.

> Propoxyphene hydrochloride, 65 mg, by mouth, every 4 hours.

> Pentazocine, 50 or 100 mg, by mouth, every 4 hours.

At times, pain may be so severe as to require morphine or similar narcotic analgesics.

> Morphine, 10 to 15 mg, by subcutaneous injection, every 4 hours.

> Hydromorphone, 2 mg, by subcutaneous injection, every 4 hours.

> Meperidine, 50 to 100 mg, either orally or intramuscularly, every 4 hours (not for long periods).

> Anileridine, 25 mg, either orally or intramuscularly, every 6 hours.

Occlusion of the Mesenteric Vessels. This is not a frequent episode, and when it occurs, it is not always a clinical picture of "acute abdomen"; however, there are instances of a sudden, agonizing colicky pain (more intense in arterial than in venous occlusion) and tender abdomen with little or no meteorism and rigidity, but with vomiting, signs of internal hemmorhage, rapidly progressing shock, and death. The diagnosis is suspected in the elderly, arteriosclerotic patient who shows suggestive vascular symptoms. It may occur after abdominal surgery.

As soon as the diagnosis is made, the help of a surgeon experienced in vascular surgery will be requested, and the administration of procaine, papaverine, and an anticoagulant will start.

> Procaine, 1.5% solution, to give an epidural injection of 25 ml of the solution.
>
> Papaverine hydrochloride, 10 to 30 mg, by intravenous injection.
>
> Heparin, 10,000 units, given intramuscularly or intravenously, every 6 hours—check clotting time, to be no less than 20 minutes. Together with heparin, start:
>
> Bishydroxycoumarin (25, 50, 100 mg tablets), 300 mg the first day, 200 mg the second, and 50 to 100 mg thereafter—check prothrombin time, 15 to 30% of normal; and discontinue heparin when this becomes effective.

Diseases of the Hematopoietic System

Rupture of the Spleen. The first sign is a very intense pain in the left side of the abdomen, with or without radiation to the left (rarely to the right) shoulder. This occurs following trauma to the region, or following palpation of an enlarged spleen (mononucleosis, abscess, malaria, endocarditis). Symptoms of internal hemmorhage (hypotension, tachycardia, shock) and muscle rigidity are present, together with symptoms of peritoneal irritation (peritonitis). It should be kept in mind that following trauma or pressure over the spleen, the capsule sometimes ruptures later, and the symptoms and signs of splenic rupture become delayed.

Pain shall be treated only under very special circumstances, since immediate splenectomy is mandatory as soon as the diagnosis is made.

> Meperidine, 100 mg, by intramuscular injection.
>
> Morphine sulfate, 10 to 15 mg, by intramuscular injection.

Spleen Infarction. Only exceptionally, splenic infarction will provoke symptoms of "acute abdomen." Together with pain, there is tenderness on palpation over the organ. It may follow septicemia complicating endocarditis.

A patient with infarction of the spleen will be put to bed rest and will receive sedatives.

> Meperidine, 100 mg, by subcutaneous injection, every 4 to 6 hours.
>
> Methadone, 10 mg, by subcutaneous injection, every 4 to 6 hours.
>
> Morphine sulfate, 10 or 15 mg, by subcutaneous injection, every 4 to 6 hours; 5 to 10 mg, by intravenous injection, the first dose, if the pain is severe enough.

Splenectomy will be performed as soon as possible.

Mesenteric Adenitis. Occasionally, the inflammation with suppuration of the mesenteric lymph nodes will provoke an "acute abdomen." The diagnosis can be made only after surgery.

Since in acute mesenteric adenitis (or lymphadenitis) the rule is a complete resolution, treatment should be as conservative as possible. Only in cases of disturbing pain or diarrhea should analgesics be given:

> Acetylsalicylic acid, 300 or 600 mg, in tablets, every 4 to 6 hours.
>
> Codeine, 30 to 60 mg, by mouth, every 4 to 6 hours.

and also cholinergics:

> Belladonna tincture, 10 to 20 drops in water, every 6 hours.
>
> Atropine, 0.5 mg, tablets; one-quarter or one-half of a tablet, every 6 hours.

Hemolytic Anemia Colic. In hemolytic anemia there may occur an acute abdominal syndrome very similar to a biliary colic followed by increasing jaundice and worsening anemia. Other symptoms may be: fever and chills, malaise, generalized aches, prostration, and even shock.

The treatment of pain is of little or no importance in the abdominal crises of hemolytic anemia, since the main objectives are to eliminate the causative factor, when known, or to remove the spleen (splenectomy) in spherocytic anemia. Blood transfusion and the use of corticoids are advisable. The rest of the therapy will comply with the requirements of each particular disease.

Endocrine and Metabolic Diseases

Diabetic Acidosis. The onset is gradual, but as soon as symptoms become obvious and the patient looks extremely ill because of the acidotic condition, "acute abdomen" may become apparent, and more than one case has been erroneously sent to the operating room. There are a violent abdominal pain, vomiting, meteorism, fever, and leukocytosis. Of course, a genuine "acute abdomen" may develop in a diabetic patient, but the first thought whenever this situation occurs (that is, the sudden onset of a violent pain together with other specific symptoms) is that a diabetic acidosis is present. All other symptoms of diabetic acidosis can be detected: dry and flushed skin, dry mouth and intense thirst, hyperventilation (air hunger) with acetone odor of breath, tachycardia with weak pulse and the characteristic laboratory findings of hyperglycemia, glycosuria, and decreased CO_2 combining power of the blood serum.

When diabetic acidosis provokes pain resembling an abdominal emergency, no special effort will be made to give analgesics, since they are of very little avail. The physician will start immediately the specific treatment and will refer the patient to a specialist in diabetes for further care. All efforts will be made to diagnose the exact metabolic situation by thorough laboratory studies of the urine and the blood. Insulin is to be given from the very beginning. Also, an intravenous infusion will be started immediately with hypotonic saline with sodium bicarbonate. The rest of the treatment belongs in specialized antidiabetic techniques.

> Regular insulin, 200 to 700 units, or even somewhat more, during the first 24 hours; starting with 50 units by subcutaneous injection together with 50 units by the intravenous route, particularly if there is any sort of circulatory collapse; and repeating 75 to 100 units every hour until reaching any beneficial effect, and then decreasing the frequency.

Hypoglycemia. More rarely, acute abdominal pain may also be a part of the hypoglycemic syndrome, generally developing after excessive injection of insulin (even more rarely, spontaneously). The symptoms are moist and pale skin, frequent hunger, shallow respirations, full and bounding pulse, frequent tremors, and possibly convulsions. The pathognomonic is hypoglycemia, below 60 mg in 100 cc of blood. Appendicitis or cholecystitis may be taken for hypoglycemia.

There is no need for analgesics under these circumstances, since the objective of the treatment is to restore immediately the lost balance of blood sugar concentration. A patient yet alert, or semialert, will take any form of sugar by mouth: a few teaspoonfuls of sugar (sucrose) or glucose (dextrose) fruit juices (better with sugar), honey, candies, etc. All patients potentially subject to hypoglycemia (insulin users, patients with hyperinsulinism, etc.) must always carry lumps of sugar with them. If the patient is not able to swallow, use:

Dextrose, 25% solution, inject intravenously, 40 to 80 ml— equivalent to 10 to 20 g of glucose.

The patient should be referred to a diabetes specialist for further treatment.

Adrenal Crisis. The syndrome of adrenal insufficiency, showing the characteristic helpless asthenia with, possibly, severe acute abdominal pain radiating to the back and/or legs, vascular collapse, and renal shutdown, might suggest gastric or intestinal perforation. These symptoms of adrenal failure may occur in acute overwhelming infective conditions (particularly in younger people and children) or follow surgery, trauma, or dehydration.

As with other acute crises due to endocrinopathies, in cases of acute hypoadrenalism, analgesics are of no use. As soon as the diagnosis is made, the patient will receive hydrocortisone (of the sodium succinate or phosphate, 100 mg by intravenous injection, given at a rapid rate of 30 seconds), followed by 1000 ml of 5% glucose in isotonic saline with an additional 100 mg of hydrocortisone, given in a 2-hour period. The total 25-hour dose of hydrocortisone should reach 300 mg or more, and additional saline will be given to restore to normalcy hydration and natremia. At times, vasopressor drugs are needed; but at this point the patient will be referred to an endocrinologist for further treatment.

Hyperthyroidism. If hyperthyroidism leads to acidosis, the "acute abdomen" may occur. Other symptoms of hyperthyroidism may give the diagnostic clue.

Basically, the endocrine condition has to be treated either with surgery, radioactive drugs, or antithyroid agents, as propylthiouracil. Symptomatic treatment may be helpful, particularly with adrenergic blocking agents.

Guanethidine, 50 mg, by mouth, once a day.

Propanolol, 20 mg, by mouth, every 8 hours.

Tetany. In spasmophilia or frank tetany there may occur acute abdominal painful crises of a colicky type encouraging a diagnosis of cholecystitis, appendicitis, or the like. Also, there are circulatory and nervous symptoms, such as excessive irritability of the nerves, tonic or clonic contractures, and always a very low concentration of calcium in blood.

In hypoparathyroidism, the painful tetanic spasms will respond very well to the intravenous injection of:

>Calcium gluconate, 10% solution, 10 to 30 ml, at a very slow rate; to be repeated after 6 hours, if needed.

Once the patient is relieved of muscle contractures, the rest of the treatment will be evaluated and carried out by an endocrinologist.

Pituitary Cachexia. In either Simmond's or Sheehan's disease, acute abdominal pain (like paralytic ileus) may be a part of a varied symptomatology which leads to the diagnosis of pituitary insufficiency, namely, extreme loss of weight, asthemia, dehydration, and lowered metabolism.

When abdominal pain occurs in hypopituitaric patients, it may be due not only to the hypophyseal deficiency itself, but also to secondary deficiencies of the depending glands. The general treatment of this condition is better handled by an experienced endocrinologist. To relieve pain, temporally, analgesics may be used, namely:

>Codeine, 30 or 60 mg, by mouth, every 4 to 6 hours.

>Propoxyphene hydrochloride, 65 mg, by mouth, every 4 hours.

Parasympathomimetics (anticholinergic drugs) might be used cautiously.

>Belladonna tincture, 10 to 20 drops in a little water, repeated every 6 hours, or as tolerated.

>Atropine, 0.5 mg, tablets; one-half tablet, every 6 hours, or as tolerated.

>Paregoric elixir, up to 4 ml, in little water.

Porphyria. In erythropoietic porphyria the skin lesions on exposed surfaces are of paramount diagnostic interest, but hemolytic anemia may occur, which also may give rise to acute abdominal crises (q.v.). In hepatic porphyria colicky acute abdominal crises occur together with vomiting and other abdominal symptoms. The urine of these patients will darken when exposed to sunlight. The other forms of porphyria (heredity or symptomatic photosensitive hepatic porphyria) will rarely provoke any abdominal crisis.

In hepatic porphyria, crises of abdominal pain are common complaints. They respond very well to the administration of:

Chlorpromazine, 25 mg, by intramuscular injection, repeated every 4 hours while the pain is uncontrolled; shift to 25, 50, or 100 mg, by mouth, every 6 hours, thereafter.

Barbiturates are contraindicated, because they may trigger an attack. Other analgesics will be given at small doses.

Codeine, 30 mg, by mouth, every 4 to 6 hours.

Meperidine, 50 mg, by mouth, every 4 to 6 hours.

Diet, water intake, and other measures will follow the regular pattern for the treatment of porphyria.

Nervous Diseases

Radiculitis. A characteristic combination of symptoms, both sensory and motor, constitutes a syndrome, according to the nerve roots involved. It is not rare that fulgurant pains radiate from the back to the abdomen, simulating in some instances an "acute abdomen." Nevertheless, most cases will show a radicular distribution of pain, which helps to make a correct diagnosis.

For the symptomatic treatment of pain due to radiculitis, analgesics and muscle relaxants are of important help in aiding the general physical measures that are to be taken in all cases not subject to surgery. Among the analgesics are:

Acetylsalicylic acid, 600 mg, in tablets, every 4 to 6 hours.

Propoxyphene hydrochloride, 65 mg, by mouth, every 4 hours.

Codeine, 30 or 60 mg, by mouth, every 4 to 6 hours.

Muscle relaxants to be used are:

Meprobamate, 400 mg, by mouth, every 6 hours.

Carisoprodol, 350 mg, by mouth, every 6 or 8 hours.

Summon the help of a specialist to decide on the management of the frequently found herniated disc, traction and massage. Rest on a firm, flat bed is helpful.

Tabes Dorsalis. In tabes dorsalis the acute crisis is characteristic: an intense fulgurant epigastric pain (radiating or not to other regions of the abdomen or the rest of the body), together with a relatively well-tolerated vomiting, which simulates an "acute abdomen"; but other painful crises are equally frequent. The diagnosis is made after a neurological examination and the finding of other tabetic manifestations (ataxia, a particular gait, paresthesia, incontinence of urine, arthropathy, perforating ulcers, abnormal pupillary reflexes, etc.).

Acute abdominal crises are not rare in patients with tabes dorsalis. The treatment, of course, is that of late syphilis, mainly with penicillin at high dosage.

> Procaine penicillin, 600,000 units, every 12 hours, to reach a total of 7 million to 10 million units.

Patients sensitive to pencillin will receive, instead, erythromycin or a tetracycline.

> Erythromycin, 500 mg or 1 g, every 6 hours, for a total of 10 to 15 days.

> Tetracycline, same dosage as above.

If needed, the symptomatic relief of headache will be accomplished with any of the usual analgesics.

Surgery

Postsurgical Acidosis. This is a rarity nowadays, but was a deadly complication in the past. Because of an acidotic imbalance (q.v.), symptoms of "acute abdomen" (pain, vomiting, hiccup, meteorism) may appear suddenly during the first 2 days following surgery, notably abdominal procedures, and particularly operations on the liver. Care should be taken not to diagnose a nonexistent peritonitis.

This is almost always a respiratory acidosis due to impairment of the normal excretion of CO_2 through the lungs. To aid in this, oxygen is administered by mask or by intranasal tube. This condition is also combatted by intravenous infusion of glucose and sodium bicarbonate solutions. Do not give sedatives or narcotic analgesics. This situation is to be solved by the surgeon in charge of the operation.

> Sterile solution, 5% sodium bicarbonate, 5% glucose in Ringers solution. Give 1 liter intravenously over a period of 1 or 2 hours. Repeat if necessary.

Torsion of Pedunculated Tumors. This is a very rare occurrence but sometimes occurs with pedunculated abdominal tumors—fibromas. Most frequently, there is not usually any previous diagnosis of a tumor. A syndrome of "acute abdomen" of unidentified etiology will justify a laparotomy, which will be both diagnostic and curative.

The pain may need to be allayed by the use of narcotic analgesics.

Meperidine, 100 mg, by subcutaneous injection.

Methadone, 10 mg, by subcutaneous injection.

Morphine sulfate, 10 to 15 mg, by subcutaneous injection; or even 5 to 10 mg, by intravenous injection, if needed.

But restoration of normal position of the tumor (better, its removal) is an emergency procedure.

Torsion of Pedunculated Cysts; Rupture of Cysts. Ovarian cysts are most frequently found, and there is almost always a previous diagnosis of the cyst. Pain due to its torsion is of the type of the "acute abdomen" syndrome: it is very sharp, and may simulate appendicitis, peritonitis or even perforation of an organ, ectopic pregnancy, and the like. Many diagnostic clues are uncovered by a good anamnesis; but because this is an accident subject to surgery, the operation will solve the problem in all its aspects. Rupture of cysts (folicular or lutein) will give similar symptoms, but they are milder. Bimanual examination will be helpful in these cases.

This, also, is an emergency situation, and as such must be treated by a surgeon. The only help to be given to the patient is the administration of a narcotic analgesic, as stated in the above paragraph.

Torsion of the Pedicle of the Spleen. An "acute abdomen" syndrome suddenly appears, with fever, rapid increase of spleen volume, and black feces (melena).

There is no tumor. This is an extremely rare occurrence, always requiring surgery. If needed, give analgesia as stated above for "Torsion of pediculated tumors."

Poisoning

The great majority of poisons taken either accidentally or voluntarily are taken by mouth and swallowed. Many of them, like corrosive substances, will provoke immediate pain. The clinical picture will be that of intestinal colic (q.v.). Anamnesis, when available, will solve the diagnostic problem; when no direct clues are at hand, indirect investigation will be carried out: with bottles, drinking glasses or cups, etc. Do not forget the legal implications involved in all cases of poisoning. A rapid review of the most important forms of poisoning that may develop an "acute abdomen" syndrome (intestinal colic) follows:

Lead Colic. Abdominal colicky pains, epigastric in origin but radiating to the rest of the abdominal walls, the limbs, and the thorax, are the most important symptoms. During the acute stage there is also a bout of hypertension. The kind of work, medication, or any other circumstance related to the use of lead, and the other symptoms and signs of lead intoxication (dark line on the gums, anemia with basophilic punctuate, red and white blood cells in the stained blood smear, neurological findings, etc.), will help confirm the diagnosis.

There is always some discomfort, which may become severe pain if the intoxication is great. Analgesics of the type of:

> Codeine, 30 mg, by intramuscular injection,

may be of some help, but the basic treatment consists of the intravenous infusion of:

> Calcium disodium edetate, 15 to 25 mg for each kg of body weight, repeated every 12 hours during 5 days; series to be repeated following 2 days of rest, as needed,

either alone or together with:

> Dimercaprol, 3 to 5 mg for each kg of body weight, by intramuscular injection, every 4 hours at the start, for 2 days, and decrease to 6 hours the third day, and every 12 hours to complete about 10 days of therapy.

Copper Colic. The symptoms are like those for lead colic (q.v.). The bloody stools may appear green; and mouth structures, blue. In acute intoxication the patient deteriorates rapidly (shock, coma, death).

The severe abdominal pains need analgesia by means of narcotics, such as:

> Morphine, 10 to 15 mg, by subcutaneous injection.

Of course, gastric lavage is mandatory (use potassium ferrocyanide, 0.1% solution; or milk, white of eggs, etc.), and artificial respiration might be required. The use of calcium disodium edetate (see "Lead Colic" for details) is advisable.

Mercury (Acrodynia). There are good reasons to imply that acrodynia is the result of an excessive reactivity to mercury. The syndrome is characterized by acral pain (thus the name), but crises resembling "acute abdomen" are not rare. The pink colored fingers and toes, buttocks, nose, and cheeks are essential for diagnosis. In acute mercury poisoning, the symptoms are like those due to corrosive substances, such as acids and alkalies (q.v.). Salivation, stomatitis, diarrhea, and vomiting are prominent features.

The abdominal cramps of mercury poisoning most frequently require the administration of:

> Morphine, 10 to 15 mg, by subcutaneous injection, to be repeated as needed.

The ingestion of the poison can be treated by means of gastric lavage with sodium formaldehyde sulfoxalate (5% solution) or, at least, sodium bicarbonate (5% solution), because it will be ready at hand, in most instances; also milk and whites of raw eggs for stomach lavage.

> Dimercaprol, 3 to 5 mg for each kg of body weight, by intramuscular injection, every 4 hours at the start for 2 days, and decrease to every 6 hours the third day, and every 12 hours to complete about 10 days of treatment.

Other measures will be taken, as needed.

Acids and Alkalies. The diagnosis of acute intoxication after swallowing strong acids and alkalies is obvious: burns and scars are seen in the mouth and pharynx and indirectly detected in the esophagus, stomach, and even intestines. Vomiting is colored with transformed hemoglobin ("coffee ground" or black vomit). Deterioration is very rapid, and signs of peritonitis will rarely be absent.

For acids, as soon as possible give milk, white of eggs, milk of magnesia, or magnesium oxide to neutralize the acid at the earliest possible moment. The pain provoked by the corrosive activity upon the gastric mucosa can be treated with:

> Codeine, 60 mg, by intramuscular injection, repeated as needed.

> Morphine sulfate, 10 to 15 mg, by intravenous or intramuscular injection, repeated as needed.

Do not forget that sodium bicarbonate in these cases will liberate great amounts of carbonic gas, and should not be given.

For poisoning by alkalies, as soon as possible, give about 500 ml of a solution of equal parts of vinegar and water, or citrus fruit juice. Perhaps a better activity might be shown by citric acid (2 to 4 g) or tartaric acid (2 to 4 g). A good protection to the gastric mucose is afforded by olive oil, margarine, or butter. If the pain is severe give:

> Meperidine, 100 mg, by intramuscular injection, every 3 or 4 hours, as needed.

> Morphine sulfate, 10 to 15 mg, by subcutaneous injection, as needed—the initial dose could be 5 to 8 mg, by intravenous injection.

Corticoids may help for a better healing.

Nitrates. Intestinal colic is associated with flushed face, and throbbing headache, muscle relaxation and tremors, dilated pupils, cyanosis and irregular respirations, and finally shock.

For pain give:

> Morphine sulfate, 10 to 15 mg, by subcutaneous injection is most frequently needed.

Gastric lavage or induced vomiting are to be advised. Other injuries caused by the poison must be treated accordingly (hemodialysis, transfusions, etc.).

Insecticides. Chlorinated organic insecticides of the type of DDT and chlordane do not incite abdominal pains; but organic phosphate insecticides of the parathion type will induce colicky pains with diarrhea, headache, weakness, hypersecretion of saliva, tears, and pulmonary exudates (edema). Blurred vision and miosis are suggestive clues.

Organic phosphate insecticides and paradichlorobenzene may incite abdominal pain, which should *not* be treated with morphine sulfate. Give:

> Atropine, 1 to 4 mg, by intramuscular—or intravenous—injection; repeat 1 or 2 mg every 20 or 30 minutes, not to surpass 15 or 20 mg in 24 hours,

as the first choice. Other measures are to be taken, as needed.

Arsenic. Colicky pains are outstanding symptoms, in association with cramps and a characteristic diarrhea, always compared with "rice water." There are also found: thirst, a burning sensation from the esophagus to the stomach, dry mouth, a characteristic garlic odor to the breath, and finally shock. Fine, red skin eruptions also occur. Give:

> Morphine sulfate, 10 to 15 mg, by subcutaneous injection,
> repeated as needed;

as the best analgesic for the abdominal colic provoked by arsenic poisoning. The drug:

> Dimercaprol, 3 to 5 mg for each kg of body weight, by
> intramuscular injection, every 4 hours for the first 2 days,
> to be decreased to every 6 hours the third day, and then
> every 12 hours to complete about 10 more days of therapy,

is the best drug against arsenic toxicity. Other measures (gastric lavage, intravenous infusions, etc.) are to be taken, as needed.

Antimony. Symptoms are like those in arsenic intoxication (q.v.). Antimony poisoning also incites abdominal pain which needs:

> Morphine sulfate, 10 to 15 mg, by subcutaneous injection,

as the palliative of choice. Other measures are to be taken, as needed (gastric lavage, milk, intravenous infusions, etc.). Start as soon as possible:

> Dimercaprol, 3 to 5 mg for each kg of body weight, by
> intramuscular injection, every 4 hours during the first 2
> days, every 6 hours the third day, and every 12 hours thereafter to complete about 10 more days of therapy.

Cadmium. Violent, painful cramps, with diarrhea and vomiting, follow swallowing of cadmium compounds.

The ingestion of cadmium provokes severe abdominal pains, which may require the use of analgesics. It is best to use:

> Codeine, 60 mg, by intramuscular injection, to be repeated
> as needed.

In spite of its being irritating to the kidney (watch for symptoms, if it is used!), the best chelating drug is:

> Calcium disodium edetate, 15 to 25 mg for each kg of body
> weight, repeated every 12 hours during 5 days; the series to
> be repeated following 2 days of rest, as needed.

Other measures are to be taken, as needed.

Barium. Symptoms are similar to those of cadmium intoxication, plus hypertensive bouts with extrasystoles and convulsions. There are also hypertensive bouts as in lead colic, but the distribution of pain is different.

The pains require administration of:

Morphine sulfate, 10 to 15 mg, by subcutaneous injection, repeated as needed.

Gastric lavage should be started immediately. The substances:

Sodium sulfate, 30 to 60 g, by mouth;

Magnesium sulfate, 30 to 60 g, by mouth,

are of much help, as sedatives may also be:

Sodium amobarbital, 300 to 500 mg, by intravenous injection.

Chloral hydrate, 2 g in 100 ml of olive oil, by the rectal route.

Phenols. The abdominal pain is associated with salivation, a characteristic phenolic odor to the breath, local necrosis of lips and mouth (first white and then brown), burning sensation from mouth to stomach, and a very intense depression with hypotension. Renal symptoms are rarely absent (oligo- or anuria, hematuria, etc.).

Pain is severe enough to require:

Morphine sulphate, 10 to 15 mg, by subcutaneous injection, repeated as needed.

Immediate oral administration of olive or cottonseed oil (large quantities!) or activated charcoal, if available (also large quantities!), is necessary. As soon as possible, pass a stomach tube and use olive oil for gastric lavage. Water may be used for lavage, but other oils, mineral oils, fats, or alcohol are not to be used. Other measures will be taken as needed.

Alcohol. Following intoxication by either ethyl or methyl alcohol, abdominal pain may be an important symptom, together with the characteristic hyperactivity of "drunkenness." Methyl alcohol has been used as a substitute for ethyl alcohol and has provoked even more violent abdominal crises than ethyl alcohol, with pain in the eyes and sudden blindness.

In the case of *ethyl alcohol* intoxication, for pain do not give strong narcotic analgesics. Use mainly:

Codeine, 30 to 60 mg, by intramuscular injection, repeated as needed.

Gastric lavage (or emetics, except for apomorphine) and other measures will be applied as needed (aided respiration, intravenous glucose in cases of hypoglycemia, cathartics, frequent change of position in bed, etc.). In the case of *methyl alcohol* intoxication, codeine (as above) may be given for pain. Gastric lavage will be started immediately with sodium bicarbonate (3% solution), as well as an intravenous injection with the same agent.

> Sodium bicarbonate, 4 mEq solution for each kg of body weight, repeated every 4 hours, as needed.
>
> Ethyl alcohol, 0.75 mg per kg, to follow every 4 hours, during 4 days.

Also, other measures will be taken as their need arises.

Fluorides. Poisoning by fluorides also provokes pain, excessive secretions, hypotension, dyspnea, convulsions, and coma.
The immediate administration of:

> Calcium gluconate, 10% solution, up to 10 ml, by intravenous injection,

and early gastric lavage with large quantities of milk, or with calcium chlorate, calcium gluconate, lime water, etc., will help to control abdominal cramps, in most cases. Other measures will be taken as their need arises.

XI. CHRONIC ABDOMINAL PAIN

Perhaps second to headache is chronic abdominal pain, which includes not only ailments of the gastrointestinal tract, but also diseases of other systems, such as the circulatory, the urinary, the gynecologic, the osteomuscular, etc. These will be dealt with in this section.

Except in the cases of catastrophic events resulting from very acute reactions and incidents occurring during specific stages of certain diseases, which culminate in the "acute abdomen" syndrome, all those diseases that may provoke an acute pain may also be the cause of chronic abdominal suffering. From the diagnostic point of view there are two main differences: in the case of chronic abdominal pain there is no immediate need for determining the nature of the clinical picture, and there is almost always a better determination of the painful area. Only a few instances of diffuse pain will occur. The great majority of cases will fall into some of the following divisions: (1) epigastric pain, (2) pain in the right flank, (3) pain in the left flank, (4) pain in the right iliac fossa, (5) pain in the left iliac fossa, (6) pain in the hypogastrium, (7) pain of circulatory origin,

(8) pain from the urinary system, (9) pain of gynecologic origin, and (10) pain of osteomuscular origin.

Diffuse Abdominal Pain (Umbilical)

A diffuse abdominal pain is mainly referred to the umbilical region, extended in a more or less definite manner to the neighboring regions. It may be due to any cause which may also be the basis of a localized pain, or its diffuseness may precede its limitation to a circumscribed area.

Tuberculosis of the Intestines. Ordinarily, a patient with known pulmonary tuberculosis will complain of crampy pains and diarrhea associated with anorexia and a permanent sensation of discomfort when there is an enterocolitic spreading of the infection.

In addition to the basic care with tuberculostatic drugs, abdominal pain may be treated with the following:

Codeine, 30 or 60 mg, by mouth, every 6 hours.

Belladonna tincture, 10 to 20 drops, in water, every 6 to 8 hours, according to tolerance.

Similar medications could also be used. Irritant foods (spices, roughage, liquors, etc.) are to be avoided; and rest, encouraged.

Tuberculosis of the Peritoneum. The symptoms will be similar to those ascribed to the original abdominal complaints: a diffuse pain all over the abdomen, that may be crampy on occasions and associated with cachexia, tenderness, and ascites. The examination of peritoneal fluid may give the diagnosis.

The treatment will be the same as stated above.

Chronic Peritonitis. The symptoms are essentially the same as those discussed in the foregoing lines. The etiological factor should be found from the anamnesis or from examination of the peritoneal fluid.

Chronic peritonitis may produce abdominal pain, which appears diffuse, dull, and constant. The basic treatment will be to find and control the source of the infection (antibiotics, surgery); but the patient has to be relieved of the discomfort produced by the disease—namely, he must receive analgesic medication.

Meperidine, 100 mg, every 4 to 6 hours, either by mouth or by intramuscular injection.

This might be the first choice, but the following may also be used:

> Codeine, 60 mg, by mouth, every 4 hours.

Other analgesics may be tried.

Porphyria. The painful abdominal crises that occur in porphyria may be of a diffuse character. Other symptoms of the disease will be also present (constipation, skin eruption, change of color of the urine, etc.).

Most cases of porphyria will present chronic abdominal pain. A diet high in proteins and carbohydrates will help to controll all symptoms, including pain. If really needed, give the following:

> Codeine, 30 mg, by mouth, every 6 hours.
>
> Meperidine, 50 mg, by mouth, every 6 hours.
>
> Propoxyphene hydrochloride, 65 mg, by mouth, every 6 hours, but stop as soon as possible.
>
> Chlorpromazine, 50 or 100 mg, by mouth, every 8 to 12 hours.

All of these may help to control pain as well as possible mental symptoms.

Epigastric Pain

Peptic Ulcer. In general, the pain shows a very clear relationship to the timing of feeding: it is relieved by the ingestion of food, and recurs with the emptying of the stomach (hunger pains). There is a tender spot in the painful region. Esophageal ulcers have pains at a higher location than those with duodenal ulcer. Patients with gastric ulcers may have lower secretion of acid, not always high amounts as generally expected. Other symptoms are nausea and vomiting (may be bloody), anemia, heartburn, etc. The final diagnosis is made by X-ray examination.

Chronic epigastric dull pain is the most frequent manifestation of peptic ulcer, and as such should be treated. Of course, the general treatment will be that designed for peptic ulcer. As in the case of acute attacks, the basic drugs will be antacids and parasympatholytics (anticholinergics). The one favored by a large number of patients is sodium bicarbonate.

> Sodium bicarbonate, less than half a teaspoonful, every 3 hours; but never to be used for a relatively long-term therapy.

For a longer-term therapy, use instead a mixture of magnesium oxide and calcium carbonate.

> Magnesium oxide, 15 to 60 g (according to individual reaction to avoid constipation) plus calcium carbonate, the amount needed to complete 120 g; to give of the mixture half or one level teaspoonful in half a glass of water, every 2 or 3 hours.

Since the use of calcium may induce hypercalcemia, check for the event and act accordingly. Other pharmaceutical preparations and even OTC remedies could be of help. The first trial for anticholinergic medication will be given to tincture of belladonna.

> Tincture of belladonna, 10 to 20 drops, in water, half an hour before meals and at bed time; the dosage adjusted to individual reactions.

> Atropine, 0.5 mg, tablets; half a tablet 30 minutes before meals and at bedtime, watching for individual reactions.

> Dicyclomine hydrochloride, 20 mg, in tablets, before meals and at bedtime.

> Propantheline bromide, 7.5 or 15 mg, in tablets, before meals and at bedtime.

Similar products could be used; and a general treatment should be completed for each particular patient.

Cancer. Pain in cancer of the stomach may be of the same type as in peptic ulcer, though its aggravation by the ingestion of food is a frequent finding. Low gastric acidity is a differential sign from the high acidity found in most cases of peptic ulcer. Other symptoms are: anorexia, with a special dislike for meats; vomiting, with coffee-ground appearance and resultant or independent weight loss; and characteristic findings on the X-ray plate. Epigastric pain is also felt in cancer of the ascending colon.

No matter that the abdominal pain provoked by cancer can reach acute, catastrophic proportions, it has to be considered as a chronic pain. Of course, when this pain occurs, morphine sulfate is the analgesic of choice.

> Morphine sulfate, 5 to 10 mg, intravenously, repeated in 15 to 30 minutes.

Otherwise, morphine will be used subcutaneously, or alternate drugs administered, instead.

Morphine sulfate, 10 to 15 mg, by subcutaneous injection, repeated as needed and tolerated.

Meperidine, 100 mg, by subcutaneous injection, repeated every 4 hours, or as needed and tolerated.

Codeine, 60 mg, by subcutaneous injection, repeated as needed and tolerated (average: every 4 hours).

In the case of carcinoid syndrome, abdominal pain may be treated with paregoric elixir or belladonna tincture, whenever it accompanies diarrhea.

Paregoric elixir, up to 4 ml in water, repeated as needed and tolerated.

Laudanum (opium tincture), 20 to 30 drops, in water, repeated as needed and tolerated.

Tincture of belladonna, 10 to 30 drops, in water, repeated as needed and tolerated.

For this disease, corticoids might be of help, and serotonin antagonists are useful at times. But surgery is the last resort, whenever advisable.

Hyperchlorhydria will rarely incite epigastric pain, but it may be present. Heartburn is the main symptom.

Together with remedies for pain and cough, the free market is overrun with OTC medications for hyperchlorhydria ("heartburn"). None is better than the other, and some may provoke untoward effects in certain individuals, if taken indiscriminately. Since the essential of the treatment of hyperchlorhydria does not differ too much from that for peptic ulcer, we refer the reader to the corresponding paragraph, calling attention particularly to antacids and anticholinergics. (See above, "Peptic ulcer".)

Peptic Esophagitis and Diaphragmatic (Hiatal) Hernia. Peptic esophagitis may cause epigastric discomfort, pain, and heartburn. The diagnosis becomes firmer if diaphragmatic hernia is found in the X-ray. In diaphragmatic (hiatal) hernia a dull, postprandial, retrosternal pain may appear together with hiccough or belching and subside spontaneously in a short time. This is indicative of hiatal hernia. Ordinarily, these hernias are small; when they are larger, other symptoms may be present, such as dyspnea, cough, etc. The diagnosis depends on roetgenologic studies.

In both instances the treatment is practically the same, antacids being of paramount importance in most cases.

> Bismuth subgallate, 500 mg or more, by mouth, every 4 to 6 hours.
>
> Bismuth subcarbonate, 500 mg or 1 g in capsules; 300 or 600 mg, in tablets; take from 500 mg up to 4 g a day.
>
> Sodium bicarbonate, less than half a teaspoonful, every 4 to 6 hours.

Neither of the above-mentioned drugs should be used for long-term therapy. For this purpose, use instead the following:

> Magnesium oxide, 15 to 60 g (according to individual reaction to avoid constipation) plus calcium carbonate, the amount needed to complete 120 g; to give half or one level teaspoonful in half a glass of water, every 4, 6, or 8 hours.

To avoid pain, these patients should lose weight if they are over the average for height and age, should not have tight belts or tight clothes of any kind, and should sleep with the head of the bed elevated (about 10 inches). For better results, surgery is needed for many patients, particularly those with small sliding hernias.

Chronic Gastritis. Patients with chronic gastritis of the hypertrophic type may show symptoms suggestive of peptic ulcer. The diagnosis depends on gastroscopy, biopsy, and gastric secretion analysis.

If it is due to iron deficiency anemia or pernicious anemia, the adequate treatment will solve the problem. If it is associated with excessive production of gastric juice (hyperchlorhydria), antacids and anticholinergics are of some help in most instances (see "Peptic ulcer"). Patients with hypochlorhydria may benefit from the administration of agents capable of liberating hydrochloric acid, plus the treatment of the basic cause. In general, the patient will be advised to avoid gastric irritants (alcohol, spices, salicylates, coffee, tea, etc.). Some symptomatic relief should be offered by the use of tranquilizers and anticholinergics.

> Glutamic acid hydrochloride, 340 mg pulvules, one to three, before meals.
>
> Phenobarbital, up to 50 mg, every 6 to 8 hours, by mouth.
>
> Chlorpromazine, 50 mg, by mouth, every 6 to 8 hours.
>
> Diazepan, 2 to 5 mg, by mouth, every 4 to 6 hours.

Tincture of belladonna, 10 to 30 drops, in water, every 6 hours.

Atropine, 0.5 mg, tablets; half a tablet every 6 hours.

Perigastritis. Pain is permanent, perhaps diffuse over the epigastric region, and frequently preceded by ulcer-like symptoms. A diffuse mass may be felt on palpation, easily taken for a cancer. A diferentiation may be attempted when pain subsides or is alleviated by a change in position; but the final diagnosis is made by roentgenographic examination.

This is a circumscribed form of peritonitis, either acute or chronic, and is to be treated as such. As for chronic peritonitis, find the source of the infection, and use antibiotics and surgery. In addition, administer analgesics. The first trial will be with meperidine.

Meperidine, 100 mg, every 4 to 6 hours, by mouth or subcutaneously, as convenient.

Codeine, 60 mg, by mouth, every 4 hours.

Cholecystitis. Pain may be felt at the epigastrium, with the same characteristics that will be discussed under "Pain in the Right Flank," q.v.

Surgical treatment is ordinarily the final solution for the great majority of cases of cholecystitis and cholelithiasis. In the meantime antacids, anticholinergics, and sedatives will be useful, particularly in the absence of stones.

Sodium bicarbonate, less than half a teaspoonful, every 4 to 6 hours.

Magnesium oxide, 15 to 60 g (according to individual requirements to avoid constipation) plus calcium carbonate, amount needed to complete 120 g; give half or one level teaspoonful in half a glass of water, every 6 to 8 hours. Watch for hypercalcemia, when the treatment is prolonged enough.

Tincture of belladonna, 10 to 30 drops, in water, every 4 to 6 hours.

Atropine, 0.5 mg, tablets; one-half tablet every 4 to 6 hours.

Phenobarbital, up to 50 mg, by mouth, every 6 to 8 hours.

A low-fat diet should be given, and overweight persons should lose weight to reach the normal level for height and age.

Hepatomegalia. An enlarged liver, because of circulatory failure, may give epigastric pain; but the main symptoms occur at the right flank (q.v.).

Most patients with an enlarged liver will complain of visceral pain. Because this is usually due to congestive heart failure, the logical approach is to treat the heart following the regular routine of rest, reduction of sodium and water retention, treatment of the causative factor (if any), oxygen therapy if there is respiratory distress, and the use of cardiotonics (digitalis, in the first place). Analgesics are of no use.

Colitis. In any form of colitis, but particularly in mucomenbranous colitis (irritable colon), pain may be felt also in the epigastrium. Other symptoms will be the same ones associated with pain in the flanks (q.v.).

In the case of pain due to mucous colitis (spastic or irritable colon), anticholinergic drugs will be the first choice for treatment.

> Tincture of belladonna, 10 to 20 drops, in water, every 6 to 8 hours, or according to effect and tolerance.
>
> Atropine, 0.5 mg, tablets; half a tablet every 6 to 8 hours, or according to effect and tolerance.

Opiates will also be of help in a large number of patients, who respond well to laudanum or paregoric, particularly when pain is accompanied by diarrhea.

> Laudanum (opium tincture), 20 to 30 drops in water, repeated as needed and tolerated.
>
> Paregoric elixir, up to 4 ml in water, repeated as needed and tolerated.

The rest of the treatment will follow the accepted rules: diet, sedatives or tranquilizers (together with psychological reassurance), adequate physical activity, etc.

Chronic ulcerative colitis will be treated following the general rules stated for the acute attacks (q.v., in the corresponding paragraph of the "Acute Abdomen" section). Paregoric elixir, or a combination of paregoric and tincture of belladonna, will be used during the chronic stages. Also, anticholinergics (belladonna tincture, atropine) are of help. As stated in the corresponding paragraph, corticoids and salicylazosulfapyridine are to be given to these patients.

Appendicitis. It is by no means infrequent that the appendicular pain is referred to the epigastric region, particularly among young people. Pressure over the appendicular points will exacerbate the pain. The symptoms are the same as for a usual appendicitis attack.

A clinical picture of chronic appendicitis (which is a nonexistent disease) may be a serious situation, because the need for surgery will not always be apparent—although surgery is practically the only solution to the problem. Analgesics will do their work to allay pain, and may be used temporarily, until the surgeon takes care of the patient.

> Propoxyphene hydrochloride, 65 mg, by mouth, every 6 hours.
>
> Codeine, 30 or 60 mg, by mouth or subcutaneous injection, every 4 to 6 hours.
>
> Meperidine, 50 mg, by subcutaneous injection, every 4 to 6 hours.

Pancreatitis. Both acute and chronic pancreatitis may provoke epigastric pain, without the catastrophic characteristics of "acute abdomen." The painful sensation will be somewhat shifted towards the right side of the epigastrium in the case of lesions of the head of the pancreas, or toward a lower area, in the case of lesions of the body and tail of the gland; it may also radiate to the back, or the right flank; it may occur late after ingestion of food; and, finally, it may mimic the pains found in peptic ulcer, cholelithiasis, and cholecystitis (particularly when pancreatitis is associated with any of these diseases, which is not a rare event). The diagnosis will usually be obtained by exclusion of all other more frequent diseases with the same symptoms. Signs pointing to the pancreas would be: pancreatic insufficiency, increased amylase in the urine, steatorrhea, hypo- or hyperglycemia, palpation of the pancreatic gland as a hard transverse elongated tumor, and, in many instances, the evident scar of a laparatomy. The diagnosis of cancer or cysts of the pancreas would depend on the microscopic findings of an immediate section of an epigastric tumor taken in the operating room.

During recurrent attacks, the pain is acute and severe; during the chronic stage, dull and boring. Since narcotic addiction is easy with these patients, morphine and similar drugs should be avoided. It is better to use the following:

> Codeine, 60 mg by subcutaneous injection, every 4 to 6 hours, or as needed and tolerated.
>
> Meperidine (with caution), 100 mg by subcutaneous injection, as needed and individually tolerated.

Surgical procedures (cholecystectomy, subtotal pancreatectomy, bilateral sympathectomy, etc.) will be decided by the specialist.

Radiculitis is marked by paroxysmal pains, as in tabes dorsalis, superficially located, spontaneous or following any sort of stress upon the vertebral column, frequently associated with paresthesias and more rarely with motor impairment or trophic changes. Dorsal radiculitis may give origin to intercostal neuralgia, or to neuralgia in the epigastric region.

Surgery will be considered as the basic treatment, as well as other physical resources; and the use of analgesics and muscle relaxants will be of help in many instances.

> Acetylsalicylic acid, 600 mg, in tablets, every 4 to 6 hours, preferably with meals.

> Codeine, 30 or 60 mg, by mouth, every 4 to 6 hours.

> Propoxyphene hydrochloride, 65 mg, by mouth, every 4 hours.

> Meprobamate, 400 mg, by mouth, every 6 hours.

> Carisoprodol, 350 mg, by mouth, every 6 to 8 hours.

Pleuritis. Ordinarily, this shows a characteristic chest pain aggravated by motion. Frequently, the pain will center in the epigastric region. All other details are similar to pleural chest pains (q.v.)

Treat the infection (if any) with the adequate antibiotic, and give analgesics for chronic pain, chosen in the following sequence:

> Codeine, 60 mg, by mouth, every 4 hours.

> Codeine, 30 mg, by intramuscular injection, every 4 hours (shift to oral administration as soon as possible).

> Meperidine, 50 to 100 mg, by intramuscular injection, four to six times a day.

> Morphine sulfate, 10 or 15 mg, by subcutaneous injection, repeated as needed and tolerated.

If analgesics cannot control pain, intercostal nerves can be blocked by paravertebral infiltration.

> Procaine, 2% solution, use up to 5 ml by injection.

Hypoglycemia. In the preceding pages we discussed the frequency of "acute abdomen" associated with hypoglycemia (q.v., for more complete information on the subject). But often there is only a dull epigastric ache, like hunger pains, that might encourage the wrong diagnosis of peptic ulcer. The accompanying symptoms may help in the final diagnosis (sweating, weakness, tremor, behavioral changes, dizziness, and even convulsions leading to coma).

Rarely, abdominal pain is felt in hypoglycemia. The use of mild analgesics will suffice in most intances.

> Acetylsalicylic acid, 600 mg, in tablets, every 4 to 6 hours, preferably, with meals.
>
> Codeine, 30 or 60 mg, by mouth, every 4 to 6 hours.
>
> Acetaminophen, 600 mg, by mouth, every 6 hours.
>
> Propoxyphene hydrochloride, 65 mg, by mouth, every 6 hours.

The administration of glucose by mouth or intravenously is critically needed at times, when indicated by a low blood sugar. The rest of the treatment will follow established rules (corticoids, diazoxide, zinc glucagon, diet, sedation, etc.).

Pain in the Right Flank

Duodenal Ulcer. Peptic ulcers located in the duodenal region show the classic sequence of symptoms: characteristic pain, principally felt on an empty stomach and alleviated on the ingestion of food, with periodic exacerbation and amelioration; vomiting, with or without bloody contents; and hyperchlorhydria in most instances. An X-ray examination is needed to establish the diagnosis.

The treatment of duodenal ulcer does not differ basically from the treatment of peptic ulcer (q.v.), except that in patients with duodenal ulcer bed rest for 1 or 2 weeks is advisable, but not always mandatory as it is with gastric ulcer, when the 2 or 3 initial weeks should be spent in the hospital. Rest at home is enough, and relative activity can start as soon as the control of pain is obtained. This laxity does not preclude the needed use of antacids, anticholinergics, and the general care of the condition.

Cholecystitis. When there is a pure cholecystitis, without lithiasis, there are no biliary colics, but a vague ache on the right flank is frequently (not always) present. Tenderness of the region is constantly found. Other symptoms may be dyspepsia and fever. The diagnosis depends on the laboratory and the roentgenologic examination of the biliary function. In biliary lithiasis there is almost always a cholecystitic component, which gives the clinical picture of cholecystitis between the acute colicky pains. Radiologic examination is essential for diagnosis.

If the patient also has stones, most probably surgery will be needed. But all cases will follow the general routine, which includes the use of antacids, anticholinergics, sedatives, and a low-fat diet (which will also help him to regain the desirable normal weight).

> Sodium bicarbonate, less than half a teaspoonful, every 4 to 6 hours.

> Magnesium oxide, 15 to 60 g (depending on individual reactions to avoid constipation) plus calcium carbonate, amount needed to complete a total of 120 g; give half or one level teaspoonful in water, every 6 to 8 hours; and watch for hypercalcemia if the treatment is prolonged enough.

> Tincture of belladonna, 10 to 30 drops, in water, every 4 to 6 hours, according to effect and tolerance.

> Atropine, 0.5 mg, tablets; one-half tablet every 4 to 6 hours.

> Phenobarbital, up to 50 mg, by mouth, every 6 to 8 hours.

Congestion of the Liver. Patients with congestive heart failure very frequently complain of pain in the right flank, and on palpation they ordinarily feel an increase in the constant dull ache. The liver is enlarged, and liver function tests may be altered. The hepatic symptoms commonly increase or decrease with worsening or improvement of the primary heart condition.

Analgesics are of little advantage in cases of pain due to congested liver. Since this condition is usually due to congestive heart failure, that condition must receive the basic care (rest, decrease of sodium and water retention, treatment of known causative factor, oxygen therapy for respiratory distress, and the use of cardiotonic drugs).

Hepatitis. In viral hepatitis (formerly called catarrhal jaundice) there is a more or less marked infective syndrome (fever) associated with pain in the right flank. The liver is tender and enlarged to palpation. There are gastrointestinal symptoms and a characteristic jaundice. The principal diagnostic problem is with diseases that also cause jaundice. The acute increase of transaminse (SGOT) favors the diagnosis of viral hepatitis. Similar symptoms may be due to homologous serum jaundice, but in this case there is the antecedent of blood transfusion, the use of intravenous plasma, unsterile instruments, or other means for transfer of the virus.

Pain is mostly mild in hepatitis, and very rarely will need any special care. If it does, corticoids are preferred.

> Prednisone, 20 mg, three to five times a day; with gradually decreasing dosage.

Corticoids are not to be used indiscriminately, since they should be reserved only for the severely ill patient. The rest of the treatment will follow the generally accepted rules.

Subphrenic Abscess (Subdiaphragmatic). There is pain in the right flank or low chest, radiating to the corresponding shoulder; and there are symptoms of a septic condition (fever with spikes or continuous). It follows a surgical procedure or a perforation of a neighboring organ. Elevation and immobility of the right hemidiaphragm, with or without gas, is diagnostic.

There is no better choice than to drain the abscess, but symptomatic care will help. Give analgesics, as needed.

> Acetylsalicylic acid, 600 mg, in tablets, every 4 to 6 hours, preferably with meals.
>
> Codeine, 60 mg, by mouth, every 4 to 6 hours.
>
> Meperidine, 100 mg, by subcutaneous injection or by mouth, every 4 to 6 hours; but do not keep patient on this drug for long periods.

Cancer of the head of the pancreas causes pain in the right flank radiating to the back or the epigastrium. Rarely, there will be no pain. There is obstructive jaundice with dilatation of the gallbladder.

Pain is the most important symptom, and as such should be treated. The sequence of use of the adequate drugs for pain is as follows, using the next step only after a trial of the preceding one:

> Codeine, 60 mg, by intramuscular or subcutaneous injection, every 4 to 6 hours.
>
> Meperidine, 100 mg, by subcutaneous injection, every 4 to 6 hours.
>
> Morphine sulfate, 10 or 15 mg, by subcutaneous injection, as needed and tolerated.

Surgery is the final remedy for this disease.

Colitis. In rare instances the inflammatory diseases of the colon are limited to the ascending portion and its hepatic curvature. In general, these will cause pain in the right flank, and even objective signs (masses, tenderness, etc.). If colic cancer attacks this segment, pain is frequently referred to the epigastrium.

No matter how or where pain from colitis is present, the treatment will be the same, according to its kind: mucous colitis or ulcerative colitis. For mucous colitis anticholinergics will be the first, and opiates the second choice. For ulcerative colitis, also opiates or a combination of paregoric elixir and tincture of belladonna is of help. For more details, see corresponding paragraphs above and below.

Heterotopic Pain from the Right Iliac Fossa. Any disease of the organs located in this region may radiate pain to the right flank. These diseases will be discussed in the following paragraphs.

Referred pain felt in the periumbilical or epigastric areas may come from: nervous diseases or diseases of the spine, pleuritic reactions, dilation of the right heart, hypoglycemia, etc., which conditions will be treated specifically.

Pain in the Right Iliac Fossa

Pain in the right iliac fossa is also an extremely frequent complaint in human pathology, and a frequent cause of diagnostic problems. It will include, as well, pain from genitourinary organs, which will be discussed separately because it may occur in either the right or the left side.

Appendicitis. Chronic appendicitis is no longer considered a surgical problem, at least in the United States. There may be continuous pain over the region, more exquisitely felt over the appendicular points. The pain may increase at times in an acute form. Objective findings (a mass in the appendicular region) are more rarely encountered, except for pain elicited on pressure over the classical points. But things are a little different when the above symptomatology occurs in a patient who has previously suffered a well-proved acute appendicitis attack. In these cases, there are some strong bases for speaking of chronic appendicitis. Even the layman will think of appendicitis when experiencing pain in the right iliac fossa.

While surgery is performed—and the patient should be referred to the surgeon from the first—some help will be afforded by the following:

> Propoxyphene hydrochloride, 65 mg, by mouth, every 6 hours.

Codeine, 30 or 60 mg, by mouth or subcutaneous injection, every 4 to 6 hours.

Meperidine, 50 mg, by subcutaneous injection, every 4 to 6 hours.

Colitis. Lesions limited to the cecum are not exceptional. The symptomatology is almost an exact copy of chronic appendicitis, perhaps more diffuse. There may be also symptoms of a more generalized colitis, less marked than those found in the right fossa. Tuberculosis of the cecum may occur in patients with tuberculosis elsewhere in the body, particularly pulmonary tuberculosis. When it affects the colon, the cecum is the most affected segment. In these patients the symptoms of greatest importance are: profuse diarrhea, fever, and more or less marked cachexia. Locally, a mass may be palpated. The exact diagnosis is obtained only after biopsy is performed. There is also a cecal localization of actinomycosis, but its diagnosis depends on the finding of the Actinomyces. Diverticulosis of the cecal region brings on a symptomatology entirely similar to that discussed in the above lines: the diagnosis will be made after surgery or roentgenological studies. Intestinal obstruction (cecal obstruction) may also occur at this location, and may produce only a minor pain.

For treatment, see the corresponding paragraphs in other sections.

Cancer. There is often slight pain in cancer, generally disproportionate to the large mass that can be palpated. The general condition of the patient is good for long periods of time. The differentiation from benign tumors or other lesions of the region depends, in the great majority of cases, upon surgery and biopsy.

Surgery is the final solution for cancer in the abdominal cavity, except for those cases in which chemotherapy is the best election. To allay pain, we should give codeine first, meperidine second, and resort to morphine only as a last choice. Otewise, the regular treatment with morphine might be supplemented with meperidine or codeine, to avoid large doses of morphine.

Codeine, 60 mg, by subcutaneous injection, every 4 to 6 hours.

Meperidine, 100 mg, by subcutaneous injection, every 4 to 6 hours.

Morphine sulfate, 15 mg, by subcutaneous injection, as needed and tolerated.

Crohn's Disease. The acute form may simulate an appendicular attack. The chronic form also provokes crampy pains in the abdomen, particularly in the right iliac fossa. Other important symptoms are fever and diarrhea. On examination, few signs are elicited, but tenderness on pressure over the terminal ilium in the right iliac fossa and even muscle rigidity (of a voluntary type) may be found. In the case of a diffuse form of the disease, signs and symptoms of malnutrition will predominate; in the inflammatory form, fever and appendicular-like symptoms; in the obstructive form, symptoms and signs of incomplete intestinal obstruction; and in complicated forms, abscesses with or without fistulae. The final diagnosis depends on X-ray examination.

Pain is not an important feature of regional enteritis, and should not receive any special attention except the general treatment already scheduled for this disease. Only anticholinergics should be used, since abdominal cramps are almost always coincident with diarrhea.

> Tincture of belladonna, 10 to 30 drops, in water, before meals and at bedtime.

> Atropine, 0.5 mg, tablets; half or one tablet, according to effect and tolerance, before meals and at bedtime.

Pain in the Left Flank

Pancreatitis. The principal location of pancreatic pain is epigastric (q.v.). In some instances there is a more or less marked shift of the pain toward the left flank, with little or no variation of the remaining symptomatology.

The dull and boring pain of the chronic stages of pancreatitis may respond well to codeine or meperidine. Morphine is better avoided, because of the risk of addiction.

> Codeine, 60 mg, by subcutaneous injection, as needed and tolerated (average: every 4 or 6 hours).

> Meperidine (with caution), 100 mg, by subcutaneous injection, as needed and individually tolerated.

Refer the patient to the specialist for further care.

Gastric Diseases. Again, the main location for gastric pain is the epigastric region (q.v.), although not rarely, when the disease centers by choice in the greater curvature or close to the cardias, it may shift toward the left flank. This holds true for peptic ulcer, chronic gastritis, gastric dilatation, aerophagia, gastric tumors (cancer), and even merely dyspepsia. This pain, when localized in the left flank, does not differ at all from the pain regularly felt about the epigastric area.

By the same token, treatment will not differ, either, and the reader is asked to consult other adequate paragraphs in the book.

Enteritis and Colitis. The pain in chronic ulcerative colitis is of a crampy nature and centers toward the left flank, though it cannot be specifically located at this site, since it may be more diffusely extended. The main symptomatology consists of the numerous bowel movements (to 20 or more, a day) associated with crisis of cramps and accompanied by rectal tenesmus. Tenderness is found in both flanks, but particularly at the left side. The stools are bloody and may contain pus. X-ray and proctosigmoidoscopy examinations will establish the diagnosis. In mucous colitis the symptoms are much less conspicuous. Patients who complain of chronic constipation or frequent diarrhea, whose feces may be covered or mixed with mucus, also refer to pain over the left flank and left iliac fossa. The pain may be relieved by gentle manual pressure over the region, but may also cause some tenderness over the area. There are no other symptoms, except for some neurotic conditions (anxiety, tenseness). In Whipple's disease there are also fever and arthritic symptoms, together with a possible polyserositis. Megacolon is more common among children, who show also constipation, abdominal distension, and a rectum either empty or filled with feces. In diverticulitis there is frequently a "left sided appendicitis."

Pain due to intestinal lipodystrophy (Whipple's disease) may be treated with codeine or belladonna.

Codeine, 30 or 60 mg, by mouth, every 6 hours.

Tincture or belladonna, 10 to 15 drops, in water, before meals and at bedtime.

But the basic treatment will be carried out with the appropriate antibiotic, in most instances for a long period of time.

In tuberculous enterocolitis, the same help as above can be given, but the basic treatment is with tuberculostatic medication.

In ulcerative colitis (for more complete information, see the corresponding paragraph in the acute abdominal pain section) pain may be relieved with opiates and belladonna.

Paregoric elixir, up to 4 ml in water, every 4 to 6 hours.

Laudanum (opium tincture), 20 to 30 drops, in water, repeated as needed and tolerated.

Paregoric elixir and tincture of belladonna, equal parts (or paregoric 2, belladonna 1); give 1 or 1.5 ml every 4 to 6 hours, as tolerated.

Opium, 65 mg, plus belladonna, 8 mg, for one suppository; insert one every 4 hours.

Tincture of belladonna, 10 to 30 drops, in water, before meals and at bedtime, as tolerated.

Atropine, 0.5 mg, tablets; half or one tablet before meals and at bedtime, as tolerated.

Propantheline bromide, 15 mg, tablets; one tablet every 6 or 8 hours.

Tranquilizers or sedatives are good for these patients, corticoids are of good use, and salizylazosulfapyridine is advised.

Salizylazosulfapyridine, 500 mg, tablets; two or four tablets (individualized dosage) every 6 hours.

Pain due to megacolon may respond well to parasympathomimetic drugs, such as the following:

Neostigmine, 15 mg by mouth, every 8 hours.

Betanechol, 10 mg, tablets, every 6 hours.

Also, administer enemas frequently.

If pain is due to diverticular problems, anticholinergics—as described above—will result in good help to the basic therapy.

Diseases of the Spleen. Most of the diseases of the spleen provoke a painless increase in size of the organ. In some instances, when there is a perisplenitis, a mild pain may be felt. It may happen to patients with chronic malaria (hard, tender, enlarged spleen, with mild pain in the left flank); aseptic infarction of the organ (moderately enlarged spleen, with pain in the left flank and mild peritonitic symptoms); splenic abscess (moderately enlarged spleen, mild pain in the left flank); cysts (only moderately painful when they reach a large size); and cancer (rapid enlargement, pain, tenderness on palpation). Rupture of the spleen will provoke pain mainly in the left upper side of the abdomen, which at times spreads to the left shoulder, with muscle rigidity and tenderness; in severe cases shock may result. Rupture of the spleen most frequently occurs because of trauma (an excellent guide point for the majority of cases), infectious mononucleosis, leukemia, malaria, typhoid fever, etc.

In all instances the basic condition will be treated, and in cases of rutpure surgery has to be carried out immediately. Analgesics do not have use in these conditions.

Pain in the Left Iliac Fossa

Appendicitis. The possibility of an attack of appendicitis in a person with situs inversus viscerae should always be kept in mind. The symptoms are exactly the same, but the location of pain and of the objective findings are at the left side, as also happens in attacks of Meckel's diverticulitis, as stated lines above. A roentgenologic examination will establish the diagnosis in cases of these rare occurrences.

Surgery is the rational approach for both diseases. In the meantime, pain may be alleviated by analgesics and parasympatholytic drugs.

> Paregoric elixir, up to 4 ml in water, every 4 to 6 hours.

> Tincture of belladonna, 10 to 20 drops, in water, before meals and at bedtime.

> Paregoric elixir and belladonna tincture, equal parts (also, paregoric 2, belladonna 1); give every 4 to 6 hours, as tolerated.

Colitis. As stated before, under the heading "Pain in the Left Flank" (q.v.), both ulcerative and mucous colitis may show pain extended to, or primarily located in, the left iliac fossa. This occurs more frequently when the sigmoid or the rectosigmoid are locally involved in infective or parasitic diseases, as in any other form of ordinary colitis. There is not a frank pain in the left iliac fossa, but some sensation of discomfort, with local tenderness, and muscular rigidity is found on palpation. Diarrhea (with mucous or mucosanguinolent stools), or constipation, in some women signs of left adnexitis, may also be present. A direct examination, by rectoscopy or sigmoidoscopy, together with roentgenological studies, will establish the diagnosis.

For treatment, see paragraphs above dealing with "Colitis."

Diverticulitis. Symptoms are very similar to an appendicitis attack located at the left side (q.v., above); or better, to the possible stage of chronic appendicitis. There is pain in the left iliac fossa, a palpable mass is found, the stools are diarrheic, rectal hemorrhages are not an exception; but only a good radiologic examination will establish the diagnosis.

See adequate paragraphs, above, for diverticulitis ("appendicitis," "intestinal perforation").

Cancer of the Sigmoid. Pain is crampy or mild, or even absent: it is not a reliable symptom for diagnosis. Other suggestive symptoms are: constipation, feces with an abnormal form, dyspepsia, hemorrhages, mucus, anemia; but only after a time the patient will deteriorate. The diagnosis depends on rectosigmoidoscopy and roentgenological examination.

Surgery is the final outcome in most instances, either immediate, or following some initial procedures, or together with appropriate chemotherapy. Pain, when present, mostly requires the use of morphine.

> Morphine sulfate, 10 or 15 mg, by subcutaneous injection, repeated as needed and tolerated.

Whenever possible, instead of morphine, or as an alternate, other drugs might be tried.

> Meperidine, 100 mg, by subcutaneous injection, every 4 hours, or as needed and tolerated.

> Codeine, 60 mg, by subcutaneous injection, every 4 hours, or as needed and tolerated.

Intestinal Occlusion. Occasionally, the first symptom of sigmoid cancer is a bout of intestinal occlusion, or the occlusion may be due to a strangulated hernia, volvulus, or fecal impaction in the terminal portion of the colon. Intestinal occlusion will give, in the great majority of cases, the clinical picture of "acute abdomen," but it should always be kept in mind that the symptoms may only be of subacute intensity with not too marked pain in the left iliac fossa.

Acute organic intestinal obstruction has been reviewed above (see the section on acute abdominal pain), where the use of meperidine, codeine, or papaverine hydrochloride was advised, together with other adequate measures, before surgery is performed. When the situation is not acute, these medications can be tried before operation.

> Meperidine, 100 mg, by subcutaneous injection, every 4 to 6 hours.

Codeine, 60 mg, by intramuscular injection, every 4 to 6 hours.

Papaverine hydrochloride, 60 to 100 mg, by intramuscular injection, every 4 to 6 hours.

If the problem refers to a paralytic ileus, particularly post-surgery, instead of the above drugs food restriction will be ordered; and if the symptoms are severe enough, the restriction will be total, and gastrointestinal suction will be started. In this instance, intravenous infusions are needed, and the patient will be referred to the surgeon for evaluation and action. Paralytic ileus due to injuries, infections, metabolic derangements, etc., requires the additional treatment of the causative factor. It is not to be forgotten that in the case of paralytic ileus the main symptoms are pain, distension, and absence of sounds.

Hypogastric Pain

Any of the diseases discussed in the foregoing lines may accompany an inferiorly located pain, but true hypogastric pain is mainly due to diseases of the urinary bladder or the prostate.

Cystitis. Pain in the hypogastrium together with frequent and urgent urination are typical indications of cystitis. The condition may be either acute or chronic, in the first instance associated with chills and fever. The second diagnostic step is to disclose the causative factor: gonococcus, *Escherichia coli*, tuberculosis, cancer, and others. Pus in the two glasses used for collecting urine is suggestive of cystitis. For a more accurate diagnosis, specialized urologic techniques are needed. Terminal hematuria is also a sign of cystitis, but plain hematuria will suggest cancer. Bladder irritability is also suggestive of hypertrophy of the prostate. Urinary retention is frequently accompanied by pain and tenderness in the hypogastrium. The dilated hard bladder is felt on palpation. This is one of the first symptoms of an enlarged prostate.

The basic treatment is that of the bacterial cause by specific antibiotherapy, including chemotherapeutic agents more adequate for use against urinary infections (rapidly excreted sulfonamides, nitrofurantoin, methenamine mandelate, etc.). The following medications have a particularly soothing effect on cystitis pains.

Trimethoprin, 160 mg, plus sulfamethoxazole, 800 mg, by mouth, every 12 hours, for no more than 10 or 14 days.

Methylene blue, 65 to 130 mg, by mouth, every 8 hours (warn about discoloration of urine and staining of clothes).

Phenazopyridine hydrochloride, 200 mg, by mouth, every 8 hours (warn about discoloration of urine and staining of clothes).

Sulfisoxazole, 500 mg, tablets; six to eight tablets at once, then two to four tablets every 4 to 6 hours until temperature is normal for 48 hours.

In addition, antispasmodics are also helpful for the irritated urinary mucosa.

Tincture of belladonna, 10 to 20 drops, in water, every 4 to 6 hours.

Atropine, 0.5 mg, tablets; half or one tablet, every 4 to 6 hours.

Sedatives are frequently welcomed by patients.

Prostate. There is a group of characteristic symptoms suggesting prostatic lesions: abnormal micturition, hypogastric and perineal pain together with a sensation of pressure, symptoms of cystitis (see above), and other general signs depending on the extension of the lesions. In the case of inflammatory changes (prostatitis) there may be fever. In prostatic adenoma the symptoms are milder (dysuria, nocturnal erections, etc.). In prostatic cancer the symptoms are not present for long periods, though hematuria might be among the early symptoms.

When pain is present because of chronic prostatitis, it may be treated as for cystitis (see above), since it is usually due to this cause. Prostatic massage, repeated twice a month, may also be of help. The rest of the treatment should be carried out by a urologist.

Gynecologic diseases might cause hypogastric pain. For diagnosis and treatment see, in the following pages, the section devoted entirely to gynecologic diseases.

Diseases of the Circulatory System

Aneurism of the Abdominal Aorta. A pulsating mass may be the only symptom of aneurism, but it is not rare that there is pain in the medial segment of the abdomen. The pain may radiate or be referred to the back or the groin and pudendal parts. Also, the pulsating mass may or may not be tender on palpation; when tender, ordinarily it is fixed and not movable. Because most of these aneurisms are atherosclerotic in nature, they are easily visualized in the X-ray film.

Pain is felt by many patients with aortic aneurism, particularly if it is of the dissecting type. Surgical treatment is the most rewarding therapeutic approach, and with the facilities available in some highly specialized centers results are good. Cases with normal blood pressure may benefit from the use of propanolol hydrochloride.

>   Propanolol hydrochloride, 20 mg, by mouth, every 6 hours.

>   Propanolol hydrochloride, 1 mg (1 ml) or 2 mg (2 ml)
>   by intramuscular injection, every 6 hours.

Patients with elevated blood pressure will be treated to reduce the hypertension if after study of the various factors involved it seems likely to be of benefit.

Aneurism of the Iliac Arteries. The obvious aneurismatic symptomatology is plain to see: a pulsating mass in either the right or the left iliac fossa, which does not suggest relationship with the digestive system. There is an intense pain radiating to the corresponding muscle.

For treatment, see above.

Occlusion of the Pelvic Arteries. This episode starts with severe pain, with numbness of the lower limbs and lack of pulsations with changes of color of the sites, depending on the obstructed blood supply. In case of doubt, the help of a specialist will be required.

The treatment for occlusion of arteries is largely surgical. As palliative remedies—only for prevention and amelioration of effects—vasodilators may be given to soothe pain and increase the nutrition of tissues suffering from slow occlusion.

>   Papaverine hydrochloride, 60 to 100 mg, by intramuscular
>   injection, every 6 hours.

>   Nylidrin hydrochloride, 6 mg, tablets; one or two every
>   6 hours (or 8 hours).

>   Nicotinic acid, 50 mg, tablets; one, two, or three every
>   8, 12, or 24 hours.

>   Isoxsuprine hydrochloride, 10 or 20 mg, tablets; one or two
>   every 6 to 8 hours.

Cyclandelate, 200 mg, tablets, every 6 hours, before meals and at bedtime.

Thrombosis of the Pelvic Veins. This venous lesion does not cause spontaneous pain, but is revealed by tenderness on palpation, together with fever, if inflammation of some significance is present.

The two main steps in treating thrombosis of the pelvic veins are anticoagulant therapy and surgery whenever possible. No efforts should be made for an isolated control of pain.

Diseases of Metabolism

Diabetic Acidosis. In diabetic acidosis, abdominal pain (sometimes leading to the erroneous diagnosis of "acute abdomen") is extremely frequent. This occurs in a known (rarely an unknown) diabetic patient who slowly deteriorates, and then appears extremely ill, with dry and flushed skin (important symptom), breath with acetone odor (also, an important symptom), and with exaggerated hyperglycemia and decreased CO_2 combining power of the plasma (which are diagnostic).

In diabetic acidosis, pain may be extremely severe, or only a moderate dull discomfort. Regardless of its nature, no direct treatment for pain is advisable; but antidiabetic therapy should be started and a diabetologist called immediately. First make a thorough test of the urine (sugar, albumin, diacetic acid, acetone), draw blood for laboratory procedures (glucose, cholesterol, SGOT, BUN, electrolytes), and inject in the vein 50 units of regular insulin, particularly if there is any suspicion of circulatory collapse. With some extra 50 units injected subcutaneously, the initial 100 units required will be completed. Thereafter, repeat 75 to 100 units subcutaneously every hour until the symptoms and the blood and urine chemistry have impoved; then, decrease the amount of insulin, to reach a 24-hour amount of 200 to 700 units. At times, much larger amounts are needed! Also, intravenous infusions will start promptly with hypotonic saline and sodium bicarbonate. The rest is up to the specialist.

Hypoglycemia. In rare occasions, epigastric pain may accompany hypoglycemic crises, but it is not diagnostic, not even suggestive of diagnosis. Other signs and symptoms of hypoglycemia are to be considered and confirmed with the finding of low levels of blood glucose. Other symptoms are: sweating, tremor, weakness, behavioral changes, dizziness, convulsions, and even coma.

No analgesia is needed. The objective is a rapid restoration of blood sugar concentration, which is easily achieved with sugar. Most cases who fall under the present classification are still alert enough to swallow a few spoonfuls or lumps of sucrose (plain sugar), honey, or candy, or to drink fruit juices and sweet beverages. It must always be remembered that all persons subject to hypoglycemic attacks (insulin users, patients with hyperinsulinism) must carry lumps of sugar with them at all times, to be taken at the first warning. If the patient is not able to drink or swallow, give an intravenous injection of dextrose.

> Dextrose, 25% solution (1 g = 4 ml); inject intravenously 40 ml (10 g) or 80 ml (20 g).

Refer the patient to an endocrinologist or a diabetologist.

Diseases of the Urinary System

Pyelitis and Pyelonephritis. An acute differentiation between pyelitis and pyelonephritis is rarely accepted on clinical grounds, because in what could be considered a pure pyelitis there is almost always involvement of the renal tissue. Many cases are secondary to a previous infection, others follow a pregnancy, and only rarely the primary infective foci are unknown. The main symptoms are dysuria and frequent urination; the urine is turbid, with pus; chills and fever occur; and abdominal pain is felt in the corresponding flank, with or without radiation to the pudendal parts. Pain may be dull or show acute crises; also the general symptoms may be more or less marked or even absent (in these last cases, pyuria is the only symptom). Tenderness is found in the corresponding costovertebral region. Some abdominal rigidity may be present in more acute cases, and there may be felt an enlarged renal mass. Chronic cases may run prolonged courses, even for years, with occasional recrudescence of more acute symptoms with practically an asymptomatic interval between the crises. Pyuria is characteristic in all instances; X-ray pictures are revealing only when dilatation of the renal pelvis occurs.

Specific antimicrobial therapy will be carried out in each case. To alleviate pain, advise bed rest, force ingestion of fluids (even give intravenous infusions whenever needed), and prescribe any of the following drugs:

> Acetylsalicylic acid, 600 mg, in tablets, every 4 to 6 hours, preferably with meals.

Acetaminophen, 600 mg, by mouth, every 6 hours.

Acetophenetidin, 300 mg, by mouth, every 4 to 6 hours.

The patient should be sent to a urologist for evaluation, since surgical procedures are needed at times.

Hydronephrosis. In hydronephrosis almost always a tumor is felt on palpation. The tumor may or may not provoke some discomfort as dull abdominal pain; and may or may not be constantly present, because it may disappear between the crises of pain (Dietl's crises). Fever and pyuria may be concomitant symptoms, particularly the latter. The diagnosis depends on the recurrence of Dietl's crises or the persistent tumor with some discomfort in the corresponding flank, and on radiologic studies and other urologic examinations (ureteral reflux, rapid drip from a ureteral catheter).

Treatment of pain in cases of hydronephrosis is a very minor thing. Either codeine or papaverine can be used, but employment of any such drug will be occasional, since while the obstruction is present, there is always the threat of impairment of renal function.

Codeine, 30 or 60 mg, by mouth, every 6 to 8 hours.

Papaverine hydrochloride, 150 mg, in slow-release capsules, one every 12 hours.

The patient must be referred immediately to a urologist for further treatment.

Perirenal Abscess. In most instances of perirenal abscess there is dull pain in the corresponding flank, but pain may be either acute or absent. There is also pain, and tenderness, in the costovertebral region. Muscle rigidity may be present. The general syndrome of fever may be present, and a mass may be palpated. When the abscess irritates the psoas muscle, there is some flexion of the leg upon the body. X-ray examination adds more diagnostic evidence (the kidney shows less mobility, and its shadow is obliterated).

Pain will be treated with analgesics of the type of codeine, methylene blue, or phenazopyridine hydrochloride.

Codeine, 60 mg, by mouth, every 4 hours.

Methylene blue, 65 or 130 mg, by mouth, every 8 hours (inform about discoloration of urine and staining of clothes).

Phenazopyridine hydrochloride, 200 mg, by mouth, every
8 hours (inform about discoloration of urine and staining
of clothes).

Anticholinergic or parasympathomimetic drugs, of the type of atropine and its compounds and derivatives, may also be of help.

Tincture of belladonna, 15 to 30 drops in water, every 4
to 8 hours, according to tolerance.

Atropine sulfate, 0.5 mg, tablets; half or one tablet every
8 hours, according to tolerance.

These patients should be referred to the urologist as soon as possible, since the basic treatment depends on the adequate selection of the antimicrobial therapy and the indicated surgical procedures.

Kidney Abscess. This is also known as renal carbuncle or cortical abscess. The symptoms are identical with symptoms of perinephritic abscess (q.v.). The diagnosis may be made by pyelography, showing distortion of the calyces.

As is done for perirenal abscesses, in the case of abscess of the kidney the patient should be referred to the urologist at the earliest possible moment, because the basic treatment here also depends on the adequate selection of drugs to combat the infection or to protect surgical procedures. To allay pain, on a temporary basis, the following may be used:

Methylene blue, 65 or 130 mg, by mouth, every 8 hours
(inform of discoloration of the urine and staining of
clothes).

Phenazopyridine hydrochloride, 200 mg, by mouth, every
8 hours (inform of discoloration of the urine and staining
of clothes).

Codeine, 60 mg, by mouth, every 4 hours.

Parasympathomimetic drugs (anticholinergics) can also be used.

Tincture of belladonna, 15 to 30 drops, in water, every
4 to 8 hours, according to individual tolerance.

Atropine sulfate, 0.5 mg, tablets; half or one tablet every
8 hours, according to individual tolerance.

Movable Kidney. A movable kidney will not produce any substantial symptomatology per se, except intermittent hydronephrotic crises (q.v.) and the possible palpation of the movable organ. Some cases will refer a dull, vague abdominal pain.

Viscerae which can be easily displaced from their normal position do need surgical fixation as the only solution to the problem. At times, pain may be felt and help requested; but since in many instances this complaint is mainly psychological, before injecting an analgesic give a placebo, such as the injection of sterile water. If it does not work, give the following medication:

> Meperidine, 100 mg, by subcutaneous injection; follow with same dose by mouth every 4 hours.

> Morphine sulfate, 10 or 15 mg, by subcutaneous injection; of half the dose by the intravenous route, if so needed; follow with meperidine by mouth, as stated above.

Tuberculosis of the Kidney. Dull pain is very frequently felt in the area of the diseased kidney (flank and costovertebral region). The outstanding symptom is frequency with terminal painful dysuria. The diagnosis depends on urine cultures (should be repeated, if negative) and the X-ray film showing the characteristic moth-eaten areas together with the irregularly narrowed and dilated ureters.

The basic care for tuberculosis of the kidney depends on a long-standing antituberculous drugs administration and performance of any form of needed surgery. Treatment of pain is a serious problem for the patient. Use for this purpose any of the following.

> Codeine, 60 mg by mouth, every 6 to 8 hours.

> Meperidine, 50 (or 100) mg by mouth, every 4 to 6 hours.

> Propoxyphene hydrochloride, 65 mg, by mouth, every 6 hours.

Cancer of the Kidney. Dull pain in the corresponding flank is associated with a palpable mass, hematuria (the most important symptom) that on occasion may provoke colicky pain because of clot formation, and fever. Radiologic studies are essential for diagnosis (irregular shape, distortion, displacement). Surgery may be both diagnostic and curative or, at least, palliative.

As usual, chemotherapy and surgery are the essentials of the treatment. Allaying pain is only a palliative measure.

> Morphine sulfate, 10 to 15 mg, by subcutaneous injection, repeated as needed and tolerated.

Meperidine, 100 mg, by subcutaneous injection, every 4 to 6 hours, as needed and tolerated.

Codeine, 60 mg, by subcutaneous injection, every 4 to 6 hours, as needed and tolerated.

Polycystic Kidneys. Suggestive symptoms are: pain located in one or both flanks and costovertebral areas, either dull and constant or of an intermittent colicky character; palpation of a tumor, sometimes giving the impression of a bunch of grapes; and hematuria. When the findings are bilateral, the diagnosis of polycystic kidneys is easier; otherwise pyelograms are needed for better accuracy.

There is very little to do relating to polycystic kidneys, except to protect against infection, or to treat it if it develops, and to treat hypertension whenever it appears. Pain in the flanks is only episodic and not always intense enough to command special care. If necessary, it can be treated with any of the following drugs:

Papaverine hydrochloride, 150 mg, in slow-release capsules, one every 12 hours.

Codeine, 60 mg, by mouth, every 4 to 6 hours.

Meperidine, 50 to 100 mg, by mouth, every 4 to 6 hours.

Propoxyphene hydrochloride, 65 mg, by mouth, every 6 hours.

Renal Lithiasis. A dull, constant pain in the corresponding flank is suggestive of lithiasis when there is an evident history of renal colics or the pain follows a recent attack. The diagnosis depends on radiography.

Not all patients with renal stones suffer agonizing colic, but they may complain of backaches. These are due to impacted stones or infection. The treatment, therefore, has to be surgical or dependant on antimicrobial drugs. Nevertheless, discomfort may be allayed with the following drugs.

Codeine, 60 mg, by mouth, every 4 to 6 hours.

Papaverine hydrochloride, 150 mg, in slow-release capsules, one every 12 hours.

Propoxyphene hydrochloride, 65 mg, by mouth, every 6 hours.

252 DIAGNOSIS AND TREATMENT

If the pain is not relieved with the above or similar drugs, before giving morphine try pentazocine hydrochloride.

>   Pentazocine hydrochloride, 50 mg, tablets; one every 4 hours.

Adrenal Tumors. Although this is not, exactly, a disease of the urinary system, it is placed here for anatomical reasons. These tumors are rare, and pain is ordinarily very mild. The main symptomatology is endocrinological in nature, and the diagnosis is made by visualization of an enlarged adrenal by radiology.

Nonmalignant tumors of the adrenal glands will rarely need help for pain. If they do, any analgesic can be used as a palliative measure.

>   Acetylsalicylic acid, 300 or 600 mg, in tablets, every 4 to 6 hours, preferably with meals.
>
>   Acetophenetidin, 300 mg, by mouth, every 4 to 6 hours.
>
>   Acetaminophen, 600 mg, by mouth, every 6 hours.
>
>   Codeine, 60 (or 30) mg, by mouth, every 4 to 6 hours.

The choice of the treatment depends on whether the tumor is a functioning gland or not.

Gynecologic Diseases

Dysmenorrhea. Only rarely, dysmenorrheic pains will provoke symptoms of "acute abdomen" (q.v.). Ordinarily, menstrual pains, in spite of being cramplike, are moderate or even mild. The location is in the hypogastric region, and the occasion is the menstrual period, either the hours preceding the menstrual flow or during the already established menstruation. The duration may vary from a few hours to several days.

Among women, this is one of the most common pains of which they complain. Of course, the basic treatment depends on the evaluation of its cause, and that, in turn, will decide what will be effective against the pain. Considering premenstrual tension as an early stage of dysmenorrhea, we may say here that in most instances common analgesics will be of sufficient help.

>   Acetylsalicylic acid, 600 mg, every 4 hours, in tablets; preferably with meals.
>
>   Acetaminophen, 600 mg, by mouth, every 6 hours.

Codeine, 60 mg, by mouth, every 4 to 6 hours.

Propoxyphene hydrochloride, 65 mg, by mouth, every 6 hours.

If these do not work, sodium restriction and diuretic agents can be added, or used by themselves.

Chlorothiazide, 500 mg, by mouth, every 8 to 12 hours.

Hydrochlorothiazide, 50 or 100 mg, by mouth, every 12 hours.

Acetazolamide, 250 mg a day, by mouth, in divided doses.

The above regimen is advised to start a few days (about 1 week) before the expected menstruation. When dysmenorrhea appears after the first menstruation, it is preferable to use one of the following drugs:

Codeine, 30 or 60 mg, by mouth, every 4 to 6 hours.

Tincture of belladonna, 10 to 20 drops, in water, every 4 to 6 hours, according to tolerance.

Atropine, 0.5 mg, tablets; half or one tablet (according to effect and tolerance), every 4 to 6 hours.

Papaverine hydrochloride, 150 mg, in slow-release capsules, one every 12 hours.

When menstrual pain persists for more periods than expected, a consultation with an endocrinologist or a gynecologist is advisable, particularly if it resists additional trials with hormonotherapy. Also, this holds true for dysmenorrhea appearing later in life. Keep in mind recent warnings against the use of these hormones.

Conjugated estrogens, about 1 mg a day, for 20 days preceding the expected menstruation; together with:

Ethisteron, 10 to 20 mg a day, for the last 10 days of the preceding cycle; or:

Hydroxyprogesterone, 2.5 mg a day, the last 10 days of the estrogen cycle as listed above.

Abortion. Intermittent abdominal pain associated with vaginal bleeding in a known pregnant woman is suggestive of abortion. The symptoms will progress and increase in cases of imminent and inevitable abortion.

This is a condition to be treated by a gynecologist, who will be called immediately. The only help to be offered, while he takes care of the case, is to start antibiotic therapy, in the case of infection, or to start treatment with progesterone (or its derivatives) if deficient corpus luteum function is suspected. Also, sedation should be offered to these patients. No serious effort should be made to treat pain itself.

Adnexitis. Inflammation of the adnexa uteri may provoke both acute and chronic syndromes. The acute syndromes have been discussed in the section on "Acute Abdomen" (q.v.). Chronic diseases of the adnexa will cause a more or less moderate pain in the corresponding iliac fossa, with little or no muscle rigidity. Tenderness on palpation, which is better elicited and detected on bimanual palpation, will also detect an enlarged tube or ovary. There will be increased dysmenorrhea and symptoms of fever. If there is a suppuration, most probably some remittance will be found and the fever will adopt the characteristic spiked curve. The second stage of diagnosis, as in all infective diseases of this sort, is to determine the causative factor (gonococcal, tuberculosis, streptococcal). In gonococcal salpingitis there is a greeninsh leukorrhea and intense pain. Streptococcal salpingitis is usually a consequence of septic abortions. Tuberculosis of the adnexa gives very mild local symptoms.

Surgery and antibiotics are essential for the treatment of salpingitis (including tuberculous salpingitis). The first step will be to delay menstruation with a contraceptive pill.

> Norethindrone plus mestranol tablets, one a day.

Then, treat pain with regular analgesics.

> Codeine, 60 mg by subcutaneous injection, one every 6 hours, or as needed and tolerated.

> Meperidine, 100 mg by subcutaneous injection, one every 6 hours, or as needed and tolerated.

Finally, start antibiotic therapy and refer the patient to the gynecologist for evaluation of the desirability of surgery.

Ovarian Cysts. Ovarian cysts produce mild, dull pain in the corresponding iliac fossa. The symptoms may be tumoral or of an endocrine nature.

Follicular cysts commonly disappear in about 2 months. If pain disturbs, give diathermy and administer progesterone.

> Progesterone, 50 mg, by intramuscular injection, once a day, for 10 days.

Also, analgesics can be added to the treatment.

> Acetylsalicylic acid, 600 mg, in tablets, every 4 to 6 hours, preferably with meals.
>
> Codeine, 60 mg, by mouth, every 4 to 6 hours.

Luteal cysts also disappear in about 2 months, and the only treatment they need is the use of analgesics as stated above. Severe pain ordinarily points to more important complications requiring surgery. Other types of cysts are also dependent on surgery, and will be referred to the gynecologist.

Ovarian Cancer. There may be a dull pain in the corresponding iliac fossa, but it is of no diagnostic help. Most frequently, it is a metastasis from a cancer located in the digestive system.

Ovarian cancer is always the subject of surgical removal. The pain is not severe and usually responds to regular analgesics.

> Codeine, 60 mg, by subcutaneous injection or by mouth, every 4 to 6 hours.
>
> Meperidine, 100 mg, by mouth, every 4 to 6 hours.

Ectopic Pregnancy. In rare instances, symptoms similar to those of adnexitis may exist before rupture of an ectopic pregnancy. The diagnosis may be difficult, except for the data of missed menstruations preceding symptoms of adnexial involvement: there is no increase of the uterine volume, but there are an enlarged adnexum and a positive pregnancy test.

Surgery is the only treatment. The gynecologist should be called immediately. Blood replacement will be done whenever necessary: start blood infusions and give some sedation.

Diseases of the Osteomuscular System

Osteitis and Periostitis. Very rarely, the inflammation of the iliac bone will be the clinical picture of an infective process in the iliac fossa (appendicitis, diverticulitis).

Infections of the bones may affect locally the bone structure or only the periostium, but in any instance the logical approach is the same as stated for osteomyelitis. The basic treatment consists of the use of proper antibiotic therapy and the performance of adequate surgery. Treatment of pain is only a minor part of the problem.

> Acetylsalicylic acid, 600 mg, in tablets, every 4 to 6 hours, preferably with meals.

Acetophenetidin, 300 mg, by mouth, every 4 to 6 hours.

Acetaminophen, 600 mg by mouth, every 6 hours.

Tumors of the Iliac Fossa. Bone tumors, like sarcomas, chondromas, etc., are also rare diseases and may bring on a dull pain in the corresponding iliac fossa. The tumor is detected on palpation and confirmed radiologically.

Benign tumors which reach a size sufficient to cause pain, or malignant tumors, have to be removed. But, in the meantime, proper analgesia should be offered to the patient, ranging from common analgesics to narcotics.

Codeine, 60 mg, by subcutaneous injection or by mouth, as needed, every 4 or 6 hours.

Propoxyphene hydrochloride, 65 mg, by mouth, every 4 hours.

Meperidine, 100 mg, by subcutaneous injection or by mouth, as needed, every 4 to 6 hours.

Morphine sulfate, 10 to 15 mg, by subcutaneous injection, as needed and tolerated.

Floating Ribs. The floating ribs of thin, asthenic tall persons may incite a dull, vague pain in the epigastric region.

Rarely, this discomfort will require treatment; but, when needed, some support, as directed by the specialist, will be given. The use of common analgesics may also help.

Codeine, 60 mg, by mouth, every 4 to 6 hours.

Papaverine hydrochloride, 150 mg, in slow-release capsules, one every 12 hours.

Spondylitis. Either tuberculous or rheumatic spondylitis may cause pain radiating to the iliac fossae. The symptomatic complex may be similar to other infective diseases of the corresponding side (if radiation is unilateral); but there are other symptoms of a spondylitic nature that will help to establish the correct diagnosis, particularly with the help of radiography.

Each type of spondylitis—ankylosing, degenerative, etc.—will receive the adequate care for the individual disease. The abdominal pain referred to by some patients has to be treated only symptomatically, with analgesics or with antispasmodic drugs.

Acetylsalicylic acid, 300 or 600 mg, in tablets, every 4 to 6 hours, preferably with meals.

Codeine, 60 mg, by mouth, every 4 to 6 hours.

Tincture of belladonna, 10 to 30 drops, in water, as needed and tolerated.

Papaverine hydrochloride, 150 mg, in slow-release capsules, one every 12 hours.

Psoitis. Only exceptionally, psoitis will be an independent clinical feature. Ordinarily, it is a complication secondary to a perinephritic abscess, appendicitis, adrenal tuberculosis, and most frequently tuberculous spondylitis. There is pain in one or both of the iliac fossae, either spontaneous or on palpation, and there may even be some muscle rigidity. A typical position of the leg will reveal inflammation of the psoas: the leg is both flexed and abducted, and the patient walks bent forward. The diagnosis is made by the superimposition of psoitic symptoms to those of the primary disease.

When there is an infection of the psoas muscle, most commonly it is the consequence of an infection from the spine, ordinarily tubercular in nature. The infection has to be treated with chemotherapy and surgery, as needed. But some help will be given by analgesics.

Codeine, 60 mg, by mouth, every 4 hours.

Papaverine hydrochloride, 150 mg, in slow-release capsules, one every 12 hours.

Meperidine, 100 mg, by mouth, every 4 hours.

Poisoning

When we were discussing poisoning capable of causing "acute abdomen" symptoms, a series of substances was mentioned, which may also prompt less acute symptoms of abdominal pain. To the formerly discussed substances (q.v.), the following may be added.

Ammonia (gas). Abdominal pain, mucosal irritation, cough, and even pulmonary edema are symptoms. Shock or convulsions may also ensue.

Do not ever use narcotic analgesics with these patients. For the pain following gastrointestinal irritation give weak acid solution, like that of citrus fruit. The rest of the treatment will be to prevent or cure pulmonary edema (artificial respiration, oxygen therapy under positive pressure, etc.) and to wash the eyes with water.

Benzene. Benzene and related substances (gasoline, kerosene, etc.) cause stomach pain, headache, cold skin, tremors, and a state of drunkeness.

If the substance is inhaled, give fresh air or oxygen therapy, and if there is pain, give morphine.

> Morphine sulfate, 15 mg, by subcutaneous injection, repeated if needed.

If it is swallowed, give also morphine for pain, gastric lavage (not if it is inhaled), artificial respiration (oxygen therapy), and other measures that may arise in individual cases. In benzene poisoning emetics and sympathomimetics are contraindicated.

Bismuth. Symptoms are abdominal pain associated with other gastrointestinal symptoms, headache, and fever. A characteristic bismuth stomatitis will help in diagnosing this poisoning.

Analgesics can be used for pain, but always by injection.

> Codeine, 30 or 60 mg, by subcutaneous injection, repeated as needed and individually tolerated.

> Meperidine (with caution), 50 or 100 mg, by subcutaneous injection, repeated as needed and individually tolerated.

These patients also need gastric lavage, cardiac and respiratory stimulation, and in severe cases dimercaprol.

> Dimercaprol, 3 to 5 mg for each kg of body weight, by intramuscular injection, starting with shots every 4 hours; the third day, every 6 hours; thereafter, to complete about 10 days of therapy, now with one injection every 12 hours.

Bromates, Nitrates, and Chlorates cause abdominal pains associated with other digestive symptoms, including diarrhea and jaundice. There are also headache, hypotension, anuria, dyspnea, collapse, delirium, and coma with or without convulsions.

Pain may be severe enough to require the use of morphine.

> Morphine sulfate, 10 or 15 mg, by subcutaneous injection, repeated as needed and tolerated.

Remove the poison from the stomach (gastric lavage, emetics). If methemoglobinemia develops, give blood transfusions.

Caffeine. Symptoms are abdominal pain associated with insomnia, restlessness, headache, tremors, palpitation, tachycardia with irregular pulse, convulsions, and possibly collapse.

If pain is severe, morphine might be needed to allay discomfort. (See prescription above.) Short-acting barbiturates are to be given intravenously in the great majority of cases.

Sodium pentobarbital, 300 mg, by intravenous injection.

If the patient is seen within half an hour of the ingestion of caffeine, gastric lavage will be performed, or emetics will be given. If collapse supervenes, give intravenous supportive fluids.

Cantharides. Symptoms are burning pain in the stomach, blisters in the mouth, dyspepsia, and a severe gastroenteritis. Delirium, tetanic convulsions, and coma may also occur.

The pain provoked by the ensuing severe gastroenteritis will be treated with morphine (see above, for prescription). To remove as much poison as possible, give apomorphine by injection, but do not use a different emetic or stomach tubing.

Apomorphine, 5 mg, by subcutaneous injection.

The rest of the treatment should follow the accepted lines for this kind of poisoning.

Carbon Tetrachloride. When swallowed, it provokes abdominal pain associated with headache, mental confusion, dysarthria, dilated pupils, and jaundice after a few days.

No efforts are required to treat pain—which is not always severe. Remove the patient from the site of exposure and give oxygen therapy. Other measures will be carried out as generally accepted and advised.

Colchicin causes gastric pain, vomiting, diarrhea, hematuria, prostration, then convulsions, and finally paralysis.

As soon as the diagnosis is made, induce vomiting or give a gastric lavage, followed immediately by a cathartic. Give oxygen, and treat the oliguria present in most cases. When these measures are applied, there is very little need of analgesia.

Digitalis. Symptoms are abdominal pain, headache, dilated pupils with disordered vision, protruding eyeballs, violent heart beats with extrasystoles, lethargy, and convulsions. An electrocardiogram may solve the diagnosis (digitalis intoxication pattern).

No direct efforts will be made to treat abdominal pain, which is not too severe in most instances. Immediately after the poison is swallowed, gastric lavage will be made or emetics given. Absorption can be delayed by giving milk or activated charcoal before the lavage. Potassium is the best antidote.

Potassium chloride, 2 g in water, every hour, by mouth, until the electrocardiogram shows improvement or potassium intoxication supervenes.

> Potassium chloride, 15% (2 mEq/ml) or 22.3% (3 mEq/ml) diluted and injected intravenously, 10 to 15 mEq every hour, also monitored as above.

The patient should be referred immediately to a heart specialist.

Formaldehyde. Symptoms are gastric pain with bloody vomiting on occasion, irritation of the gastrointestinal tract, and final collapse and coma.

If it is inhaled, give fresh air or oxygen therapy, and ammonia vapors (with care). If it is swallowed, give ammonia water, probably the best drug.

> Ammonia, 0.2% solution in water, to take 240 ml.

When this is not readily available, give milk or egg white, followed as soon as possible by gastric lavage with ammonia.

> Ammonia, 0.1% solution, q.s.

Acidosis, if present, requires intravenous infusion of bicarbonate or sodium lactate. No other efforts to treat pain are required.

Gasoline and Kerosene. See "Benzene," above.

Phosphorus. Symptoms include pain from an extensive gastrointestinal irritation; garlic-smelling, bloody vomitus (with phosphoric luminescence in the dark); and bloody diarrhea.

Emesis is to be induced by means of tap water, a half or one liter, repeated at least three times. Following the lavages, give sodium sulfate and liquid petrolatum.

> Sodium sulfate, 30 g in 200 ml of water.

> Petrolatum, liquid, 120 ml.

Instead of plain water for emesis, a solution of copper sulfate can be used.

> Copper sulfate, 0.2% solution, half a liter, for repeated gastric lavage.

If pain still continues after the lavage and administration of sodium sulfate and petrolatum, morphine can be given.

> Morphine sulfate, 15 mg, by subcutaneous injection.

The rest of the treatment will follow according to established rules.

Thallium salts may cause abdominal pain, neuritis with paresthesias and paralysis, characteristic alopecia, dyspnea, and convulsions.

The gastric irritation may be relieved by gastric lavage with iodides.

> Sodium iodide, 1% solution, for gastric lavage.
>
> Potassium iodide, 1% solution, for gastric lavage.

Emetics can also be given, followed by activated charcoal. The rest of the treatment will be according to established rules (intravenous infusion of sodium iodide, and chelating agents—sodium diethyldithiocarbamate or diphenylthiocarbazone—given by mouth, as suggested recently).

Turpentine Oil. Symptoms are extensive gastrointestinal irritation with pain, vomiting, diarrhea, painful urination, characteristic odor of breath and urine, dilated pupils, and coma.

Pain can be treated by subcutaneous injection of morphine.

> Morphine sulfate, 15 mg, by subcutaneous injection, repeated as needed and tolerated.

Perform a gastric lavage or give emetics. Also, give copious amounts of water and sodium sulfate.

> Sodium sulfate, 30 g, in water.

Nephritis has to be treated in most instances.

XII. LIMBS

Pain in the limbs results from a great number of diseases and injuries, is a frequent complaint presented by patients, and at times is a challenge to the diagnostician. For the purpose of clarity, two main sections will be included here: one, for the upper limbs, including shoulders, arms, and hands; the other, for the lower limbs, including hips, legs, and feet. Each of these sections will consider articular, muscular, and vascular pain, pain in the bones, neural structures, and heterotopic pain; plus pain in the shoulder and elbow for the upper limbs and pain in the feet for the lower.

PAIN IN THE SHOULDERS, ARMS, AND HANDS

Articular Pain

Any joint may be affected by arthritic or rheumatic pains. Perhaps, the most frequently affected, or at least, the joints that provoke more complaints from the patients, are those corresponding to shoulders, arms, and hands. But the most important and disabling arthropathies are those corresponding to the inferior limbs, which have to bear the weight of the whole body, and thus become more easily injured.

Arthritis. The invasion of a joint by gonococci or tubercle bacilli, which are the most frequent invaders (others may also be etiological factors, such as staphylococcus, streptococcus, pneumococcus, etc.), will cause symptoms similar to those of rheumatism. The main one is acute arthritis in a joint that becomes red, hot, and swollen. In tuberculous arthritis the symptoms are confined to one joint and show a chronic course. In gonococcal arthritis, there is a previous urethritis, and the local symptoms are intense and occur with fever and malaise. Other infective agents also cause acute together with systemic symptoms. The diagnosis is mainly made by isolation of the causative germ from the synovial fluid.

In the case of gouty arthritis, the local symptoms will refer mainly to the great toe, but tophi are found in any tendon, joint, or bursa. From longstanding, prominent tophi, discharge of urates may take place, particularly in the hands and feet. Symptomatology may show an acute or chronic course. The acute attack usually involves one joint; the pain reaches excruciating intensity (with shiny, red, hot, and tender skin), and may last a few days, at the beginning, but recur in a chronic form. Gout brings on limitation of movements and distortion of shape of the joint. The diagnosis is made by detection of high levels of uric acid in the blood (over 8 mg/100 ml) and the response to the use of colchicine internally.

Cases of acute septic arthritis will be treated with adequate antibiotic therapy, aspiration and irrigation of the infected joint, and drainage whenever it is indicated. These measures will allay pain; but it can be helped with immobilization (using splints, if necessary) and elevation of the joint, the application of hot compresses, and the use of analgesics.

> Acetylsalicylic acid, 600 mg, tablets, every 4 to 6 hours, preferably with meals.
>
> Propoxyphene hydrochloride, 65 mg, by mouth, every 4 hours.

In chronic septic arthritis, surgery and antibiotic therapy are the most important measures to be taken. The use of analgesics may help a little for the comfort of the patient. Use acetylsalicylic acid or propoxyphene hydrochloride, as above; or any other similar analgesic.

The treatment of gouty arthritis will be handled with more detail under the headings of "Articular Pain" and "Pain in the Feet," both in the section devoted to "Pain in the Hips, Legs, and Feet." Here we will summarize: keep weight within normal limits and avoid prolonged fastings and dehydration; use anti-gout agents, such as colchicine, sulfinpyrazone, allopurinol, phenylbutazone, indomethacin, and also ACTH or corticoids. Codeine or meperidine are to be given whenever needed.

Other forms of arthritic pains, like Reiter's syndrome, sarcoidosis, neurogenic, chondrocalcinosis, etc., have to be treated symptomatically, for pain or for the basic cause (also specifically, if such a treatment is available). In these cases, use acetylsalicylic acid, codeine, meperidine, propoxyphene hydrochloride, etc. (see above lines).

Rheumatoid arthritis. There is pain in several joints, all of them swollen and tender on palpation. In the adult type, smaller joints (fingers, wrists, feet) are affected more frequently than the larger joints (hips, shoulders, knees, elbows), the reverse of the juvenile type. Pain is worse after periods of inactivity. The muscles corresponding to the diseased joints are stiff, and the stronger flexors produce the characteristic cramped position of the affected parts. In the adult type, muscles become atrophied and give a noticeable fusiform shape to the fingers. In children, growth and general development are impaired.

Bed rest will be encouraged, but only to a limit, alternating with well-planned physical activity (progressive increase of exercises, to a reasonable working ability, always below the actual tolerance of the affected joints). Rest refers to bed rest (additional 4 to 8 hours, increasing the regular 8-hour night rest) and articular rest (with use of splints, etc., whenever advisable). Also, moist or radiant heat will help to relax muscles and allay pain. But the use of salicylates will be the initial cornerstone of therapy, before resorting to crysotherapy, corticoid therapy, or other drugs.

> Acetylsalicylic acid, 600 mg, tablets, every 4 hours; preferably after meals, and accompanied by a small daily dose of thyroid extract (15 to 30 mg a day, by mouth).
>
> Sodium salicylate, 600 mg, by mouth, as above.
>
> Sodium salicylate, larger doses; 1200 mg by mouth, every 4 to 6 hours, to increase to 2 g every 4 hours. Those who do not tolerate salicylates well should receive the help of antacids, to protect against local irritation (sodium bicarbonate, 300-mg tablets or the amount of

powder taken with the point of a knife); also, the use of small amounts of thyroid extract (30 mg a day) will increase tolerance in many cases.

Whenever the patient does not benefit from salicylates, corticoids will be tried next.

Prednisone, 5 to 10 mg every 6 hours. As soon as the patient improves, but not later than by 3 weeks, the dosage should be decreased, so that the compete treatment lasts for about 6 weeks, or less. Intra-articular injections (hydrocortisone, 25 to 50 mg) may be given.

If the use of corticoids is not beneficial for some patient who also does not benefit from salicylates, gold therapy might receive a trial.

Gold sodium thiomalate, in increasing dosages of 10, 25, 50, and 100 mg for each ml. To use 10 mg, once the first week; 25 mg, once the second week; thereafter, 50 mg once a week, to reach a total administration of 1 g (19 injections of 50 mg). If the response is good, decrease the dosage to 50 mg every 2 weeks; then, every three weeks; and finally maintain (tolerance permitting) 50 mg once a month for a long time.

Gold thioglucose (aurothioglucose), 10, 50, and 100 mg for each ml. To be used as above.

The use of antimalarials, phenylbutazone, indomethacin, and cytotoxic drugs will be evaluated by a specialist.

Degenerative arthritis. The joints are painful, but there is no involvement of muscles or swelling of the joints. This form of arthritis ordinarily begins after 40 years of age; the patients are mostly obese and do not complain of systemic symptoms.

Both the obese and the hyperactive patient should avoid unnecessary stress on the affected joints, or even have the aid of supportive devices. It also means that the obese must regain normal weight for age and height. Application of heat, locally, also helps. Orthopedic measures are needed, at times. The rest of the treatment will follow the same steps as for rheumatoid arthritis (q.v.).

Rheumatic fever. The articular symptoms, almost identical with rheumatoid arthritis, commonly follow a bout of pharyngitis and are associated with heart murmurs, precordial pain, arrhythmia, pericardial friction rub, and even heart failure. Some patients also show skin rashes or chorea. The detection of beta-hemolytic streptococci is an important diagnostic datum.

Salicylates are almost specific for rheumatic fever, and will be given from the very beginning of the disease, at an average dose in mild cases, or in large amounts in severe ones.

> Acetylsalicylic acid, 600 mg, tablets, every 4 hours, preferably with meals.

> Acetylsalicylic acid, larger doses; to start with 60 mg for each kg of body weight, in four or six doses given during the 24-hour period; to increase to 90, 120, and 180 mg for each kg of body weight, also in six divided doses during the day. The medication will be given with meals, whenever possible, or accompanied by sodium bicarbonate, 300-mg tablets or the amount of powder taken with the point of a knife. A small amount of thyroid extract (30 to 60 mg a day) may be given to increase tolerance.

Patients with rheumatic fever will also receive antibiotics (penicillin) and corticoids (prednisone), the latter to be replaced by salicylates if they prove ineffective after a trial of about 5 days. By this time, the patient should be treated by a specialist; but if care is needed, start corticoids immediately.

> Prednisone, 5 to 10 mg, by mouth, every 6 hours. After 3 weeks the dosage should be gradually decreased, to come to a total treatment of about 6 weeks. At times, higher doses are needed, up to 20 mg or even 40 mg every 6 hours; withdrawal will take a longer time.

Additional treatment, particularly in case of complications, will be advised by the specialist.

Muscular Pain

Bursitis. The inflammation of the bursae surrounding muscle tendons brings on very intense pain when the corresponding muscle is in motion and its tendon presses over its bursae. In acute bursitis, the symptoms appear suddenly, with pain, local tenderness, and limitation of movement. In chronic bursitis the symptoms are similar and the muscle becomes atrophic because of lack of exercise. The most frequently involved bursa is the subdeltoid, and the pain is referred to the shoulder. Pressure on the bursa causes pain.

Within the first few hours of the beginning of symptoms, radiotherapy usually gives very good results. Also, the early administration of corticoids will control symptoms rapidly in many instances.

> Prednisone, 5 mg, every 8 hours; decrease the dosage as soon as the effects are noted, and discontinue gradually over a period of 15 or 20 days.

For well-established cases, rest, immobilization, local heat applications, and the use of analgesics are needed:

> Acetylsalicylic acid, 600 mg, tablets, every 4 hours, preferably with meals.

> Codeine, 60 mg, by subcutaneous injection, every 6 hours; or by mouth, every 4 hours.

> Meperidine, 100 mg, by mouth, every 4 to 6 hours.

These patients also may need the intra-articular injection of corticoids.

> Hydrocortisone acetate, 25 mg in 1 ml, suspension; inject from 1 to 5 ml into the bursa.

Stress myalgia. A normal, healthy person may complain of stress myalgia ordinarily some hours (next day) after any strenuous or prolonged unaccustomed use of muscles. Pain will occur in the muscles used for that kind of exercise: arms and back after shoveling snow; legs and waist after climbing a mountain, etc. Perhaps the most frequent form of stress myalgia is that following exercising beyond present capability, as happens after the first day of a new variety of gymnastics. Rest, massage, heat applications, and the use of muscle relaxants together with analgesics will help.

> Meprobamate, 400 mg, by mouth, every 6 hours, for a total of 2 or 3 days.

> Acetylsalicylic acid, 600 mg, in tablets, every 4 or 6 hours, preferably with meals; for a total of 2 or 3 days.

Myositis. Muscle pain and inflammation are the common symptoms in trichinosis. There are initial gastrointestinal symptoms. Then, fever and edema of the eyelids. All muscles may be involved, but most frequently the abdominal muscles are. Suggestive, for diagnostic purpose, are an early eosinophilia and the history of ingestion of poorly cooked pork.

Several entities, not related to each other, can be included here, as follows:

Polymyositis will receive a basic treatment with corticoids and analgesics, as required, during the acute episodes of pain. Physical therapy is also helpful.

> Prednisone, up to 60 to 80 mg a day for as long as needed, or until symptoms of hyperdosage appear.

> Codeine, 60 mg, by mouth, every 4 or 6 hours.

Fibromyositis requires rest, heat, massage, splints, hard mattress, salicylates, and local injection of anesthetics.

> Acetylsalicylic acid, or sodium salicylate, 600 mg, by mouth, every 4 to 6 hours, preferably with meals.

> Procaine, 1% solution, to inject 0.5 or 1 ml into the nodules.

For the stiff-man syndrome: avoid any stimulation likely to provoke spasms; give myoneural blocking agents, such as:

> Succinylcholine, 20 mg in 1 ml solution; inject intravenously 10 to 30 ml.

Peripheral nerve blocking is advisable in many cases.

> Lidocaine, 1 or 2% solution, to inject on affected areas, up to 1 to 4 ml each.

Diazepam is useful, at times.

> Diazepam, 5 to 10 mg, by mouth, every 8 hours.

Cramps. The characteristic clinical complex is the extremely painful involuntary muscle contraction. They may be due to an unknown cause: nocturnal cramps; or they may be due to insufficient blood flow to a muscle. Common causes are pregnancy and dehydration. They may also have a neurologic etiology. The most important association is tetanus, in which cramps are the outstanding symptom.

Most muscle cramps are due to either hypocalcemia (tetany) or muscle anoxia (night cramps of vascular origin). In the first instance, the treatment depends on the administration of calcium salts, together with vitamin D, dihydrotachysterol, or parathyroid hormone.

> Calcium chloride, 10% solution, inject 5 to 10 ml intravenously.

> Calcium gluconate, 10% solution, inject 10 to 20 ml.

Calcium lactate, powder, 1 level teaspoonful three times a day.

Dihydrotachysterol, 0.125 mg in capsules; give 0.75 to 2.5 mg a day, in divided doses.

Parathyroid hormone, 50 to 100 units by subcutaneous or intramuscular injection, repeating every 6 to 8 hours, for not more than 1 week.

Cramps due to poor vascular supply may be improved by massage, hot applications, and the use of vasodilators, like papaverine.

Papaverine hydrochloride, 150 mg in slow-release capsules, every 12 hours.

Tetany. In tetany there is also a muscle contraction, not always like a cramp, but more suggestive of ordinary muscular contractions. Muscles of the upper limbs and face are more frequently involved. Pain may accompany tetanic crises, which are characteristically associated with a proven hypocalcemia.

See "Cramps," above, for the treatment of acute conditions. For maintenance, use the following.

Calcium lactate, powder, 1 level tablespoonful once or twice a day.

Calciferol, 40 to 200 units a day.

Dihydrotachysterol, 0.75 to 1 mg a day.

In all instances, check blood calcium frequently and adjust dosage.

Infectious Diseases. Generalized pain in most of the muscles in the body, particularly the limb muscles, is frequently associated with infectious diseases. The most common example is influenza; the most excruciating, dengue. The upper limbs may hurt because of infection, which must be treated etiologically with specific therapy, principally antibiotics. Most frequently causes will be: trichinosis, poliomyelitis, tabes dorsalis, gonococcal or tubercular invasions, localized osteomyelitis, etc. The reader is referred to each one of the corresponding paragraphs.

Vascular Pain

Polyarteritis Nodosa. This infrequent disease is characterized by attacks in which muscular pain in the extremities (or in the abdomen) and arthralgias are associated with fever, malaise, a moderate hypertension, and an elevated eosinophilia. But the symptomatology is extremely variable, depending on the location of the arterial lesions, and may refer to the heart (cardialgia or any other heart disease), kidneys (glomerulonephritis), gall bladder (hepatic colic), or gastrointestinal tract (appendicitis, proctitis, etc.). The diagnosis is established by biopsy.

Fever and pain may respond to acetylsalicylic acid, acetaminophen, etc.

> Acetylsalicylic acid, 600 mg, tablets, every 4 to 6 hours, preferably with meals.

> Acetaminophen, 600 mg, by mouth, every 6 hours.

> Acetophenetidin, 300 mg, by mouth, every 4 hours.

The basic treatment will be carried out with corticosteroids.

> Prednisone, 5 to 10 mg, two or three times a day; to decrease dosage, but not stop its use.

Erythromelalgia. The hands become painful and red; the attack may follow heating, and also a dependent position of the arms, arm swinging or exercise; it is relieved by cooling or elevation of the limb.

If erythromelalgia accompanies organic neurologic diseases, hypertension, gout, or polycythemia vera, any of these diseases have to be treated. If not (primary erythromelalgia), acetylsalicylic acid should be tried first (which drug should also be used as pain reliever for secondary erythromelalgia).

> Acetylsalicylic acid, 600 mg, tablets, every 4 hours; to continue two or three doses after the attack is over.

It is beneficial to cool and elevate the affected limb. Severe, unresponsive cases have to be treated surgically (crushing or sectioning the nerve).

Acrodynia. The symptoms are similar to erythromelalgia—hands are painful and red; the difference consists of chronicity. Sweating and bothersome paresthesias are accompanying symptoms. Children are especially affected. Most cases are due to mercury poisoning, which condition is the one to be controlled: avoid further contamination, which step may be enough for recovery; give pyridoxine; and detoxify with dimercaprol (BAL) or penicillamine.

> Pyridoxine, 50-mg tablets, two a day.

> Dimercaprol (BAL), 100 mg for each ml solution: give 3 to 5 mg for each kg of body weight; every 4 hours the first two days, every 6 hours the following day, and every 12 hours thereafter, for a total of 10 to 15 days.
>
> Penicillamine, 250 mg in capsules, to start taking this dosage every 6 hours on an empty stomach. The dosage may be increased up to a total of 4 or 5 g a day, in divided doses.

Raynaud's Disease. Pain is located in the tips of the fingers associated with blanching or cyanosis in the same area. The attack lasts for a few minutes, rarely more than 1 hour. Repeated attacks give origin to local, painful ulceration that may end in gangrene. Women are more frequently affected than men. The typical attack may also occur in the toes, the nose, and the ears. Smokers have to give up the habit; and the hands (and all the body) must be kept warm, at all times. Surgery is the last resort, when the use of vasodilators fail.

> Papaverine hydrochloride, 150 mg, slow-release capsules, one every 12 hours.
>
> Nicotinic acid, 50- or 100-mg tablets, to take 50 to 150 mg, one to three times a day.
>
> Reserpine, 0.25-mg tablets; start with one dose a day; increase up to four or eight tablets a day (in divided doses), as needed; to establish a maintenance therapy of one tablet a day.

Gangrene. In dry gangrene, the necrotic tissues show a black appearance; in wet gangrene the color is grayish and the tissues show edema, blisters, and necrosis. Gangrene occurs more frequently in the fingers and toes, but other parts of the body can be affected. For a more detailed discussion see this heading under "Pain in the Skin."

Any of the diseases that are prone to cause gangrene (diabetes, etc.) has to be aggressively treated. Once gangrene is established, pain must be relieved by means of analgesics and the patient referred immediately to a surgeon for further evaluation and action.

> Meperidine, 100 mg, by subcutaneous injection.
>
> Methadone, 10 mg, by subcutaneous injection.

The patient must be at bed rest, the limb placed horizontally or slightly elevated, the lesion covered with wet dressing (sterile saline), and antibiotics used either locally or systemically whenever indicated.

Pain in the Bones

Traumatic. The diagnosis is obvious in the great majority of instances. There may also be accompanying skin lesions. A contusion can produce a subperiosteal hematoma. Luxations and fractures give origin to characteristic signs and symptoms. Contusions, dislocations, and fractures are the common injuries to the upper limbs.

Contusions, with or without hematoma, are treated at the start with ice packs for 20 minutes. Thereafter, hot compresses could be used; and very rarely analgesics will be needed.

Dislocations are also treated with ice packs at the start. Apply to the site for 20 minutes, every 6 to 8 hours; hot packs or compresses would be useful only after the second day, but with care not to cause a burn. If the pain is severe enough for more drastic measures, infiltrate the painful area with:

Procaine hydrochloride, 1% solution; inject up to 10 ml.

Fractures will be sent to the orthopedic surgeon, but the first aid will include relief of pain and apprehension with:

Codeine, 60 mg, by subcutaneous injection, repeated as needed.

Meperidine, 100 mg, by subcutaneous injection, repeated as needed.

Methadone, 10 mg, by subcutaneous injection, repeated as needed.

Morphine, 5 to 10 mg, by intravenous injection; or 10 to 15 mg, by subcutaneous injection. If more analgesia is required, it is better to resort to any of the above analgesics.

Osteomyelitis. The first symptom is pain in the affected bone, associated with fever. The bone is tender on palpation, which may also show some swelling over the bone (and also over the adjacent joints). Fluctuation may be present. Because motion is painful, movements are restricted by the patient. The diagnosis depends on X-ray examination, but this evidence might appear late.

To soothe pain is only a minor part in the treatment of osteomyelitis, either acute or chronic. Pain shall be relieved, but not abolished, by means of analgesics.

Acetylsalicylic acid, 600 mg, every 4 to 6 hours, preferably with meals.

Acetophenetidin, 300 mg, by mouth, every 4 to 6 hours.

Acetaminophen, 600 mg, by mouth every 6 hours.

The rest of the treatment is designed to manage properly the bone (or generalized) infection, basically with adequate specific antibiotics and surgery.

Tuberculosis of the Bones and Joints. Pain is mild in the great majority of cases, particularly at the early stages of the disease. Limitation of movement may be the first symptom, which might be caused by muscle spasm. Any bone may be affected, particularly the spine and legs. The clinical course is intermittent, and the diagnosis depends on the finding of tuberculosis elsewhere in the body (lungs) and the X-ray picture.

Associated lesions of lungs or other body areas are important requirements for the total therapy, which includes rest, diet, chemotherapy, and surgery. The general care given will diminish pain, but whenever further help is needed, analgesics can be given.

Codeine, 30 or 60 mg, by mouth, every 4 to 6 hours.

Meperidine, 50 mg, by mouth, every 4 to 6 hours, but do not keep the patient on this medication for too long a time.

Osteosis. Both Paget's and Recklinghausen's diseases may involve pain, but it is not intense. The diagnosis depends on X-ray examinations, and the bone deformities, when they are present. Parathyroid osteosis due to hyperfunction of the gland requires the surgical removal of the excessive glandular tissue. Following the operation there is frequently a need to give vitamin D. In all instances, the administration of analgesics will only give transient alleviation of the pain.

Acetylsalicylic acid, 600 mg, in tablets, every 4 to 6 hours, preferably with meals.

Propoxyphene hydrochloride, 65 mg, by mouth, every 4 hours.

Bone Cysts. Bone cysts may be mildly painful, and the deformity poorly marked. There are, ordinarily, X-ray findings. Curettage is the only good approach for treatment of bone cysts, whenever it is possible. If there is pain, some relief may be obtained with analgesics.

Codeine, 60 mg, by mouth, every 4 hours.

Meperidine, 100 mg, by mouth, every 4 to 6 hours.

Acetylsalicylic acid, 600 mg, in tablets, every 4 hours, preferably with meals.

Propoxyphene hydrochloride, 65 mg, by mouth, every 4 hours.

Osteomalacia. Intense bone pains usher in the clinical picture of osteomalacia. They are more intense at night and during exercise. Spontaneous fractures and deformities of the bone suggest the diagnosis, which is confirmed radiographically.

Annoying or even severe pain may be present, and should be relieved, at times; but the basic treatment depends on the cause of the osteomalacia.

Acetylsalicylic acid, 600 mg, tablets, every 6 hours, preferably with meals.

Acetaminophen, 600 mg, by mouth, every 6 hours.

Acetophenetidin, 300 mg, by mouth, every 6 hours.

Osteomalacia of the adult responds almost specifically to vitamin D given in large doses.

Vitamin D, 100,000 units, once a day. If larger doses are needed, check blood calcium levels periodically.

Osteomalacia due to pancreatic insufficiency requires not only higher calcium intake, but also vitamin K, and, more importantly, pancreatic enzymes.

Calcium lactate, powder, 1 level teaspoonful, three times a day.

Calcium gluconate, 10% solution; inject 10 to 20 ml, intravenously.

Pancreatin; take 250 or 500 mg with meals.

In cases of sprue, a special diet, vitamin B_{12}, and folic acid are essential for recovery.

All patients with osteomalacia will receive calcium therapy by mouth, and will be checked for blood calcium levels periodically.

Calcium lactate, powder, 1 level teaspoonful, one to three times a day.

Calcium gluconate, 1-g tablets; take two to five tablets, 1 hour after each meal.

Milkman's Disease. Milkman's disease may cause pain in the arms, but the main symptomatology is found in the legs (q.v.).

Actually, it is a special form of osteomalacia, and should be treated as such (see above).

Pernicious Anemia. Bone pains may be present in pernicious anemia, but there are other more important symptoms on which diagnosis depends (lingual, gastrointestinal, and, most importantly, degenerative changes in the nervous system). The blood picture will show a macrocytic anemia, the stomach contents will be achlorhydric, and the therapeutic trial (vitamin B_{12} or radioactive vitamin B_{12}) will be positive.

Relief of pain, on a temporary basis, will be achieved by means of analgesics; but the treatment of the disease depends on the use of cyanocobalamin injections.

> Acetylsalicylic acid, 600 mg, in tablets, every 6 hours, preferably with meals.
>
> Acetaminophen, 600 mg, by mouth, every 6 hours.
>
> Propoxyphene hydrochloride, 65 mg, by mouth, every 4 hours.

The use of vitamin B_{12} will be regulated according to accepted routine.

Polyglobulia. In polycythemia vera there are painful muscles in the limbs, particularly the legs (q.v.), but other signs and symptoms are more important for diagnosis.

A number of patients suffer from pain similar to gout, and will be treated as such (see discussion of arthritis, above). All the rest will depend on phlebotomies, chemotherapy, or radiophosphorus.

Myeloma. Multiple myeloma, as the name implies, causes scattered skeletal lesions. Pain in the bones is the most important symptom, and it may occur in the limbs or the trunk. Other symptoms may be headache, malaise, and loss of weight. The diagnosis is made by radiography and biopsy of a lesion.

Radiotherapy, surgery, and chemotherapy may ameliorate the disease. For pain, radiotherapy is the best approach. But analgesics may be used, including narcotics.

> Acetylsalicylic acid, 600 mg, in tablets, every 4 to 6 hours, preferably with meals.
>
> Codeine, 60 mg, by mouth, every 4 hours.

Meperidine, 100 mg, by subcutaneous injection, every 4 to 6 hours.

Morphine sulfate, 10 or 15 mg, by subcutaneous injection, every 6 to 8 hours; or as needed and tolerated.

Neoplasms of Bones. The most important symptom in the great majority of bone tumors, particularly malignant tumors, is pain. In osteoid-osteoma, pain increases during the night hours. In osteogenic sarcoma, pain is followed by swelling, and so happens in Ewing's tumor. Metastasis from the breast, prostate, lungs, thyroid, and kidney also begins with pain. The diagnosis mainly depends on a good X-ray examination.

The essentials of the treatment depend on surgery, chemotherapy, and radiotherapy, the latter being capable of allaying pain to a great extent. Whenever necessary, the use of analgesics will be considered.

Codeine, 60 mg, by subcutaneous injection, repeated as needed and tolerated.

Meperidine, 100 mg, by subcutaneous injection, repeated as needed and tolerated.

Methadone, 10 mg, by subcutaneous injection, repeated as needed and tolerated.

Morphine sulfate, 10 or 15 mg, by subcutaneous injection, repeated as needed and tolerated.

Neurogenic Pain

Brachial Neuralgia. Pain, numbness, and weakness variably distributed along the arm (from shoulder to fingers) characterize brachial neuralgia, also called brachio-cervical neuralgia or cervical root syndrome. In a way, it is to the arm as sciatica is to the leg. Some times, brachial neuralgia is preceded by a crisis of wryneck; on other occasions, pain in the arms comes first. Pain increases with coughing and motion of the head. There are paresthesias, hyperesthesia, and worsening of pain when one is stretching the nerve (the arm in a 90° angle in relation to the trunk, a little forced to the back and the hand facing upwards). As a result of pain, a change in posture may result ("leading chin"). On palpation, pain is elicited by pressure over the involved roots, in the cervical region, or over the nerves in the arm.

Pure brachial neuralgia is rare. Most cases are due to disk diseases in the spine, heart troubles, arthritis, neoplasms, and cervical rib.

Each of these conditions will receive adequate treatment, and the use of analgesics will be common to all:

> Acetylsalicylic acid, 600 mg, in tablets, every 4 hours, preferably with meals.
>
> Codeine, 60 mg, by mouth, every 4 hours.
>
> Meperidine, 100 mg, by subcutaneous injection or by mouth, every 4 to 6 hours.

Scalenus Anticus Syndrome. Pain of a neuralgic type is felt in the arms, at times together with edema. It is worse during the night and improves after the arm is moved. The scalenus anticus syndrome seems to be due to anomalies of the cervical column, and is more frequent among women. (See the discussions of cervical rib in the sections on "Pain in the Neck" and "Pain along the Spine," above.)

Surgery applied to cervical ribs, fibrous bands, or the muscle itself is the only means to a complete cure. Otherwise, bed rest, with traction on the neck; a sling, to support the arm; and pillows to support the shoulders—all of these will be of help. Pain can be relieved temporarily with analgesics.

> Acetylsalicylic acid, 300 or 600 mg, in tablets, every 4 to 6 hours.
>
> Codeine, 60 mg, by mouth, every 4 to 6 hours.
>
> Propoxyphene hydrochloride, 65 mg, by mouth, every 4 hours.

Polyneuritis. Polyneuritis is characterized by the involvement of multiple nerves, with pain scattered over all involved areas. Ordinarily, they are symmetrically distributed, and affect mainly the limbs. In the arms, pain may affect the portion closer to the shoulder (brachial), the forearm (antebrachial), or the hand (inferior). Muscular atrophy, particularly of the hand, may be another symptom.

The patient will stay in bed and receive analgesics for pain.

> Codeine, 60 mg, by subcutaneous injection, repeated as needed and tolerated.
>
> Meperidine, 100 mg, by subcutaneous injection, every 4 to 6 hours.
>
> Methadone, 10 mg, by subcutaneous injection, repeated as needed and tolerated.

As soon as pain is relieved, massage and passive motion will start. Splints and stretching will be used.

Causative agents will be treated, accordingly (poisoning, infections, nutritional and metabolic causes, cancer).

Give a high calorie diet and vitamins of the B complex.

Causalgia. This syndrome frequently follows a traumatic lesion of the affected nerve. Pain is excruciating and associated paresthesias worsen the situation, particularly cutaneous hyperesthesia. The slightest touch to the skin triggers an attack of pain. Patients keep the limb motionless, and a secondary muscle atrophy may supervene. Vasospasm may be severe: dystrophies may be a consequence.

In mild cases, keep the extremity cool and well-protected against any sort of stimulus. With this protection and the use of analgesics, the disease may subside in a few months.

> Acetylsalicylic acid, 600 mg, in tablets, every 4 to 6 hours, preferably with meals.
>
> Acetaminophen, 600 mg, by mouth, every 4 to 6 hours.
>
> Acetophenetidin, 300 mg, by mouth, every 4 hours.
>
> Propoxyphene hydrochloride, 65 mg, by mouth, every 4 hours.

Severe cases, or those which do not improve from the above care, will be treated by sympathectomy, in most instances.

Glomus Tumor. Most of these tumors (over 30% of all the cases) originate beneath the fingernails. There is a bluish mark in the skin or nail over the tumor. Pain radiates to the arm, and increases with the slightest stimulation.

The only hope for abolishing the exquisite pain caused by glomus tumors, particularly on an unguinal site, is their surgical removal. There is no other method to give results; and the use of analgesics is poorly rewarding.

Pain in the Shoulder

Bursitis. This has been discussed under "Muscular Pain," under the heading "Bursitis" (q.v.).

Heterotopic Pain. Pain in the shoulder may reflect several different diseases with no interrelationship among them. Only a mention of each will be made, and the reader is referred to the sections where each particular disease is studied: diseases of the ribs and the sternum, pleuritis, pleurodynia, pneumonia and other lung diseases, mediastinal diseases, biliary lithiasis and colic, and the heterotopic pain that follows the ingestion of large quantities of food. The referred pain is but a small part of each particular clinical picture, but it will be kept in mind that in rare instances it may be the only symptom, as may happen in chronic calculous cholecystitis.

It is frequent that the pain provoked by diseases of the mediastinum and of the aorta and particularly angina pectoris radiate to the shoulders and even the whole arm. Each of these diseases will be treated specifically. As a palliative for pain, acetylsalicylic acid and similar analgesics might be used.

> Acetylsalicylic acid, 600 mg, in tablets, every 4 to 6 hours, preferably with meals.

> Codeine, 60 mg, by mouth, every 4 hours.

> Meperidine, 100 mg, by mouth, every 4 to 6 hours.

Pain in the Elbow

Any bone or joint lesion will cause pain localized in the elbow, but other symptoms will help to establish the correct diagnosis.

Tennis Elbow. This radiohumeral bursitis, like subdeltoid bursitis in the shoulder, causes a very intense pain at the slightest movement of the involved muscles. It occurs more frequently among tennis players, but may be brought on by other motions, like using a screwdriver or the like, whenever violent movements of the wrist are performed. The pain centers over the lateral epicondyle of the humerus, which is tender on pressure. Violent dorsiflexion of the hand aggravates the pain, and the local injection of an anesthetic will abolish it—the correct diagnosis can be based on this information.

At the beginning, pain may be relieved, if the patient is a tennis player, by the use of a racket with a heavier frame, massage of the painful area, application of heat, and the administration of analgesics.

> Acetylsalicylic acid, 600 mg, in tablets, every 4 hours, preferably with meals.

> Codeine, 60 mg, by mouth, every 4 hours.

Nonplayers will observe the same routine, including any change in procedure that could be equivalent to the change in the handle of the racket.

Chronic, established pain will be relieved with analgesics, as above, and by avoiding the offending movements or even having the arm immobilized in a brace or a splint. The so-called trigger points may be infiltrated by using corticoids or corticoids with local anesthetics.

> Hydrocortisone acetate, 25 mg in 1 ml, suspension; inject about 1 ml, or less, into each point.

> Procaine, 1% solution; inject 1 ml into each point.

Heterotopic Pain in the Arm

As in the case of pain referred to the shoulder, a succinct mention of the principal causative diseases will be made, and the reader asked to refer to other sections: infections (a large number of infections, such as influenza, dengue, typhoid fever, etc., cause pain in the limbs, some times more marked in the arms), cardiovascular diseases (angina pectoris, myocardial infarction, aortitis), mediastinal diseases (mediastinitis, tumors, etc.). A more detailed discussion will follow only for a few endocrine diseases that may manifest themselves in pain to the limbs.

Climacterium. The cessation of estrogen activity brings on a rich symptomatology. Pain in the bones, particularly in the limbs, may suggest the erroneous diagnosis of rheumatism. Actual bone lesions may accompany these climacterium pains.

Since rheumatism-like pains are frequent during the climacterium, they should be treated as such, in addition to the regular treatment of their stage of human life. The basic therapy will be similar to that of osteoporosis. Regular analgesics will help.

> Acetylsalicylic acid, 300 or 600 mg, in tablets, every 4 to 6 hours, preferably with meals.

> Acetaminophen, 600 mg, by mouth, every 6 hours.

> Acetophenetidin, 300 mg, by mouth, every 4 to 6 hours.

> Propoxyphene hydrochloride, 65 mg, by mouth, every 4 hours.

> Codeine, 30 or 60 mg, by mouth, every 4 to 6 hours.

Codeine together with acetylsalicylic acid is, at times, of better effect. Estrogens and progesterone are to be given to balance the endocrine deficiency.

Acromegaly. When pain is present, other less conspicuous symptoms become evident. Nevertheless, in some special circumstances, these pains in the limb bones may be the first symptoms of the disease.

Pain is not a special feature of acromegaly; but when it is present, it should be treated in the usual way, with common analgesics, if it is nonspecific, or not related to the causative factor.

> Acetylsalicylic acid, 300 or 600 mg, in tablets, every 6 hours, preferably with meals.
>
> Propoxyphene hydrochloride, 65 mg, by mouth, every 6 hours.

Regular treatment for acromegaly will be carried out with all patients.

Cushing's Disease. In both Cushing's disease and Cushing's syndrome, bone pains are felt in the areas where osteoporosis is found in the X-ray films. The diagnosis cannot be based on these pains alone.

In most instances, pain affects the head or the back; but it may also involve the limbs. Nevertheless, it is of minor degree, and treatment can be carried out with acetylsalicylic acid or similar drugs.

> Acetylsalicylic acid, 300 or 600 mg, in tablets, every 4 to 6 hours, preferably with meals.
>
> Acetaminophen, 600 mg, by mouth, every 4 to 6 hours.
>
> Propoxyphene hydrochloride, 65 mg, by mouth, every 4 hours.

Surgery or radiotherapy is the ultimate answer to treatment.

PAIN IN THE HIPS, LEGS, AND FEET

Articular Pain

Arthritis. Arthritis in the leg joints will show an identical symptomatology with arthritis in the upper limbs (q.v.). The characteristic of arthritis in the legs is that because of the pain the patient will limp when walking, or, because of the pain, might even be confined to bed.

Symptoms referring to the great toe are those principally found in gouty arthritis, either acute or chronic. The acute attack usually affects the metatarsophalangeal joint, which becomes swollen, tense, red, hot, and exquisitely painful. It is said that it hurts even to look at it. The first attacks last a few days; and thereafter attacks become progressively longer, even to weeks. Systemic reaction (fever, chills, malaise, etc.) are frequent. At the beginning, after the attack subsides, the use of the joint is completely regained. In chronic cases, the joint, and other joints similarly, become deformed and show the typical X-ray feature of gout. In all cases, the diagnosis is made by the clinical complex, the finding of hyperuricemia, and the good response to colchicine.

Acute septic arthritis will be treated with adequate antibiotics, and whenever needed, with aspiration, irrigation, and drainage of the joint. If pain is not controlled with those procedures, immobilize and elevate the joint (with splints, if needed), apply hot compresses, and give analgesics, of the acetylsalicylic type.

> Acetylsalicylic acid, 600 mg, in tablets, every 4 to 6 hours, preferably with meals.

Chronic septic arthritis requires antibiotics and surgery; so request the help of a specialist. Analgesics, as above, may help, but not too much is to be expected.

Other forms of arthritis (Reiter's syndrome, sarcoidosis, neurogenic, chondrocalcinosis) should be treated for the basic cause, when it does have a specific treatment, or at least symptomatically, using for pain any of the common analgesics such as acetylsalicylic acid, codeine, meperidine, etc.

Gouty arthritis requires a well-planned way of living: keeping within normal limits of weight, avoiding food or beverages known to cause individual attacks, avoiding long fasting periods, not allowing dehydration or acidosis. As a basic treatment, give colchicine together with probenecid or sulfinpyrazone.

> Colchicine, 0.5 mg, by mouth, every 8 hours; decrease to 0.5 mg once a day, after a few days.

> Probenecid, 500 mg, tablets; start with half a tablet every 12 hours, for 7 days, and then one tablet a day or as needed and tolerated.

> Sulfinpyrazone, 100 mg, by mouth, every 12 hours; increase gradually to 200 mg every 12 hours, as needed and tolerated.

Probenecid and sulfinpyrazone will not be given to those with acute attacks.

When these drugs fail to work, give allopurinol, if it is well tolerated (itching is an early sign of intolerance).

Allopurinol, 100 mg, by mouth, every 12 hours, according to blood uric acid response, or in severe cases, increase to 300 mg every 12 hours. (Do not give this in acute gout, either.)

For acute gout, colchicine is the drug of choice.

Colchicine, 0.5 mg, by mouth, every hour until the relief of pain or the appearance of nausea or diarrhea; 1 mg may be given every 2 hours; 4 to 8 mg are needed to control an atack.

As alternates, indomethacin or phenylbutazone, and corticoids are very effective drugs.

Indomethacin, 25 mg, by mouth, every 8 hours, to increase up to a total of 200 mg a day, in divided doses, but not for more than 3 days.

Phenylbutazone, 100 mg, by mouth, give 400 mg a day at the start, in divided doses; follow with 200 mg a day, in two installments, until the attack is controlled, but not for more than 3 or 4 days.

Prednisone, 5 mg a day, by mouth, together with colchicine. Decrease and discontinue administration as soon as possible

If the pain is very severe, before the anti-gout agents produce their effect, give codeine or meperidine by subcutaneous injection.

Codeine, 60 mg, by subcutaneous injection.

Meperidine, 100 mg, by subcutaneous injection.

Rheumatoid arthritis. In the juvenile type, the larger joints are mostly affected, and the invasion of the joints of the leg will also force the patient to limp when walking. In other respects, symptoms are identical with those discussed for the upper limbs (q.v.).

Bed rest together with a progressive increase of exercise (below the tolerance of the joint) will be encouraged. Moist or radiant heat will relax muscles and allay pain. Therapeutically, salicylates are the drugs of choice, before resorting to crysotherapy, corticoid therapy, etc.

Acetylsalicylic acid, 600 mg, in tablets, every 4 hours, preferably with meals and accompanied by a small daily dose of thyroid extract—15 or 30 mg a day, by mouth.

Sodium salicylate, 600 mg, by mouth, as above.

Sodium salicylate, large dosage: 1200 mg by mouth, every 4 to 6 hours, and increase to 2 g every 4 hours, together with small amounts of thyroid extract (30 mg a day) and if not well tolerated, also with sodium bicarbonate (300 mg, tablets, or the amount of powder taken with the point of a knife).

Those patients who do not benefit from salicylates will be treated with corticoids or with gold therapy.

Prednisone, 5 or 10 mg, every 6 hours, by mouth; decrease as soon as improvement begins; and discontinue slowly to terminate total treatment in about 6 weeks.

Hydrocortisone, 25 to 50 mg, by intraarticular injection.

Gold sodium thiomalate or gold thioglucose (aurothioglucose), solutions containing 10, 25, 50, or 100 mg in each ml. Use 10 mg, once the first week; 25 mg, once the second week; and thereafter, 50 mg a week, to reach a total of 1 (19 injections of 50 mg). If the response is good, decrease the dosage to 50 mg every 2 weeks; then, every 3 weeks; and finally maintain a prolonged treatment with 50 mg a month, tolerance permitting.

Specialists will evaluate possible use of antimalarial drugs, phenylbutazone, indomethacin, and cytotoxic drugs.

Degenerative Arthritis. As previously discussed for degenerative arthritis of the upper limbs (q.v.), the symptoms in cases affecting the lower limbs will be the same, plus limping.

Avoid stress on the affected joints, particularly in the hyperactive and the obese, and whenever it is needed, provide support. Apply heat, locally. At times, orthopedic measures are needed. In general, follow treatments as above, for rhumatoid arthritis.

Rheumatic Fever. The local, rheumatic symptoms are the same as discussed under "Pain in the Shoulders, Arms, and Hands" (q.v.). Ordinarily, patients are confined to bed.

Salicylates are almost specific for rheumatic fever, and should be started as soon as possible. Use large doses in severe cases.

Acetylsalicylic acid, 600 mg, tablets; or sodium salicylate, 600 mg, by mouth; every 4 hours, preferably, with meals.

For large doses of acetylsalicylic acid or sodium salicylate, start with 60 mg for each kg of body weight in 4 or 6 doses a day (4 to 5 g a day); increase to 90, 120, or 180 mg for each kg of body weight, also in divided doses. Medication will be given with meals, whenever possible, or given with sodium bicarbonate (300-mg tablets, or the amount of powder taken with the point of a knife) and a small amount of thyroid extract (30 or 60 mg a day).

If salicylates prove ineffective after a trial of about 5 days, give corticoids instead, which might also have been used at the start of therapy. Antibiotics (penicillin) might be a good adjuvant therapy after weighing the possibility of a susceptible germ as the causative factor.

Prednisone, 5 or 10 mg, by mouth, every 6 hours. Decrease dosage after 3 weeks, for another 3 weeks; discontinue slowly, for another 6 weeks. Higher dosages (20 to 40 mg each dose) may be given.

A specialist should take care of additional treatment, particularly if complications arise.

Coxalgia. Coxalgia is but a form of tuberculous arthritis in the coxal joint, which deserves a little discussion here. The initial symptom is pain and limping, the pain referred either to the hip or the knee. There is a limitation of movement, and the tendency of patients to stand on the healthy leg. The affected leg is placed in a typical position: flexed, abducted, and with external rotation. There is a muscle atrophy and, finally, a fistulization of an abscess. An early diagnosis is difficult: an adolescent or younger patient begins to limp and shows the foregoing symptoms; the X-ray examination is of little help. It shows only some decalcification, and only later on the cartilage lesions.

The treatment of coxalgia due to arthritic tuberculosis is that of tuberculosis itself, with streptomycin, isoniazid, and para-aminosalicylic acid, all three given initially for 6 months, then followed by isoniacid and para-aminosalicylic acid for 18 additional months. Secondary drugs will be used in resistant cases. For the symptomatic treatment of pain we will resort to papaverine, codeine, or meperidine.

Codeine, 60 mg, by mouth, every 4 hours.

Papaverine hydrochloride, 150 mg, in slow-release capsules, one every 12 hours.

Meperidine, 100 mg, by mouth, every 4 to 6 hours.

Pain Referred to the Knee. Not infrequently, the patient simply refers to having a painful knee, and there are no symptoms or signs of any local lesion. As stated in the foregoing paragraph, in cases of coxitis there is the possibility of pain in the knee. Also, it may be found in cases of arthritis or malformations of the feet. It is most interesting to note that a painful knee may be the only subjective symptom of flat feet.

Pain in the knee may be the consequence of any hip disease or foot problem, mostly arthritic or rheumatic in nature. Also, foot deformities may cause pain in the knee. Of course, in each instance the treatment will be focused on the causative condition.

Muscular Pain

Bursitis. Climacteric women may complain of intense pain in the medial aspect of the tibia, particularly distressing when using the stair steps. This is due to bursitis at the insertion of the sartorius muscle. Other bursitis cases will show the typical symptoms of the disease.

If it is treated at the very start with either radiotherapy or corticoids, the results are almost always gratifying.

> Prednisone, 5 mg, every 8 hours; decrease the dosage when effects are noted, and discontinue slowly for a total period of treatment of almost 15 to 20 days.

Well-established disease will require rest, immobilization, application of local heat, and intrabursal injection of corticoids.

> Hydrocortisone acetate, 25 mg in each ml, suspension; inject from 1 to 5 ml into the bursae.

The pain can be helped with regular analgesics.

> Codeine 60 mg, by subcutaneous injection every 6 hours, by mouth every 4 hours.

Stress Myalgia. There is no difference between the symptomatology discussed for the upper limbs (q.v.) and symptomatology here.

This discomfort follows unusual muscular activity (gymnastics, hiking, etc.). The remedy is massage, heat applications, and the taking of muscle relaxants and analgesics.

> Carisoprodol, 350 mg, tablets, one every 6 hours.

> Codeine, 60 mg, by mouth, every 4 hours.

Myositis. The same symptoms as those discussed for the upper limbs (q.v.) appear in the legs.

Polymyositis requires physical therapy, corticoids, and analgesics.

Prednisone, up to 60 or 80 mg a day, for as long as needed or until symptoms of overdosage appear; to be adjusted.

Codeine, 60 mg, by mouth, every 4 to 6 hours.

Fibromyositis requires rest, massage, heat, hard mattress, splints, salicylates, and local injection of anesthetic.

Acetylsalicylic acid or sodium salicylate, 600 mg, by mouth, every 4 to 6 hours, preferably with meals.

Procaine, 1% solution; inject 0.5 to 1 ml into nodules.

For stiff-man syndrome: avoid stimulation, give myoneural blocking agents, or perform peripheral nerve blocking, using procaine, as above. Diazepem is useful, at times.

Diazepam, 5 or 10 mg, by mouth, every 8 hours.

Cramps. In addition to all that was discussed for the upper limbs (q.v.), it is important to note the very frequent nocturnal cramps that particularly affect the muscles of the calves and feet. It is a sudden, painful contraction of the muscle; begins soon after the patient goes to bed; and is relieved as soon as a few steps are taken.

If it is due to hypocalcemia (tetany), give calcium salts, vitamin D, and dihydrotachysterol or parathyroid hormone.

Calcium chloride, 10% solution; inject 5 to 10 ml, intravenously.

Calcium gluconate, 10% solution; inject 10 to 20 ml, intravenously.

Calcium lactate, powder, 1 level teaspoonful, three times a day, by mouth.

Dihydrotachysterol, 0.125 mg, in capsules, from 0.75 to 2.5 mg, a day, in individualized and divided dosage.

Parathyroid hormone, 50 to 100 units, by subcutaneous or intramuscular injection, every 6 to 8 hours, for no more than 1 week.

Cramps due to poor vascular supply (anoxia) may improve by local massage, hot applications, and vasodilators.

Papaverine hydrochloride, 150 mg, in slow-release capsules, one every 12 hours.

Tetany. See above, the discussion of tetany in the upper limbs.

The acute tetanic attack is treated as stated in the above paragraph on "Cramps." For maintenance give:

> Calcium lactate, powder, 1 level teaspoonful, once or twice a day.
>
> Calciferol, 40 to 200 units a day.
>
> Dihydrotachysterol, 0.75 to 1 mg a day.

In all instances, check frequently for blood calcium levels, and adjust therapy appropriately.

Contracture of the Achilles' Tendon. The peculiar position of the foot (restricted dorsiflexion of the ankle) occurs with pain along the arch, metatarsalgia, and also pain referred to the calf. The pain is increased by walking barefooted or by using flat shoes or slippers. The contracture is found more frequently among women.

The administration of analgesics does not control the condition well, but helps to permit a better manipulation with massage, exercise, and gradual stretching of the tendon.

> Papaverine hydrochloride, 150 mg, in slow-release capsules, one every 12 hours.
>
> Acetylsalicylic acid, 600 mg, in tablets, every 4 to 6 hours, preferably with meals.
>
> Propoxyphene hydrochloride, 65 mg, by mouth, every 4 hours.

Contracture not responding to the above therapy will be treated surgically, for lengthening of the tendon, if it appears appropriate.

Infectious Diseases. In a large number of infective diseases (influenza, dengue, meningitis, yellow fever, etc.) there is marked pain of the limb muscles. It is not an important symptom, perhaps with the exception of dengue and "flu."

The reader is referred to each particular paragraph for information on the management of: trichinosis, poliomyelitis, tabes dorsalis, gonoccocal or tubercular infections, localized osteomyelitis, etc., each one to be treated etiologically.

Vascular Pain

Varices. Varicosities of the veins in the legs may cause some pain and paresthesia, together with some ankle edema, and even trophic changes in the skin (sclerosis) when circulation has been disturbed for long periods. In most instances the diagnosis is evident because of the varicosities visible under the skin.

The regular treatment of varicosities, mainly located in the legs, is to use elastic protection (stockings), intermittent elevation of the affected legs, injection of sclerosing agents, and surgery (whenever advisable). This treatment will control the pain (seldom of great importance).

Phlebitis. In phlebothrombosis pain is minimal, only elicited in the calf by dorsiflexion of the foot. In thrombophlebitis there is intense pain, tenderness on palpation, and swelling of the leg. Systemic symptoms are present (fever, malaise). The femoral and popliteal veins are the ones more frequently affected by phlebitis.

In the case of superficial phlebitis, order rest, elevation of the affected limb, application of heat, and surgery, if necessary (ligation in extensive or progressive cases; or stripping). Use anticoagulants only in rapidly progressive cases. Phenylbutazone is useful in many instances.

> Heparin (aqueous sodium), 7,000 to 12,000 units initially, by intravenous or subcutaneous injection; to be followed by three-fourths of this dosage every 4 hours, until warfarin or bihydroxycoumarin start to work. Check for clotting time.
>
> Warfarin, 30 to 40 mg, by mouth; once a day the first day; 10 to 20 mg, the second day; 5 to 10 mg (more or less, as needed), thereafter. Start at the same time as heparin, and control with prothrobin time, checked often.
>
> Phenylbutazone, 100 mg, every 8 hours, for at least 5 days. (Do not give to a patient with peptic ulcer.)

The involvement of deep veins requires bed rest, elevation of the affected limb, elastic bandage, anticoagulant therapy (as above), surgery in many cases, and gradual walking after 5 to 10 days of absolute rest. The advice of a specialist will be requested.

Polyarteritis Nodosa. See discussion for the upper limb.

Acetylsalicylic acid, acetaminophen, and similar drugs will effectively control the pain in most instances.

> Acetylsalicylic acid, 600 mg, tablets, every 4 to 6 hours, preferably with meals.
>
> Acetophenetidin, 300 mg, by mouth, every 4 hours.
>
> Acetaminophen, 600 mg, by mouth, every 6 hours.

Corticoids are the drugs that will carry out the basic treatment.

> Prednisone, 5 to 10 mg, two or three times a day; decrease—but do not stop—administration after results are obtained.

Erythromelalgia. The symptomatology is identical with that for the upper limbs (q.v.). The only difference is the lesser frequency of the disease affecting the lower limbs.

Organic neurologic diseases, hypertension, gout, or polycythemia vera accompanying erythromelalgia will be treated specifically. If it is primary erythromelalgia, cool and elevate the affected limb, and give acetylsalicylic acid, which is frequently very effective (for this as well as for secondary erythromelalgia).

> Acetylsalicylic acid, 600 mg, in tablets, every 4 hours; continue for 2 or 3 doses after the attack is over.

Severe, unresponsive cases have to be treated surgically (crushing or sectioning of a nerve).

Acrodynia. See discussion for the upper limb.

Since the great majority of cases of acrodynia are due to mercury poisoning, the treatment will be addressed to control of this condition. The steps to follow are: avoid further contamination, which step occasionally will be enough for recovery; give pyridoxine; detoxify with dimercaprol or penicillamine.

> Pyridoxine, 50 mg, tablets; two a day.

> Dimercaprol (BAL), 100 mg for each ml solution: give 3 to 5 mg for each kg of body weight; every 4 hours the first 2 days, every 6 hours the following day; and every 12 hours thereafter, for a total of 10 to 15 days.

> Penicillamine, 250 mg, in capsules, to start taking this dosage every 6 hours on an empty stomach. The dosage may be increased up to a total of 4 to 5 g a day, in divided doses.

Intermittent Claudication. A person who suddenly stops walking because of a sudden onset of pain, which increases with the exercise, is said to suffer from intermittent claudication. The pain accompanies paresthesias, muscular weakness, and/or cramps. Once he has relaxed for a few moments, all symptoms disappear, and the patient is able to continue walking until the next attack (depending on the severity of the disease). The oscillometric values are extremely lowered or even absent in these patients.

Since the pain in this disturbance lasts only seconds or minutes, there is no need of using analgesics. The aim is to prevent pain: advise the patient to walk slowly, with short steps, avoiding stairs and hills as much as possible, or to stop frequently (more often than he ordinarily would) for a few seconds before continuing walking. Exercising, by walking until pain starts, will be done every 4 or 5 hours during the day (to increase the number of new collateral vessels). Surgery (sympathectomy) is a final procedure, when conservative measures fail.

Thromboangiitis Obliterans. Pain of the type just mentioned, intermittent claudication, may be the first sign of Buerger's disease. Then, gradually or suddenly, more severe pain becomes persistent, and an area of gangrene is delineated in the toes or even the metatarsal region. Diagnostic signs of arterial insufficiency are the changes in color of the feet and toes: red (rubor) when dependent, and pale (pallor) when elevated above the level of the heart. Trophic changes of the affected area (nails and skin) may occur. The final outcome could be ulceration and gangrene.

Diphenylhydantoin very frequently will control pain, but the general management of these cases has to be followed with care.

> Diphenylhydantoin, 100 mg, by mouth, every 8 hours; in emergency situations give the first 100 mg by intramuscular injection.

The patient has to stop smoking and will take good care of the feet (cleansing with oil, if dry, or with alcohol, if soft; keep the nails soft, treat corns, keep warm but not hot, avoid garters and mycotic infections, treat abrasions, and take exercise). Vasodilators might be used, but with extreme caution, since they are of little help and may cause some harm. Treat any infection vigorously; and gangrene, if it is present. Sympathectomy is considered as a practical remedy.

Gangrene. See "Pain in the Skin."

Treat diabetes vigorously, or any other condition which might encourage gangrene. If gangrene develops, place the limb horizontally or slightly lowered, cover the lesion with wet dressing (sterile saline or antibiotics, if infected), give an analgesic and refer the patient to a surgeon for further evaluation and action.

> Meperidine, 100 mg, by subcutaneous injection.

> Methadone, 10 mg, by subcutaneous injection.

Pain in the Bones

Traumatic. Fractures, dislocations, sprains, and strains account for most of the traumatic pains in the bones of the extremities. These disturbances result from local trauma and are not concerned with any of the internal structures. Fractures and dislocations are diagnosed by inspection, manipulation, and loss of function and confirmed by X-ray. Sprains and strains occur in the joints an tendons and are the result of variable tears in the ligaments and tendons and often of accompanying blood vessels of any size. The immediate pain is due to the tissue distention or pressure of extravasated blood. The pain coming later with further swelling results from the outpouring of lymph around the injured tissues.

Perhaps ankle sprain is the number one painful trauma to the legs. Pain is best relieved by means of ice packs applied to the site for 20 minutes, every 6 to 8 hours; the following day, hot packs, or hot soaks are advisable, but with care to avoid the frequent burns induced by this practice. In case of unacceptable suffering, infiltrate the painful area with:

> Procaine hydrochloride, 1% solution; inject up to 10 ml.

Start to exercise (and use) the sprained ankle as soon as possible.

Dislocations will be treated as above, but giving more time for recovery and more attention to the healing of the most affected muscles and tendons. These cases have to be evaluated by a surgeon, because at times open surgical repair is needed.

Contusions, with or without hematoma, are also treated starting with ice packs. Analgesics are not really needed, in these cases.

Fractures require the help of the orthopedic surgeon, but for the time elapsed from the injury to the aid of the specialist, relief of pain and sedation of apprehension are necessary, making the use of narcotic and analgesics most valuable.

> Codeine, 60 mg, by subcutaneous injection, repeated as needed.

> Meperidine, 100 mg, by subcutaneous injection, repeated as needed.

> Methadone, 10 mg, by subcutaneous injection, repeated as needed.

292 DIAGNOSIS AND TREATMENT

>Morphine, 5 or 10 mg, by intravenous injection; or 10 or 15 mg, by subcutaneous injection. If more analgesia is required, it is permissible to resort to any of the above analgesics.

Osteomyelitis. See discussion under "Pain in the Shoulders, Arms, and Hands."

The basic treatment is devoted to managing the infection, which may be generalized or localized in the bone. Specific antibiotics and surgery are a must; so consult a specialist early in the disease. To soothe pain, give analgesics.

>Acetylsalicylic acid, 600 mg, every 6 hours, preferably with meals.

>Acetaminophen, 600 mg, by mouth, every 6 hours.

>Acetophenetidin, 300 mg, by mouth, every 4 to 6 hours.

Tuberculosis. See the discussion under "Coxalgia."

Treat tuberculosis as a disease of the whole body, with rest, diet, and chemotherapy. Surgery will be used whenever needed. If there is still the need to allay local pain, give analgesics.

>Codeine, 30 or 60 mg, by mouth, every 4 to 6 hours.

>Meperidine, 50 mg, by mouth, every 4 to 6 hours, but do not keep the patient on this medication for too long a time.

Epiphysiolysis of the Head of the Femur. Pain in the hip radiates to the knee as an early symptom. The patient limps and gets tired soon. Some limitation of motion is present with slight internal rotation and/or short abduction and flexion. The disease affects adolescents and produces limping. Radiographic examination is essential for diagnosis, revealing an enlargement of the juxtaepiphysary line, enlargement and irregular border of the metaphysis, together with a very small femoral head and a deformed neck.

This condition requires the help of an orthopedic surgeon, to repair the derangement to the advantage of the patient. Symptomatically, analgesics can be offered to allay pain.

>Acetylsalicylic acid, 300 or 600 mg, in tablets, every 4 to 6 hours, preferably with meals.

>Codeine, 60 mg, by mouth, every 4 to 6 hours.

>Propoxyphene hydrochloride, 65 mg, by mouth, every 4 to 6 hours.

Osteosis. For diagnosis see discussion under "Pain in the Shoulder, Arms, and Hands."

This condition, also known under the name of osteosis parathyroidea cystica, presents the problem in which the excessive parathyroid glandular tissue provokes hypersecretion, for which reason it has to be removed surgically. At times, after surgery, there is a need to give vitamin D. Analgesics will only give transient relief of pain.

> Acetylsalicylic acid, 600 mg, in tablets, every 4 to 6 hours, preferably with meals.

> Propoxyphene hydrochloride, 65 mg, by mouth, every 4 to 6 hours.

Bone Cysts. For diagnosis see discussion under "Pain in the Shoulders, Arms, and Hands."

Whenever possible, curettage is the only treatment for bone cysts. If they are painful, some relief may be obtained by analgesics.

> Codeine, 60 mg, by mouth, every 4 hours.

> Meperidine, 100 mg, by mouth, every 4 to 6 hours.

> Propoxyphene hydrochloride, 65 mg, by mouth, every 4 hours.

> Acetylsalicylic acid, 600 mg, in tablets, every 4 hours, preferably with meals.

Osteomalacia. For diagnosis see discussion under "Pain in the Shoulders, Arms and Hands."

This disease responds, almost specifically, to large doses of Vitamin D.

> Vitamin D, 100,000 units, once a day. If larger doses are needed, check blood calcium levels, periodically.

If it is due to pancreatic insufficiency, in addition to vitamin D, give pancreatic enzymes, calcium, and vitamin K.

> Pancreatin, 250 or 500 mg with meals.

> Vitamin K (menadiol or phytonadione), 5 mg, once or twice a day; check prothrombine time.

> Calcium lactate, powder, 1 level teaspoonful, three times a day.

> Calcium gluconate, 10% solution, to inject 10 to 20 ml, intravenously.

These and all patients with osteomalacia will receive a prolonged calcium therapy, and will be checked, periodically, for blood calcium concentrations.

> Calcium lactate, powder, 1 level teaspoonful, one to three times a day.
>
> Calcium gluconate, 1 g, tablets; two to five tablets, 1 hour after each meal.

In cases of sprue, a special diet, vitamin B_{12}, and folic acid are essential. Those who complain of pain will receive analgesics.

> Acetylsalicylic acid, 600 mg, in tablets, every 6 hours, preferably with meals.
>
> Acetaminophen, 600 mg, by mouth, every 6 hours.

Milkman's Disease. Bone pain may be so severe that walking is impossible. There are no other objective symptoms, except for occasional spontaneous fractures. It runs a chronic course, and the diagnosis depends on the finding of the typical bands or striae in the shaft of the long bones.

The treatment is the same as for osteomalacia, of which Milkman's syndrome seems to be a variety. See discussion of osteomalacia (above) for details.

Pernicious Anemia. For diagnosis see discussion under "Pain in the Shoulders, Arms, and Hands."

Cyanocobalamin (vitamin B_{12}) is the basic and effective treatment of the disease, and should be administered according to the accepted routine. For palliative treatment of pain, give analgesics.

> Acetylsalicylic acid, 600 mg, in tablets, every 6 hours, preferably with meals.
>
> Acetaminophen, 600 mg, by mouth, every 6 hours.
>
> Propoxyphene hydrochloride, 65 mg, by mouth, every 4 hours.

Polycythemia Vera. In this blood disease pain in the muscles of the legs occurs very frequently, but is only a minor symptom. There are: dusky-red complexion, perhaps the outstanding symptom; hemorrhages (epistaxis, hemorrhoids); hypertension; headache; dizziness; postprandial somnolence; weakness; and other less important symptoms. The hemogram reveals a red blood count over 6 or 7 million. There are other polyglobulias, besides polycythemia vera, principally in diseases of the circulatory system (congenital heart diseases, mitral stenosis, cor pulmonale) and among people living at high altitude; and a false polyglobulia in dehydration.

Patients suffering from polycythemia vera may complain of headache, but the most troublesome pain is of a gouty type. Since the general treatment for polycythemia will control headache, the only problem left is to treat the gouty attack with colchicine, probenecid, sulfinpyrazone, or allopurinol.

> Colchicine, 0.5 mg, by mouth, repeated every hour until the control of pain or the appearance of nausea or diarrhea (or 1 mg every 2 hours), to a total of 4 to 8 mg. After controlling the attack, the dose will be 0.5 mg a day; colchicine alone or together with probenecid or sulfinpyrazone.
>
> Probenecid, 500 mg, tablets, once a day or as needed and tolerated.
>
> Sulfinpyrazone, 100 mg, by mouth, every 12 hours; increase gradually to 200 mg, every 12 hours or as needed and tolerated.
>
> Allopurinol, 100 mg, by mouth, every 12 hours; if so required, according to blood uric acid levels, or in severe cases increase to 300 mg.

Note that the last three drugs (probenecid, sulfinpyrazone, and allopurinol) are not to be given in acute gout, since the acute attack is to be treated with colchicine, as stated above. See the paragraph on "Arthritis" in this section, for more details.

Myeloma. The bones of the hip are frequently involved, and the first symptom to appear is pain, severe and continuous, that may also provoke some limping. Headache, malaise, and loss of weight are accompanying symptoms; fever and spontaneous fractures may occur; and also respiratory complications (bronchopneumonia, emphysema, bronchitis), or complications of other organs, particularly the kidneys. On palpation, tenderness is elicited. Diagnostic clues are the presence of Bence-Jones albumin in the urine, and the specific radiographic intraosseous clear, round areas.

Analgesics may be useful to control pain, but radiotherapy is, perhaps, the best approach. Acetylsalicylic acid and similar agents might be used.

Acetylsalicylic acid, 600 mg, in tablets, every 4 to 6 hours, preferably with meals.

Codeine, 60 mg, by mouth, every 4 hours.

If needed, narcotic analgesics may be administered.

Morphine sulfate, 10 or 15 mg, by subcutaneous injection, every 6 to 8 hours, or as needed and tolerated.

Meperidine, 100 mg, by subcutaneous injection, every 4 to 6 hours.

Some other measures that can be taken may also help to control pain, such as the use of splints, dietetic supplements, and, particularly, alkylating agents.

Neoplasms of the Bones. For diagnosis see discussion under "Pain in the Shoulders, Arms, and Hands."

Surgery, chemotherapy, and radiotherapy are the essentials of the treatment of bone tumors. Radiotherapy may allay pain to a great extent; but whenever necessary, analgesics will be given.

Codeine, 60 mg, by subcutaneous injection, repeated as needed and tolerated.

Meperidine, 100 mg, by subcutaneous injection, repeated as needed and tolerated.

Methadone, 10 mg, by subcutaneous injection, repeated as needed and tolerated.

Neurogenic Pain

Sciatica. The neuralgic pain of the sciatic nerve extends along the posterior aspect of the leg, from the hip to the ankle. Pain may be either continuous or by crises. Numbness may accompany pain. Tenderness is elicited on palpation of the nerve, all along its course. Also, pain increases when stretching the nerve (Lasegue's sign). Ordinarily, sciatica is secondary to any disease or lesion that may injure the nerve, and must be diagnosed adequately. Eventual changes are muscle atrophy and spasm, diminished reflexes (Achilles), limitation of motion, deformities, trophic changes, and so on.

Pain along the nerve is mostly due to herniated discs or tumors, which will be treated accordingly, in most instances, by surgical means. Palliative treatment will be given by means of analgesics, including narcotics, when needed, and perhaps the use of vitamins of the B group.

> Acetylsalicylic acid, 600 mg, in tablets, every 4 hours, preferably with meals.
>
> Meperidine, 100 mg, by subcutaneous injection or by mouth, every 4 to 6 hours.

This neuralgia may also be due to general infections (treat with the adequate antibiotic), syphilis (use penicillin), poisoning (treat lead, arsenic, alcohol, etc., poisoning), or metabolic causes (treat diabetes, hypovitaminosis B, etc.). Also, in these cases, analgesics, including narcotics, are of valuable help.

Crural Neuralgia. Pain is felt along the leg, as in sciatica, but along the anterior aspect of the limb. Some call it anterior sciatica. Paresthesias are frequently associated with pain, and the quadriceps may suffer atrophy, while the patellar reflex is diminished or is absent. Crural neuralgia is almost secondary to abdominal diseases.

Most cases are due to infection or tumors of the abdominal organs. The basic treatment will be with antibiotics or surgery. To relieve pain, use analgesics and help with vitamins of the B group.

> Acetylsalicylic acid, 600 mg, in tablets, every 4 hours, with meals, preferably.
>
> Codeine, 60 mg, by mouth, every 4 hours.
>
> Meperidine, 100 mg, by subcutaneous injection or by mouth, every 4 to 6 hours.

Meralgia Paresthetica requires, very frequently, the decompression of the fascial canal of the nervus cutaneus femoris lateralis; but a trial will be given to avoidance of external pressure or constriction, the use of vitamins of the B group, and analgesics.

> Codeine, 60 mg, by subcutaneous injection or by mouth, every 4 to 6 hours.
>
> Meperidine, 100 mg, by subcutaneous injection or by mouth, every 4 to 6 hours.

Polyneuritis. For diagnosis see discussion under "Pain in the Shoulders, Arms, and Hands."
Start with bed rest and analgesics.

> Codeine, 60 mg, by subcutaneous injection, repeated as needed and tolerated.
>
> Meperidine, 100 mg, by subcutaneous injection, every 4 to 6 hours.

Methadone, 10 mg, by subcutaneous injection, repeated as needed and tolerated.

When pain is relieved, give massage and start with passive motion. Splints and stretching might be needed.

Of course, the causative factor will be found, to be treated etiologically (poisoning, infections, cancer, metabolic, etc.). Contractures are to be prevented.

Give a high calorie diet and vitamins of the B complex.

Radiculitis. The typical tabetic violent pains mainly affect the lower limbs. They are sudden in onset and persist for only a few seconds. Very frequently, these fulgurant attacks are the first and only evident symptom of tabes dorsalis. Other tabetic symptoms and signs are suggestive of the diagnosis: locomotor ataxia is the most characteristic, with its associated derangement of pupillary and tendinous reflexes, and visceral crisis. The examination of the spinal fluid is diagnostic. Vertebral diseases may also provoke radiculitis.

Many cases do need surgery, but all require the advice of the specialist to manage herniated disk, and to decide on traction and massage, and on the use of a firm, flat bed. In addition to these measures, analgesics and muscle relaxants are reliable for the relief of pain.

Acetylsalicylic acid, 600 mg, in tablets, every 4 to 6 hours, preferably with meals.

Codeine, 60 mg, by mouth, every 4 hours.

Propoxyphene hydrochloride, 65 mg, by mouth, every 4 hours.

Meprobamate, 400 mg, by mouth, every 6 hours.

Carisoprodol, 350 mg, by mouth, every 6 to 8 hours.

Multiple Sclerosis. In some instances, pains that have some likeness to those of tabes dorsalis appear in the legs or any other parts of the body. The extremely rich symptomatology of multiple sclerosis and its characteristic bouts and remissions may indicate the diagnosis.

There is no specific therapy yet known for the cause or cure of multiple sclerosis. Only symptomatic and general care can be given: maintain activity closer to normal without straining the patient; massage and passive exercise are helpful; psychotherapy is most important; and avoid or treat complications as they arise (urinary infections, ulcers, etc.). A good nutritious diet, with vitamins (mainly of the B group), is advised; and analgesics are given, when needed.

Acetylsalicylic acid, 300 or 600 mg, as tablets, every 6 hours, preferably with meals.

Causalgia. For diagnosis see discussion under "Pain in the Shoulders, Arms, and Hands."
For mild cases: keep the extremity cool and protected from stimulation in any way; give analgesics. In severe cases: try the above care, but if it fails, think about the advisability of sympathectomy.

Acetylsalicylic acid, 600 mg, in tablets, every 4 to 6 hours, preferably with meals.

Acetaminophen, 600 mg, by mouth, every 4 to 6 hours.

Acetophenetidin, 300 mg, by mouth, every 4 hours.

Propoxyphene hydrochloride, 65 mg, every 4 hours.

Pain in the Feet

Gout. The typical gouty attack occurs in the great toe. In acute gout pain appears suddenly, and the swollen joint is extremely tender. It has been said that if a tourniquet is applied until you cannot resist any more, that is an arthritic pain; and when more pressure is still applied after you cannot resist any more, that is a gouty pain. The skin over the swollen joint is red, hot, and shiny. Other joints of the feet can also be affected. During the acute attack there are fever, chills, and tachycardia. In chronic gout finally deformities develop after several acute attacks. The diagnosis is based on the transparent small areas of uric acid deposition in the bones, the high level of uric acid in the blood, and tophi in the ear.

Gouty arthritis requires prolonged treatment for the basic metabolic derangement. It is imperative to stay within correct limits of weight (limit calories and increase fluid intake, and avoid any food or beverage which individually may precipitate an acute attack), do not prolong fasting periods, and do not reach dangerous levels of dehydration or acidosis. The use of uricosuric agents is almost mandatory, particularly if there is evidence of the presence of tophi or X-ray indication of urate deposition in bones. It is advisable to use colchicine together with the uricosuric drugs, or at least at the start.

Colchicine, 0.5 mg, by mouth, every 8 hours; decrease to 0.5 mg, once a day after a few days of conjoint administration, and continue that way for a long time.

Probenecid, 500 mg, tablets, by mouth, start with half a

> tablet every 12 hours; after 7 days, increase to one tablet every 12 hours, as needed and tolerated.
>
> Sulfinpyrazone, 100 mg, by mouth, every 12 hours; increase gradually to 200 mg, every 12 hours, as needed and tolerated.

These uricosuric drugs are not recommended for patients suffering acute attacks or those who are known to have uric acid lithiasis. If the uricosuric agents fail to work, allopurinol will be tried, if well tolerated (early sign of intolerance is an itchy rash).

> Allopurinol, 100 mg, by mouth, every 12 hours; increase to 300 mg, every 12 hours, in severe cases (dosage depending on blood uric acid response).

Allopurinol is a toxic drug, which should be used cautiously. Like the uricosuric agents, it should not be given in acute gout.

In acute gout, colchicine is the drug of choice, to such an extent that if it fails to control the attack, the diagnosis of gout can be questioned.

> Colchicine, 0.5 mg, by mouth, every hour (or 1 mg, every 2 hours) until the relief of pain or until the appearance of nausea or diarrhea. Commonly, the needed amount reaches 4 to 8 mg.

Further attacks will be treated with 1 mg less than the amount needed for the previous time. Gastrointestinal intolerance will be treated symptomatically, which is better than using colchicine by intravenous injection. Some specialists prefer indomethacin or phenylbutazone to treat certain gout attacks when the diagnosis is well established.

> Phenylbutazone, 100 mg, tablets, by mouth; initially, 400 mg a day; to be followed by 200 mg, until the attack is controlled. Do not administer more than 3 or 4 days.
>
> Indomethacin, 25 mg, by mouth, every 8 hours; increase to a total of 200 mg in divided doses; not for more than 3 or 4 days.

Corticoids and corticotropin (ACTH) are also very useful to control the acute attacks, but mostly for the time they are given; after they are discontinued, colchicine has to be started. A final note: many patients with severe pain do need the use of analgesics to act before the effect of anti-gout drugs becomes noticeable.

Codeine, 60 mg, by subcutaneous injection.

Meperidine, 100 mg, by subcutaneous injection.

Tarsitis. There are pain and diffuse inflammation of the foot. A diffuse picture of the tarsal bones is obtained in the X-ray films. The etiological factor (tuberculosis, gonococcal, etc.) must be found.

The treatment depends on the causative factor, with a specific antibiotic therapy against gonococcal, tubercular, or any other type of infection. Against pain, temporary relief may be afforded with analgesics.

Codeine, 60 mg, by mouth, every 6 hours.

Acetylsalicylic acid, 600 mg, in tablets, every 4 to 6 hours, preferably with meals.

Meperidine, 100 mg, by mouth, every 6 hours.

Metatarsalgia. Pain is felt beneath the middle three metatarsal bones, most frequently associated with tender calluses in the same area.

A rubber support placed behind the heads of the metatarsal bones will help in taking off pressure from the ball of the foot. Also, a transverse bar on the outside of the shoe, or adhesive strapping applied to a pad cut in the form of a triangle, could afford the same results. In addition, advice will be given to exercise the muscles (pick up marbles with the toes). Codeine or papaverine may help a little.

Codeine, 60 mg, by mouth, every 6 hours.

Papaverine, 150 mg, in slow-release capsules, one every 12 hours.

Neuralgia of the feet. Pain may be felt in one or both feet, in the heel, in the sole, or in the metatarsal area.

If a local (or a general) cause can be found, it should be treated accordingly. Blocking of the nerve is needed, at times. The use of vitamin B_{12} might be of some benefit, if there is impairment to its absorption.

Cyanocobalamine; inject 500 μg, three to five times a week (subcutaneously).

Acetylsalicylic acid, 600 mg, in tablets, every 4 hours, preferably with meals.

Codeine, 60 mg, by mouth, every 4 hours.

Since carbamazepine has proved effective in a number of patients suffering from other types of neuralgia, it could be tried in these cases.

> Carbamazepine, 200 mg, by mouth, every 6 to 8 hours.

Painful heel. The heel pain is due to plantar periostitis or bursitis of the Achilles' tendon.

First, check shoes for proper size and shape. Correct abnormalities, such as flatfoot and strain on the Achilles' tendon; and advise the patient to keep weight within normal limits, to massage and apply warm soaks, and to use a rubber ring to protect the painful heel. Use analgesics, if they are needed; or inject cortisone locally.

> Codeine, 60 mg, by mouth, every 6 hours.

> Papaverine hydrochloride, 150 mg, in slow-release capsules, one every 12 hours.

> Hydrocortisone, 25 mg, solution, to inject into the painful area; may repeat three times a week.

Plantar Neuroma. Severe pain is felt and elicited on palpation in the web between the third and fourth toes. Ordinarily, the lesion is unilateral. In the early stages, instead of a severe pain there may be paresthesias in the adjacent toes.

Physical devices may help, such as a rubber support behind the metatarsal heads. But the best choice is radical surgery on the involved nerves (excision).

Plantar Warts. A painful wart is found beneath the metatarsal heads. Tenderness is elicited by pressure and limping may result from these plantar warts, as well as from any other painful lesion of the feet.

Since these may be very painful and mostly always very difficult to treat, it is best to send the patient to an experienced dermatologist or podiatrist. For temporary help, advise the use of a rubber ring, metatarsal pad or bar, etc., for protection, and give analgesics, if they are needed.

> Codeine, 60 mg, by mouth, every 4 to 6 hours.

Foot Abnormalities. Pain is felt from almost all foot abnormalities, namely, flatfoot, high-arched foot, bunion, hammer toe, and the like. The diagnosis is obvious at examination.

These will be corrected by an orthopedic surgeon. In the meantime, advise the use of warm baths, rubber protective padding, and analgesics for pain.

Acetylsalicylic acid, 600 mg, in tablets, every 4 to 6 hours, preferably with meals.

Codeine, 60 mg, by mouth, every 4 to 6 hours.

Heterotopic Pain in the Legs

Growing Pains. Children and adolescents often complain of pain in the joints during the stages of more rapid growth. Pains are felt in the limbs and joints, particularly the knees; and if not too intense, they are at least bothersome because of their persistence and the limitation they impose on the children's activity. In many cases there is not any discoverable cause, and they may be considered due to the active, physiologic changes in the joint. In other instances they are due to a true systemic or localized disease. Rheumatic fever should be suspected, particularly if the child appears weak, has slight fever and tachycardia, and does not gain as he should. Mild arthritis or osteomyelitis may affect the rapidly growing joints, and at a future time may develop into a fully developed disease. Aseptic osteosis (radiologically diagnosed) may occur at this age. Coxalgia may begin as a growing pain during adolescence. Any infection in the body may give origin to articular pains. In scurvy there are early pains in the lower limbs; a child with growing pains should be checked for other signs and symptoms of hypovitaminosis C.

The use of salicylates is advisable for growing pains, since most cases are due to true rheumatic fever. Please refer to the discussion of this disease, under "Rheumatic fever," for more details.

Endocrinopathies. Among the endocrinopathies, those that are more likely to cause leg pains are pituitary cachexia, gonadal insufficiency (Lawrence-Moon-Biedl syndrome), and myxedema. In these cases, joint pains are minor symptoms among the relatively abundant symptomatology of each disease.

See in the section on treatment of "Pain in Shoulders, Arms, and Hands" the paragraphs referring to "Climacterium", "Acromegaly" and "Cushing's disease," which are other common endocrinopathies accompanied by pains in the lower limbs.

XIII. MUSCLES

Most subjects included here have been dealt with in previous sections. The reader is referred to these sections for additional information, whenever it is needed.

Strain (wry neck). Because of a sudden jerk or wrenching, the muscles of one side of the neck become tense and tender. Because of this pain, the patient refuses to move the head, or any other part of the body that might also be affected by the pain. It is frequent that a person who went to bed without symptoms arises in the morning with this sort of pain. Any muscle of any body area may be affected, but the muscles most frequently involved are the sternocleidomastoid and the scalene group. If the pain follows an injury, it is important to rule out a dislocation or a fracture. The muscles are tender to touch and extremely sensitive to forced motion. The condition might also be due to exposure to cold.

In most instances, analgesics provide only modest results. Massage and heat are more effective, particularly in torticollis (wry neck). Anticholinergics are of relatively good effect.

> Belladonna tincture, five, ten or more drops, in water, three to six times a day, according to effects and tolerance.

> Atropine sulfate, 0.5 mg, tablets; half or one tablet, by mouth, every 6 hours, or according to effects and tolerance.

Tranquilizers may help, as well as muscle relaxants, the latter perhaps a little better.

> Meprobamate, 400 mg, by mouth, every 6 hours.

> Carisoprodol, 350 mg, by mouth, every 6 to 8 hours.

More severe cases will need a head halter to apply traction to the neck, and some will also need a collar, these cases being better under the care of the specialist.

Fibrositis. The clinical situation is similar to the one stated above. Pain starts suddenly and is increased with motion of the affected muscle, other symptoms depending on the involved area. Spasm and small painful nodules ("trigger nodules") are usually present. This condition may also be due to exposure to cold or dampness, prolonging the cold, or be secondary to injuries, infections, poisons, etc.

Rest, heat, and massage will be the first approach for treatment. If needed, analgesics and muscle relaxants, either alone or simultaneously, can be given.

> Acetylsalicylic acid, 600 mg, in tablets, every 4 hours, preferably with meals.

> Codeine, 60 mg, by mouth, every 4 hours.

Meprobamate, 400 mg, by mouth, every 6 hours.

Carisoprodol, 350 mg, by mouth, every 6 to 8 hours.

The small, painful nodules (trigger nodules) respond very well to the local injection of an anesthetic or a corticoid.

Procaine, 1% solution, 0.25 ml or more.

Hydrocortisone, 2.5% suspension, 0.25 ml or more.

More severe cases affecting the back have to be treated by complete bed rest, on a hard mattress, in addition to the care scheduled above. More complex treatment (plaster fixation, traction, surgery, etc.) will be evaluated and carried out by the specialist.

Myositis. As stated for fibrositis, myositis is an inflammation of a muscle or group of muscles which suddenly appear tense and tender to touch, and which are very sensitive to forced motion.

In general, myositis will be treated according to the same schedule as for fibrositis, since there are those who believe the two conditions are the same. The treatment will start with rest, heat, and massage. Analgesics and muscle relaxants will be given at the same time. More complex procedures will be decided by the specialist.

Polymyositis requires physical therapy, corticoids, and analgesics.

Prednisone, up to 60 to 80 mg a day, for as long as needed or until symptoms of hyperdosage appear; final dosage to be adjusted to requirements.

Codeine, 60 mg, by mouth, every 4 to 6 hours.

Fibromyositis requires rest, massage, heat, a hard flat bed, splints (if needed), salicylates, and local anesthesia.

Acetylsalicylic acid or sodium salicylate, 600 mg, by mouth, every 4 to 6 hours, preferably with meals.

Procaine, 1% solution; inject 0.5 to 1 ml, into nodules.

Stiff-man syndrome requires avoidance of undue stimulation, myoneural blocking agents, blocking of peripheral nerves (with procaine, as above), and diazepam.

Diazepam, 5 to 10 mg, by mouth, every 8 hours.

Trichinosis. The infection with *Trichinella spiralis* gives rise to gastrointestinal symptoms followed by fever, pain in the muscles, and periorbital edema. The latter might be the first manifestation of the disease, together with or followed by subconjunctival and retinal hemorrhages and symptoms of an allergic type, including a marked eosinophilia. As it may happen with any more or less serious infectious clinical complex, generalized muscular soreness is an important component of the picture; but in this disease it is especially violent.

No specific therapy is known. Pain is relieved with analgesics and corticoids, preferably given together.

> Prednisone, 5 mg, tablets; daily, 20 to 60 mg, in divided doses; decrease the dosage after 3 to 3 5 days; then, discontinue gradually, after 10 days of therapy.

> Acetylsalicylic acid, 600 mg, in tablets, every 4 hours, preferably with meals.

> Codeine, 60 mg, by mouth, every 4 hours, if needed, instead of acetylsalicylic acid.

It is advisable to try thiabendazole, which may give good results in some cases.

> Thiabendazole, 500 mg in 5 ml, suspension; give 25 mg for each kg of body weight, dosage to be repeated every 12 hours, by mouth, for 2 to 5 days, but never more than 10 days.

Tetany. This condition is characterized by tonic-clonic spasms of the muscles, particularly those of hands and feet ("carpopedal spasm"), which are painful in many instances though not always. The spasms persist from minutes to hours and may turn into convulsions when the causative factor—a drop in blood calcium—reaches very low limits. This hypocalcemia is mainly due to hypoparathyroidism, but it may also be provoked by a decreased absorption of calcium (ordinarily due to hypovitaminosis D), an increase of phosphorus, hypoproteinemia, or pancreatitis, or postsurgically or during pregnancy or lactation. Contraction of muscles under pressure (as with the cuff of the sphygmomanometer) or percussion (below the cheek) is suggestive, but the diagnosis is made by finding low figures for calcium in the blood.

See "Cramps," in the following paragraph, for the treatment of acute stages of hypocalcemia. After control, use the following for maintenance.

> Calcium lactate, powder, 1 level teaspoonful, once or twice a day.

Calciferol, 40 to 200 units a day.

Dihydrotachysterol, 0.75 to 1 mg a day, checking blood calcium concentration at frequent intervals.

Cramps. A cramp is a painful involuntary muscle contraction similar to tetany, but more distressing. Cramps may appear under different conditions mainly related to dehydration, pregnancy, or neurologic disorders: nocturnal cramps of the legs (perhaps the most frequent), those due to insufficient flow of blood to a muscle, heat cramps (provoking extremely painful paroxysmal cramps following any work done at elevated ambient temperature and consequent sweating), and tetanus (in which cramps are the outstanding symptom).

As is well known, most muscle cramps are due to tetany (hypocalcemia) or muscle anoxia (e.g., the night cramps from insufficient blood flow). Calcium medication is specific for hypocalcemia, and it should be given together with vitamin D, dihydrotachysterol, or parathyroid hormone.

Calcium gluconate, 10% solution; inject 10 to 20 ml, intravenously.

Calcium chloride, 10% solution; inject 5 to 10 ml, intravenously.

Calcium lactate, powder, 1 level teaspoonful, three times a day.

Dihydrotachysterol, 0.125 mg, in capsules, a daily amount of 0.75 to 2.5 mg, in individualized and divided dosage.

Parathyroid hormone, 50 to 100 units, by subcutaneous or intramuscular injection, every 6 to 8 hours, for not more than 1 week.

If the cramps are due to poor vascular supply, they may respond to massage, hot applications, and vasodilators, such as papaverine.

Papaverine hydrochloride, 150 mg, in slow-release capsules, one every 12 hours.

Psoitis. There is pain in one or both of the iliac fossae, either spontaneous or elicited on deep palpation, which may also reveal muscle rigidity. This tenseness of the psoas causes a typical position of the leg: flexed and abducted. When the patient walks, he bends forward. In most instances the diagnosis depends on the primary cause, since psoitis only rarely is an independent problem: perinephritic abscess, appendicitis, adrenal tuberculosis, or tuberculosis spondylitis.

Infection of the psoas muscle most frequently follows infection of the spine, mainly tuberculosis. This basic disease is to be treated with antibiotics and surgery. Some relief will be offered with analgesics.

> Codeine, 60 mg, by mouth, every 4 hours.

> Papaverine hydrochloride, 150 mg, in slow-release capsules, every 12 hours; additional doses of 30 mg, in tablets, will be given, if needed.

Bursitis. In acute bursitis the symptoms appear suddenly, with intense pain caused by muscular motion, the tendon pressing over its bursa, with local tenderness and limitation of motion. In chronic bursitis the symptoms develop gradually but are the same, muscles becoming atrophic because of inactivity. Any bursa might present inflammation and pain, the most frequently affected being the subdeltoid. In this case, pain is usually referred to the shoulder, and sleep is disturbed because of the lack of adequate positions in which to lie.

A very early treatment with either radiotherapy or corticoids may give really good results.

> Prednisone, 5 mg, every 4 or 8 hours, according to each individual case; to decrease the dosage as soon as effects are noted; to discontinue medication gradually, for a period of 15 or 20 days.

In other instances, advise rest, immobilization, local applications of heat, and analgesics.

> Codeine, 60 mg, by subcutaneous injection during the acute stage; to be followed by oral administration, same dosage; in both instances, to give medication every 4 to 6 hours.

> Meperidine, 100 mg, to start, by subcutaneous injection, and then follow by oral administration; every 4 to 6 hours.

> Acetylsalicylic acid, 600 mg, in tablets, every 4 hours, preferably with meals.

These patients may also benefit from intra-articular injections of corticoids.

> Hydrocortisone acetate, 25 mg in 1 ml, suspension; to inject from 1 to 5 ml into the bursa.

Infections. Local infections of the muscle are rare occurrences, but mainly staphylococcal abscesses are the type found. Trichinosis has been the subject of a special paragraph. The detection of a localized pain, an area of congestion, and the final accumulation of pus will be diagnostic. Muscular pains are, on the contrary, a frequent finding in influenza and dengue; and are not rare in meningitis, yellow fever, etc.

An infection localized in a muscle will be treated with adequate drugs, mainly antibiotics; and drainage whenever possible. Analgesics may help a little.

> Acetylsalicylic acid, 600 mg, in tablets, every 4 hours, preferably with meals.
>
> Acetaminophen, 600 mg, by mouth, every 6 hours.
>
> Acetophenetidin, 300 mg, by mouth, every 4 to 6 hours.

Contracture of Achilles' Tendon. The typical position of the foot, because of the restricted dorsiflexion of the ankle, associated with pain along the arch and the calf, will be enough to suggest the diagnosis. Pain is increased by using flat shoes or walking barefooted. This condition is more frequently found among women.

Analgesics may relieve pain, but do not control the situation.

> Acetylsalicylic acid, 600 mg, in tablets, every 4 to 6 hours, preferably with meals.
>
> Codeine, 60 mg, by mouth, every 4 to 6 hours.
>
> Propoxyphene hydrochloride, 65 mg, by mouth, every 4 hours.
>
> Papaverine hydrochloride, 150 mg, in slow-release capsules, one every 12 hours.

The administration of analgesics will help for a better manipulation, giving massage, exercises, and gradual stretching of the tendon. If the contracture does not respond to the above therapy, surgery for lengthening of the tendon has to be considered.

Tennis elbow is a frequent form of bursitis, affecting an X-ray demonstrable bursa. It is described in the section on "Pain in the Shoulders, Arms, and Hands."

At a very early stage of the disease, a change in grasping objects or moving the joint is to be advised in order to avoid the position of strain. A tennis player should use a racket with a thicker handle; for others, a change that could match the above indication should be made. In addition to this, advise massage, the application of heat, and the administration of analgesics.

Acetylsalicylic acid, 600 mg, in tablets, every 4 hours, preferably with meals.

Papaverine hydrochloride, 150 mg, in slow-release capsules, one every 12 hours.

Codeine, 60 mg, by mouth, every 4 hours.

Later stages with chronic pain will be treated with analgesics, as above, and the patient will abstain from offending movements or have the arm immobilized in a splint or brace. Find the "trigger points" and infiltrate them with corticoids, alone or with local anesthetics.

Hydrocortisone acetate, 25 mg in 1 ml, suspension; inject about 1 ml, or less, into each point.

Procaine, 1% solution; inject 1 ml into each point.

Injuries to Muscles. These lesions are easily diagnosed by the clinical history and the finding of evidence of contusions, hematomas, wounds, burns, etc.

Most injuries to muscles are accompanied by injuries to adjacent bones, and the latter will dominate the clinical picture. In general, they beong to the domain of the surgeon, to whom the case will be referred. However, to mitigate suffering, analgesia will be offered, with the strength of the analgesic related to the intensity of the damage and the pain.

Codeine, 60 mg, by subcutaneous injection.

Meperidine, 100 mg, by subcutaneous injection.

Morphine, 10 to 15 mg, by subcutaneous injection.

XIV. PAIN IN THE PERINEUM, RECTUM, AND SEX ORGANS

Perineal Pain

Perineal pain is, generally speaking, a dull ache felt deep in the area between the anus and the sex organs. It is more annoying than distressing, and some times the patients refer to it more as a sensation of heaviness than true pain. For diagnosis, it is a poor reference, and the physician must rely on other symptoms primarily.

Prostatic Diseases. In general, prostatic diseases incite perineal pain and also sensation of heaviness associated with specific urinary symptoms, namely, pollakiuria, dysuria, urine retention, and perhaps painful areas in the rectum and the hypogastrium. Several forms of prostatitis are preceded by urethritis, particularly gonococcic prostatitis. In acute prostatitis there are also systemic symptoms (fever). In both acute and chronic prostatitis the same enlarged prostate is felt on rectal examination, intensely painful in the acute, and very painful in the chronic form. By pressure over the gland, some pus can be obtained from the urethra, which will serve for etiological diagnosis. Prostatic adenomas are extremely frequent in men over 50 years of age: pollakiuria occurs mainly during the night; dysuria is manifested by a difficult onset of urine and a small, irregular flow. When the adenoma gets larger, the foregoing conditions are more marked, and there are other symptoms of the change (retention of urine and systemic symptomatology). The symptoms of prostatic cancer are similar. The difference is found by rectal palpation: the adenomatosis tumor is smoothly and uniformly enlarged: prostatic cancer is irregular and harder.

In acute prostatitis, bed rest, forcing fluids, and cool sitz baths, together with the use of analgesics, are an important help to the basic use of specific antibiotic therapy.

> Papaverine hydrochloride, 150 mg, in slow-release capsules, every 12 hours.
>
> Codeine, 60 mg, by mouth, every 4 hours.
>
> Meperidine, 100 mg, by mouth, every 4 hours.
>
> Belladonna tincture, 20 to 30 drops, in a little water, repeated as needed and tolerated.

In chronic prostatitis, if pain is bothersome, some of the above analgesics might be used, preferably in smaller amounts. Contrariwise to acute prostatitis, massage may be of help, repeated as indicated by the specialist, together with hot sitz baths and long-term antibiotic therapy. For both types of prostatitis, surgery might be indicated.

For the few occasions in which pain is felt because of prostatic hypertrophy (nonmalignant), any of the above analgesics could be tried. For malignancies, morphine and its analogues are needed, but surgery and other specialized techniques are a must.

> Morphine sulfate, 15 mg by subcutaneous injection, as needed and tolerated.

Meperidine, 100 mg, by subcutaneous injection, every 4 hours, or as needed.

Diseases of the Seminal Vesicles. Such diseases are very rare. There is pain, mainly in the perineal area. Rectal palpation will disclose distended seminal vesicles. It is very important to remember that, normally, the seminal vesicles are tender on palpation; and they are, perhaps, less tender when chronically infected.

Rarely, the seminal vesicles become infected. If this occurs, it mostly will happen in association with prostatitis (see above discussion), and the treatment for pain will follow the same lines.

Bladder Diseases. There may be some pain or distress in the perineal area, but when a diseased bladder causes pain, it usually starts in the hypogastric region. Other findings are pollakiuria, dysuria, and in acute cases also systemic manifestations (chills, fever, etc.). The foregoing symptoms are the result of acute cystitis, chronic cystitis, tumors and ulcers of the bladder, and even foreign bodies (inserted from the outside, or from renal stones).

Cystitis, either acute or chronic, will require additional help for discomfort, no matter if the pain is not too severe. Best results are obtained with the following:

Methylene blue, 65 or 130 mg, by mouth, every 8 hours (warn of discoloration of urine and staining of clothes).

Phenazopyridine hydrochloride, 200 mg, by mouth, every 8 hours (warn of discoloration of the urine and staining of clothes).

But also parasympatheticomimetic drugs such as the following may be of value:

Belladonna tincture, 15 to 30 drops, in water, repeated as needed and tolerated.

Atropine sulfate, 0.5 mg, tablets; one every 8 hours, or as needed and tolerated.

Conditions secondary to neurogenic bladder and also to infection may require analgesics and other drugs to allay pain or discomfort. Only initial control will be carried out with analgesics or parasympatheticomimetics, as stated above. The remaining treatment will be put in the hands of the specialist.

Injuries to the bladder will be helped initially with codeine or meperidine, but the urologist will complete the examination and decide on further treatment.

> Codeine, 30 or 60 mg, by subcutaneous injection.
>
> Meperidine, 100 mg, by subcutaneous injection.

Pain occurs late in cancer of the bladder. As usual, morphine and its analogues will be given for help.

> Morphine sulfate, 15 mg, by subcutaneous injection, repeated as needed and tolerated.
>
> Meperidine, 100 mg, by subcutaneous injection, repeated every 4 to 6 hours.
>
> Methadone hydrochloride, 10 mg, by subcutaneous injection, repeated as needed and tolerated.

Urethral Diseases. Pain may be perineal, but it is mainly local and increases during micturition. An associated purulent secretion is always present; it is evident when the patient is getting out of bed in the morning.

In women, urethral diseases are more frequently bothersome: the urethral caruncle may cause exquisite pain; it should be treated by the specialist (fulguration, etc.), but the use of methylene blue, phenazopyridine hydrochloride, belladonna tincture, etc., may afford temporary relief.

> Methylene blue, 65 or 130 mg, by mouth, every 8 hours (warn about discoloration of urine and staining of clothes).
>
> Phenazopyridine hydrochloride, 200 mg, by mouth, every 8 hours (warn as above).
>
> Belladonna tincture, 10 to 20 drops, in water, according to tolerance and effects.

Uterine Diseases. Most uterine diseases will induce at least some distress in the lumbar region as well as in the perineal area. These sensations may be the first symptom, but rarely an orienting one, since the patient will seek advice only when other more conspicuous symptoms appear (tumor, hemorrhage, deviations provoking rectal or vesical symptoms).

Analgesics are indicated only in the acute stage of cervicitis, but the treatment depends essentially on antibiotic therapy and specialized local techniques to be carried out by the gynecologist.

> Codeine, 60 mg, by subcutaneous injection, at least initially; thereafter, by mouth, every 4 to 6 hours.
>
> Meperidine, 100 mg, by subcutaneous injection, at least

initially; thereafter, by mouth, every 4 to 6 hours, as needed and tolerated.

Cancer of the uterus has to be treated by the gynecologist. Only in advanced stages will opiates be needed.

Morphine sulfate, 10 or 15 mg, by subcutaneous injection, repeated as needed and tolerated.

Meperidine, 100 mg, by subcutaneous injection, repeated as needed and tolerated.

Methadone, 10 mg, by subcutaneous injection, repeated as needed and tolerated.

The pain provoked by torsion of the pedicle of all uterine myomata might be relieved by any of the above-mentioned drugs (morphine sulfate, meperidine, methadone, etc.), but the treatment is basically in the surgeon's domain.

Endometriosis depends upon an endocrinological or surgical treatment, or a combination of both. The use of analgesics would be a minor help.

Acetylsalicylic acid, 600 mg, tablets, every 4 to 6 hours.

Codeine, 60 mg, by mouth, every 4 to 6 hours.

Propoxyphene hydrochloride, 65 mg, by mouth, every 4 hours.

Acute salpingitis requires the help of analgesics, but the treatment needs specific antibiotic therapy, and usually some sort of surgery. Try analgesia according to the following sequence:

Acetylsalicylic acid, 600 mg, tablets, every 4 hours.

Codeine, 60 mg, by mouth, every 4 hours.

Meperidine, 100 mg, by subcutaneous injection initially, followed by oral doses every 4 to 6 hours.

Morphine sulfate, 10 mg, by subcutaneous injection, to be followed by oral administration of meperidine or codeine.

Vaginal Diseases. Dyspareunia results in a difficult or painful intercourse, due to muscle spasm or local lesions (dryness, inflammation, anatomical defects, etc.). The main symptom is pain resulting during coitus.

Vaginitis may also cause dyspareunia, but the unpleasant sensations are more organic, and the local inflammation is evident on examination. To establish its nature is the second diagnostic step, also necessary for ordering the adequate treatment, either antiparasitic or antiinfective.

Dyspareunia is always a very unpleasant experience for a woman. The treatment may require surgery, specialized techniques, and psychotherapy, but a start with sedatives must be made.

> Sodium phenobarbital, 15 or 30 mg, by mouth, every 6 to 8 hours, according to tolerance and activity.

> Amobarbital, 30 to 50 mg, by mouth, every 8 to 12 hours, according to action and tolerance.

> Prochlorperazine, 5 to 10 mg, by mouth, every 6 to 8 hours; slow-release capsules containing 15 mg might be given at 12-hour intervals.

Most cases of vaginitis are either parasitic or infective in nature, and should receive the appropriate therapy. In addition, warm douches (either plain saline or acid douches) may give temporary help—do not repeat douches too frequently.

> Sodium chloride, 1½ level teaspoonfuls in a liter of water.

> Vinegar (white, distilled), 2 teaspoonfuls in a liter of water.

These patients will also benefit from the use of menstrual tampons, and have less itching and soiling.

For other details see below, under the heading "Pain in the Sex Organs."

Rectal and Anal Diseases. Some perineal distress or even pain will be apparent with rectal and anal diseases. These are of minor interest as compared with the local symptomatology, which is discussed in the following paragraphs. There details will be found for both diagnosis and treatment.

Rectal and Anal Pain

Hemorrhoids. Hemorrhoids are not painful, per se; hemorrhoidal crises are. The external hemorrhoids distend suddenly and become very painful. The distended vein is easily seen in the margin of the anus, and it may bleed. The internal hemorrhoids may protrude from the inside, and then are painful and also may bleed. Thrombosed hemorrhoids are extremely painful; the average hemorrhoidal volume increases and becomes irreducible. During defecation, pain from external hemorrhoids increases, and it may precipitate strangulation of the hemorrhoidal sac. The pain is intense, particularly if there is a coincident anal ficsure. When there is a clinical picture of rectal involvement (pain of either a colicky or a continuous nature in the rectal area, sensation of having a foreign body, constipation alternating with bloody or mucopurulent diarrhea, and systemic symptoms, particularly of a mental nature), the first disease to have in mind is, precisely, internal hemorrhoids.

When hemorrhoids become painful, the best thing to do is to consult a proctologist. In the meantime, prolapsed hemorrhoids will be gently replaced with the help of wet paper (toilet paper or paper towel). It is to be noted that the use of lubricated gloves will allow an easy further prolapsing. Thrombosed hemorrhoids will be treated with hot or cold sitz baths, as preferred by the patient, and analgesics.

> Codeine, 60 mg, by subcutaneous injection, repeated as needed and tolerated.

> Meperidine, 100 mg, by subcutaneous injection, repeated as needed and tolerated.

> Papaverine hydrochloride, 30 or 60 mg, by subcutaneous injection, repeated as needed and tolerated.

But the final steps will be taken by the proctologist, who will evacuate the thrombus or excise the whole tumor.

For local pain, when there are no other accompanying symptoms, the use of suppositories is advisable.

Polyarteritis. Within the extremely variable clinical picture due to periarteritis nodosa, a rare rectal location may precipitate a rectal syndrome (see above, under "Hemorrhoids"). In this situation, with rectal pain and other local symptoms, the diagnosis of periarteritis nodosa is well camouflaged. The conclusion is made by the evaluation of the rectal symptoms and exploratory findings (arterial nodosites seen by rectoscopy) associated with a febrile ailment of uncertain nature.

As expected, pain due to polyarteritis is almost always poorly amenable to therapy. So an emergency medication, meperidine or codeine might be given; but as a long-term effort, corticoids would give a better result (though overall success is not hopeful).

> Meperidine, 100 mg, first dose by subcutaneous injection; thereafter by mouth, every 4 to 6 hours.

> Codeine, 60 mg, first dose by subcutaneous injection, thereafter by mouth, every 4 to 6 hours.

Prednisone, starting with a high dosage (20 to 40 mg a day, in divided doses); after a few days, decrease dosage.

Perianal Abscess. The main symptomatology includes anal piercing pain, frequently associated with fever and urine retention. The diagnosis is made by direct examination of the area, showing localized tenderness and swelling.

The basic treatment depends on surgery and antibiotics. The use of analgesics depends on the need for temporary relief.

Papaverine hydrochloride, 150 mg, in slow-release capsules, one every 12 hours.

Codeine, 30 or 60 mg, by mouth, every 4 to 6 hours.

Meperidine, 100 mg, by mouth, every 6 hours.

Anal Fistula. A fistula in ano generally follows a perianal abscess. The first symptom is pain, together with intermittent pus discharge. An opening in the skin adjacent to the anus is diagnostic.

Palliative treatment of pain can be done with papaverine, codeine, meperidine, and suppositories; but there is no other solution for the problem except surgery.

Papaverine hydrochloride, 150 mg, in slow-release capsules, one every 12 hours.

Codeine, 60 mg, by mouth, every 4 to 6 hours.

Meperidine, 100 mg, by mouth, every 6 hours.

Anal Fissure. Anal fissures are, probably, the commonest cause of anal pain (together with hemorrhoids). There is a sharp pain, which makes defecation extremely difficult, and persists, increasingly severe thereafter. The fissure should be visualized by a careful examination.

Use anesthetic ointments to allay pain, applied particularly before and after defecation.

Lidocaine, 5% ointment; to apply locally whenever needed, particularly before and after defecation.

Antispasmodic drugs will afford some help for the treatment of this kind of pain.

Papaverine hydrochloride, 150 mg, in slow-release capsules, one every 12 hours.

Belladonna tincture, 15 to 30 drops, in water, every 4 to 6 hours, as needed and tolerated.

Rectal Prolapse. Pain is minimal, or even absent, except when there are associated hemorrhoids, inflammations, or fissure in ano. Diagnosis is made as soon as the everted mucosa is seen.

This condition has to be treated immediately, by replacing the prolapsed rectum to its proper location. Put the patient in a genupectoral position, or merely a lateral position, and then, gently, with wet gauze or cotton, push the prolapsed mass through the anal opening. When this is done, place a cotton ball firmly attached to the ano-perineal area, to avoid further prolapsing. Also, give mineral oil and instruct the patient to defecate avoiding all straining on the rectum. Treat proctitis, if it is present (see below, for details); and use sclerosing agents, if they are needed.

Trauma to Anus and Rectum. Pain and the causative injury are easily evaluated. If the injury is severe, it might have perforated the rectal walls and might provoke peritonitis and shock.

Important injuries need an immediate repair; namely, the treatment is surgical. Temporary relief might be given by anesthetic solutions.

Cocaine, 5 to 10% solution; instill a few drops on lacerated tissues.

Tetracaine, 2% solution; instill a few drops on lacerated tissues.

Lidocaine, 1 or 2% solution; inject 1 to 3 ml into lacerated tissues.

Minor injuries will be thoroughly cleansed and disinfected like those located elsewhere. Cold compresses will help.

Foreign Bodies. Pain and bleeding are the most frequent symptoms. There may be a history of the insertion of the foreign body. By rectal palpation it may be noted, and the finding corroborated by X-ray examination.

These objects are to be removed, always. Removal through the anus will be tried first; if that is not possible, a surgeon will take care of the case. To allay pain and nervousness during the procedure, give one of the following:

Meperidine, 100 mg, by subcutaneous injection.

Methadone, 10 mg, by subcutaneous injection.

Morphine sulfate, 15 mg, by subcutaneous injection.

Proctitis. An almost complete rectal syndrome develops in cases of inflammation of the rectal mucosa. Pain may be colicky or continuous, and it is accompanied by discomfort and repeated rectal tenesmus. Most efforts to defecate are fruitless, passing nothing or only mucus and gas. There is constipation alternating with bloody and/or mucous diarrhea. Dyspeptic and mental symptoms may also arise. The diagnosis is made by rectoscopy, showing a red, edematous, and even purpuric mucosa. Proctitis may be due to infection, which may be bacteriologically diagnosed; or it may be due to dysentery, tuberculosis, syphilis, or gonorrhea, or be nonspecific.

Since there is almost always pain, at least related to defecation, an effort should be directed toward softening the stools.

> Dioctyl sodium sulfosuccinate, 50 to 250 mg, in capsules; take up to 250 mg, as needed to soften stools, without provoking unpleasant side effects.

Also, to protect against ano-rectal spasm, give:

> Belladonna tincture, 10 to 30 drops, in water, according to effect and tolerance.

> Atropine sulfate, 0.5 mg, tablets; to take half or one tablet, according to effects and tolerance.

If there is additional diarrhea, which frequently increases pain, it will be necessary to add to the treatment:

> Laudanum (tincture of opium), 20 to 30 drops, in water, repeated as needed and tolerated.

> Paregoric elixir, up to 4 ml in water, repeated as needed and tolerated.

The rest of the treatment depends basically on the underlying cause of the proctitis.

Cryptitis. There are some symptoms of pain during and after defecation, generally accompanied by blood or pus discharge. The diagnosis is made by local examination, showing tenderness and thickness of the crypts of Morgagni, together with spasm of the sphincter.

To treat the causative infection is the basic purpose. Pain can be allayed with a stool softener.

> Dioctyl sodium succinate, 50 to 250 mg, in capsules, up to 250 mg in a day, according to effects and tolerance.

It is important to increase the bulk of the stool with medication and a diet with high residue.

Psyllium hydrophilic muciloid, 50% powder; 1 level teaspoonful in a glass of water, up to three or four times a day, as needed and tolerated. Additional water intake is imperative.

Methylcellulose, 500 mg, tablets; one to three tablets every 6 to 12 hours, according to effect and tolerance, accompanied with a glass of water.

Sodium carboxymethylcellulose, as above.

Perhaps methylcellulose and sodium methylcellulose are the best drugs to be used in these cases because they increase both bulk and intestinal peristalsis. But these patients should consult the proctologist.

Crypts may benefit from daily local applications, as follows:

Phenol, 5% oil solution.

Carbolfuchsin compound (Castellani's paint), solution.

Papillitis. Pain is mild, and a constant urge to defecate is the main symptom. An enlarged papilla may protrude (do not take it for a hemorrhoid!). The diagnosis is made by rectoscopy (do not take it for a polyp!).

See "Cryptitis," for details about treatment.

Lymphogranulomatosis. Pain, constipation alternating with diarrhea, and sensation of a foreign body are symptoms that gain some value when associated with other symptoms of stricture, which are dominant: more intense constipation, with thin, irregularly shaped feces, mucosanguinous diarrhea, and tenesmus. Symptoms of complicating perianal abscess and anal fistula are not rare.

Once the diagnosis is established, the patient has to be treated with either sulfadiazine or a tetracycline; but the enlarged and possibly ulcerated lymph glands are painful, requiring rest, warm compresses applied locally, and the administration of analgesics.

Codeine, 60 mg, by mouth, every 4 hours.

Meperidine, 100 mg, by mouth, every 4 to 6 hours.

Acetylsalicylic acid, 600 mg, tablets, every 4 hours.

Polyps and Benign Tumors may be accompanied by mild or no pain. The most important symptom is hemorrhage. The diagnosis is made by rectoscopy.

Discomfort, at most, is only minor; so, very rarely will analgesics be needed before excision of the masses, which is the treatment to follow. If needed, codeine or papaverine may be given.

Codeine, 30 mg, by mouth, every 4 to 6 hours.

Papaverine hydrochloride, 150 mg, in slow-release capsules, every 12 hours.

Cancer. There is no specific symptomatology for cancer; the symptoms may be any of those corresponding to proctitis. Unfortunately, pain may occur late in the disease. A rectoscopic examination is mandatory in all cases suggesting rectal involvement.

As usual, the best treatment for cancer is its surgical removal, whenever feasible, or its treatment with radiotherapy or chemotherapy, if such is needed. Palliative drugs for pain start with regular analgesics, then narcotics when the former are no longer effective.

Codeine, 60 mg, by mouth or subcutaneous injection, every 4 hours.

Meperidine, 100 mg, by mouth or subcutaneous injection, every 4 hours.

Methadone, 10 mg, by injection, as needed and tolerated.

Morphine sulfate, 15 mg, by injection, as needed and tolerated.

Rectal Spasm. This cramplike pain occurs more frequently at night, an unpleasant feeling located above the anus. It is mild at first but increases rapidly, and might be associated with abdominal symptoms and fainting, or might follow sexual intercourse. Rectal examination may reveal no abnormal findings, or at most a mild spasm of the levator ani. Sigmoidoscopic examination may reveal vascular congestion. Not rarely, patients with diseases of the uterus or the prostate might complain of rectal pain associated with spasms and the sensation of a foreign body. No lesions are found by rectoscopy.

To eat some food or drink some water may terminate the spasm (gastro-colic reflex). If not, give a small enema or dilate the anus, but only slightly and gently with one or two fingers. Give meperidine to complete the treatment.

Meperidine, 100 mg, by subcutaneous injection, followed by same dosage by mouth, every 4 hours, for one or two days.

Heterotopic Pain. Heterotopic pain is frequently felt in the rectum and anal region, either as a simple pain or as a more complex rectal spasm. The primary site for the offending lesion may be gynecologic (uterine tumors or retroversion, adnexial inflammation, cysts, etc.), prostatic (large adenomas or cancer), or originating from the seminal vesicles (vesiculitis), the urinary bladder (cystitis, tumors), or the urethra (urethritis). Each one will be treated, accordingly.

Pain in the Sex Organs

Dysmenorrhea. By far, dysmenorrhea is the commonest of all pains of the female sex organs. The menstrual pain is ordinarily felt in the abdomen; a few patients will refer their pain to a more deeply set location within the pelvic region. The diagnosis of dysmenorrhea is easy, because of its coincidence with the menstrual flow, either preceding it by a few hours or a day or two, or starting simultaneously and continuing together up to one or more days. It is a colicky pain, mainly located in the hypogastrium, or may be referred to the lumbar region or to the ovarian areas. It is to be noted that there are some cases of false dysmenorrhea, namely, chronic appendicitis, colitis, and the like, which show a recrudescence of pain during the menstrual periods (other symptoms, if carefully searched for, will show the exact nature of the pain). In cases of pure dysmenorrhea, no lesions in either the sex or the neighboring organs will be discovered on examination. Other cases will show an abnormal condition of the uterus, such as hypoplasia, retroversion, endometritis, adnexitis, etc.

Pain due to primary dysmenorrhea will respond well to codeine, belladonna, atropine, or papaverine; but if it persists for a long time, to hormonotherapy.

> Codeine, 60 mg, by mouth, every 4 to 6 hours.
>
> Belladonna tincture, 10 to 30 drops, in water, every 4 to 6 hours, as tolerated.
>
> Atropine, 0.5 mg, tablets; take a half or one tablet, every 4 to 6 hours, as tolerated.
>
> Papaverine hydrochloride, 60 mg, by mouth, every 4 hours.
>
> Conjugated estrogens, 1.25 mg, once a day, for 20 days before the expected menstruation.

Premenstrual Tension. Pains of the type of dysmenorrhea are associated with mastalgia, headache, irritability, and some edema; and the whole complex starts from 7 to 10 days before the onset of the menstrual flow, to end a few hours after it.

Common analgesics will easily control premenstrual pain.

> Acetylsalicylic acid, 600 mg, in tablets, every 4 hours, for 1 or 2 days. Preferably with meals.

Codeine, 60 mg, by mouth, every 4 hours, for 1 or 2 days.

Propoxyphene hydrochloride, 65 mg, by mouth, every 4 hours, for 1 or 2 days.

Acetaminophen, 600 mg, by mouth, every 6 hours, for 1 or 2 days.

Acetophenetidin, 300 mg, by mouth, every 4 hours, for 1 or 2 days.

But if the analgesics fail to control pain, diuretics can be given, either alone or with an analgesic, starting a few days before menstruation.

Chlorothiazide, 500 mg, by mouth, every 8 or twelve hours.

Hydrochlorothiazide, 50 to 100 mg, by mouth, every 12 hours.

Acetazolamide, 250 mg, a day, by mouth, in divided doses.

Mittelschmerz or Ovular Pain. This is a symptomatic complex of the female endocrine ovarian cycle, being one of the phenomena to be considered with premenstrual tension. It probably occurs in certain women at the time of rupture of the Graafian follicle, which occurs during the process of ovulation (14 days before the onset of menstruation).

If the pain is really severe, it will be advisable to supress ovulation with anticonceptional pills. Consider recent warnings against their use. Otherwise, regular analgesics will control ovular pain.

Acetylsalicylic acid, 600 mg, in tablets, every 4 hours, for 1 or 2 days, preferably with meals.

Codeine, 60 mg, by mouth, every 4 hours, for 1 or 2 days.

Vulvitis. In acute vulvitis there is pain associated with evident symptoms of local inflammation. The diagnosis is made on inspection of the area.

In chronic vulvitis, pruritus is the main trouble; but acute vulvitis may cause pain. When there is not too marked inflammation, cold compresses of aluminum acetate will give good results.

Aluminum acetate, 5% solution, to soak compresses.

With inflammation, sitz baths or hot compresses are of better effect. Antihistaminics and corticoids may also help.

Dyphenhydramine, 25 or 50 mg, every 6 to 8 hours.

Prednisone, 5 mg, once or twice a day.

Keep the area clean (avoid dryness caused by soaps, etc.), advise the use of absorbent and loose clothes, and treat the causative infection (specific antibiotic therapy).

Bartholinitis. The pain is located at one or the other side of the vulva. It is accompanied by local inflammation and the presence of an extremely painful tumor in one of the labia, with or without fluctuation. The diagnosis is made by inspection and palpation.

The patient should be referred to a gynecologist, since surgical drainage has to be done in most instances. Prepare the area with application of hot compresses (to hasten the collection of pus or the abortion of the abscess). Give antibiotics (specific, if known, or broad spectrum) and analgesics, if needed.

Acetylsalicylic acid, 600 mg, in tablets, every 4 hours, preferably with meals.

Codeine, 60 mg, by mouth, every 4 hours.

Meperidine, 100 mg, by mouth, every 4 hours.

Vaginitis. In the case of vaginitis, the pain is more deeply centered than in the case of vulvitis, and is accompanied by leukorrhea or frank purulent discharge. A laboratory search will be carried out for the etiological factor.

Most frequently, the cause of vaginitis is either infective or parasitic, and each case will be treated according to its etiology. Temporary relief from the local discomfort may be obtained with warm douches, which should not be repeated too frequently.

Saline solution, for vaginal douches, prepared with sodium chloride, 1½ level teaspoonfuls in a liter of water.

Acid solution, for vaginal douches, prepared with white, distilled vinegar, 2 teaspoonfuls in a liter of water.

Also see above, in the section on "Perineal Pain," under the heading "Vaginal diseases."

Balanitis. The patient will refer his pain to the glans penis or the prepuce. The diagnosis is made by inspection, and detecting the local inflammation of these parts.

Cleanse the area with hydrogen peroxide, zephyran, potassium permanganate, or boric acid with talcum. This treatment will be enough to ameliorate pain.

Hydrogen peroxide in equal parts of water, or one part for two or three of water.

Benzalkonium chloride, 1:2000 solution.

Potassium permanganate, 1:8000 solution.

Boric acid, one part, plus talcum powder, three parts, to keep area dry after cleaning with the above solutions.

Urethritis. Pain is continuous, more or less mild in intensity, but with violent burning during micturition. There is a purulent discharge, evident during the early hours of the morning, when the patient leaves his bed. The etiological factor should be isolated from the urethral discharge. Gonococcal urethritis is the commonest.

In nongonococcal urethritis, the causative germ may be unknown, but antibiotic therapy will always be carried out (of course, with the specific antibiotic, if it is known).

Tetracycline, 500 mg to 1 g, every 6 hours, for at least 2 days after all symptoms disappear.

If the tetracycline is not effective, try its combination with a sulfa, or give streptomycin.

Streptomycin, 1 g a day, by intramuscular injection, for 3 or more days.

In gonococcal urethritis, treat gonorrhea.

Trauma to Sex Organs. The diagnosis is obvious, and its main purpose will be to detect the extent of the injuries.

The injuries will be treated as are injuries inflicted on any other part of the body, with care to save redundant tissue, as found in the labia and the scrotum. For major injuries, refer the patient to a surgeon, and give:

Meperidine, 100 mg, by subcutaneous injection.

Morphine sulfate, 10 or 15 mg, by subcutaneous injection.

Foreign Bodies. The symptoms will be either those of a trauma or of an inflammation. The foreign body will be found on exploration. In most instances, the anamnesis is sufficient.

Those in the vagina can be easily removed. Those in the male urethra are to be removed by transurethral cystoscopy or suprapubic cystostomy, which is to be done by a urologist. If there is pain, give:

Codeine, 60 mg, by subcutaneous injection.

Meperidine, 100 mg, by subcutaneous injection.

Hydrocele. Pain is minimal, or limited to a sensation of heaviness. The main symptom is the mass of contained fluid on one side of the scrotum. The diagnosis is made by examination (fluctuation and positive transillumination).

In most instances aspiration will be needed; and in more advanced cases, hydroceletomy. The use of analgesics will provide little relief.

Hematocele. Here also, pain is minimal, but there is a sensation of great heaviness. The tumor in the scrotum is hard on palpation, does not transilluminate, and does not admit any differentiation of the involved structures (testis, epididymus, tunica vaginalis, etc.).

See above paragraph for information on treatment.

Epididymitis. Intense pain is present in most cases of epididymitis, except the type caused by infection with tuberculosis. Infection of the epididymus centers on the superoposterior side of the testis and forms a tender lump. Gonococcal urethritis may extend to the epididymus.

Epididymitis requires rest, cold or hot compresses (as preferred by the patient), sedation, and antibiotic therapy (specific, if known).

Codeine, 60 mg, by mouth, every 4 hours.

Meperidine, 100 mg, by mouth, every 4 or 6 hours.

Orchitis. There is an enlarged testis, tender on palpation and painful at all times. Ordinarily, it follows an infectious disease, mumps in the first place (only after puberty), but also may be associated with typhoid fever, undulant fever, etc. But it may follow also other etiological factors (surgery, stress, trauma, etc.).

In most instances, orchitis will respond well to rest, the use of a scrotal support, cold compresses, and antibiotics. Mumps orchitis also may respond to estrogens. For pain give:

Acetylsalicylic acid, 600 mg, in tablets, every 4 hours, preferably with meals.

Codeine, 60 mg, by mouth, every 4 hours.

Meperidine, 100 mg, by mouth, every 4 hours.

Orchiepididymitis. The inflammation of both the testis and the epididymis is evident. A good number of orchitis are true orchiepididymitis. The symptoms of both diseases (q.v.) are found in the same patient.

Antibiotic therapy and surgery will be evaluated by the urologist. To allay pain, advise rest (in bed, as much as possible; support of the bursae), cold compresses, and analgesics.

Acetylsalicylic acid, 600 mg, tablets, every 4 hours.

Codeine, 60 mg, by mouth, every 4 hours.

Meperidine, 100 mg, by mouth, every 4 to 6 hours.

Cancer and Other Tumors. Pain is not important as a symptom, since it appears late in the course of the disease.

Surgery, whenever possible, is the best approach for these situations. Only as palliative measures, to allay pain temporarily, opiates will be used, in the following sequence:

Codeine, 60 mg, by injection or orally, as needed; the frequency according to effects and tolerance.

Meperidine, 100 mg, as above.

Methadone, 10 mg, by subcutaneous injection, every 6 hours, or as needed and tolerated.

Morphine sulfate, 15 mg, by subcutaneous injection, as needed and tolerated.

Spermatic Vesiculitis. See above, under "Perineal Pain," and also, above, the discussion of "Orchiepididymitis."

Varicocele. Pain is mild or even absent. The mass of varicose veins is felt like a bag of worms in the external genitalia of both men and women (the latter almost only during pregnancy).

A complete plan to treat this problem includes: rest in bed during acute exacerbations, with cold compresses and elevated scrotum. The suspensory to elevate the scrotum will be used also when the patient leaves the bed (do not press against the scrotum from the borders of the suspensory). If the treatment starts soon, it may completely arrest the process. Only rare stubborn cases will require surgery.

Thromboangiitis of the Spermatic Vessels. This disease resembles symptomatologically an acute epididymitis. Care should be taken to determine exactly the site of the inflammation in the corresponding blood vessels.

It will be treated as is thromboangiitis of the legs (q.v.), but very special emphasis will be made on stopping smoking. The drug to be given is:

Diphenylhydantoin, 100 mg, by mouth, every 8 hours; in emergency situations give first dose by intramuscular injection (100 mg).

Sympathectomy will be discussed, if there is a worsening course of the disease.

Torsion of Pedicle of the Testis. Pain is extremely intense, and perhaps symptom number one. The testis is tender and swollen. Contraction of the cremaster muscle makes it stay high in the scrotum, which becomes edematous. Systemic symptoms (fever, nausea with vomiting) appear following necrosis of the gland.

Local pain is very acute, and an injection of morphine or meperidine is recommended.

> Morphine sulfate, 15 mg, by subcutaneous injection.

> Meperidine, 100 mg, by subcutaneous injection.

But the patient has to be referred immediately to the urologist or a surgeon, since surgery is the only possible way to save the testicle from gangrene unless a manual reversal of the torsion can be performed. If it occurs to the right testicle, the torsion takes place clockwise, so it has to be reversed counterclockwise; if it occurs to the left testicle, it takes place counterclockwise and has to be reversed clockwise.

Referred Pain to External Genitalia. As we have discussed in each corresponding section (q.v.), there are several diseases, particularly of the kidneys, bladder, and prostate, which may originate heterotopic pain in the external genitalia. The first to be considered is renal colic, in which pain radiated to the external genitalia of both men and women is characteristic. Its association with more important symptoms will give the exact diagnosis. Only in very rare instances will pain in the external genitalia be the dominant symptom of a renal colic. Diseases of the bladder, such as cystitis, calculi in the bladder, and vesical tumors, may also be accompanied by pain in the external genitalia; but it is a minor symptom within the general symptomatology of each disease. Also, a similar incidence may occur in cases of prostatic diseases. Finally, other diseases, including those of the digestive system, such as appendicitis, colitis, and the like, may give origin to heterotopic pain in the external genitalia; but we will say once more that it is only a minor symptom within a richer symptomatology.

It is not rare that a urethral stone causes genital pain, or other diseases of the urinary system, including the bladder. Also, an attack of appendicitis may cause pain in the penis, as well, also, as lesions of the spine. These diseases will be treated specifically; but some help will be afforded by analgesics.

> Codeine, 60 mg, by mouth, every 4 hours.

> Papaverine hydrochloride, 150 mg, in slow-release capsules, every 12 hours.

XV. PAIN IN THE SKIN

Infective Origin

Acne. Pain, usually moderate, increased by pressure over the inflamed area, is the first symptom to be noted. The characteristic lesion is superficial, in the pilosebaceous apparatus, and begins as a comedo which may develop into a true papule, then a pustule and finally a scar. Acne affects, preferentially, males during puberty, and centers on the face and the head, and the upper parts of the chest and the back. The diagnosis is obvious.

These painful lesions only rarely will require treatment for pain. Initially, warm compresses may help; but only when there is a frank collection of pus will an incision with a small scalpel be warranted. To avoid new lesions, tetracycline or clindamycin have been recommended. Also, contraceptive pills(?), keratoplastic and keratolytic agents, irradiation, dermabrasion, etc., have been advised.

Folliculitis. The clinical course of folliculitis is very similar to that of acne, with the main difference of a deeper setting. Pain is more intense, and inflammation more prominent. The lesion is a small nodule surrounding a hair; its inflammation may turn into pustulation.

Cleanse the area with sodium bicarbonate solution, and continue wet compresses for at least 15 minutes.

> Sodium bicarbonate, 3% solution (8 teaspoonfuls to 1 liter of tap water).

Use local antibiotic ointments or creams, such as neomycin or any other similar drug.

> Neomycin, 1% ointment or cream; apply locally every 6 to 8 hours.

Systemic antibiotic therapy will be used if the above measures fail.

Furuncle. The infection of the pilosebaceous apparatus is greater in furunculosis, invading the perifollicular area. There is a very painful elevated pustule with necrosis of its central portion. Pain is more intense in fingers, nose, and ears. They also center in the axillae, breasts, and buttocks, but may be found anywhere in the body.

Treat as acne. See above.

Carbuncle. When several furuncles develop in the same area and are confluent, the pain and inflammation are considerable. Cellulitis extends to the surrounding area and the tumor makes a frank elevation above the skin level. The presence of several openings draining pus is diagnostic. Systemic manifestations (fever, malaise) are the rule.

If sensitivity of causative germs is known, use the adequate antibiotic systemically; otherwise, choose the proper broad spectrum antibiotic. Moist heat may help to allay pain and localize the process. Mature lesions must be incised superficially, and the area protected with antibiotic ointments or creams (preferably, the specific one) covered with bandages. At times, analgesics are needed.

Codeine, 60 mg, by mouth, every 4 hours.

Meperidine, 100 mg, by mouth, every 4 hours.

Pustules. Pustules are small purulent lesions centering superficially in the skin. Most frequently, they start with a vesicle, but sometimes they are the initial lesion. They may be due to different clinical entities, being the late stage of acne, folliculitis, furuncle, carbuncle, chicken pox, smallpox, herpes, and the like. The most important lesion, as a pustule, is the so-called malignant pustule, or anthrax, ordinarily originating on the hand, arm, face, or neck. Anthrax presents little or no pain, but the infarcted ganglia are most frequently painful. The dark pustule surrounded by a red halo and showing vesicles is characteristic.

Treat as carbuncle, above.

Paronychia. The infection of a finger around and under the nail is very painful. Ordinarily, following a first stage of local inflammation, there is a second stage of pus formation. The diagnosis is made by the location of the infection.

The exquisite pain of paronychia would need the use of opiates, should it not be responsive immediately to incision and drainage, as soon as pus is collected. In the meantime, cold or hot compresses may be applied on the affected finger. Drainage will be aided by antibiotics and a covering bandage.

Pemphigus. The first stage of pemphigus, which is characteristic for diagnostic purposes, is the appearance of large vesicles or bullae directly arising from a normal skin or mucosa (no erythematous halo around the vesicle). As soon as the bulla breaks, there is a painful erosion in the skin. Diagnosis is suggested when the epidermis can be easily detached from the dermis by lateral pressure (Nikolsky's sign); but in cases of difficult diagnosis a biopsy of the skin is mandatory (acantholysis).

The patient should be hospitalized, for better care. Intravenous infusions (blood, feeding) may be needed. Bed rest is imperative. Local skin lesions will be treated with wet dressings.

Sodium bicarbonate, 3% solution (8 teaspoonfuls in 1 liter of tap water).

Neomycin, 1% solution; use as such.

Mouth lesions will be treated with anesthetic preparations, particularly before eating.

Tetracaine, 2% solution; instill a few drops.

The basic treatment requires massive doses of corticoids, and should be better managed by a specialist.

Prednisone, up to 150 mg, by injection, the first day; to be continued by oral administration, decreasing the dosage rapidly to maintenance levels.

Immunosuppressive drugs might be used if the above treatment fails (methotrexate, etc.).

Impetigo. In a way, impetigo runs a clinical course similar to that of pemphigus; namely, in a first stage the vesicles are swollen, and the erosive surface is frankly purulent. As soon as the vesicle breaks, the lesion becomes painful.

Keep the area clean, using:

Sodium bicarbonate, 3% solution (add 8 teaspoonfuls to 1 liter of tap water),

and maintaining it wet with compresses, for at least 15 minutes, every 12 hours. Larger lesions must be opened, and the necrotic tissue trimmed away; then cover the lesion with antibiotic ointments or creams.

Neomycin, 1% ointment or cream, to apply every 6 to 8 hours.

Other topical antibiotic ointments or creams can also be used.

Ecthyma. The characteristic lesion is a painful, shallow ulcer covered with a crust and surrounded by an erythematous halo. There may be a history of a previous impetigo, or the lesions follow a trauma. Ecthyma frequently occurs on the lower parts of the legs.

It will be treated as impetigo. See above paragraph.

Cellulitis. The lesion consists of a regional inflammation with induration, swelling, heat, and pain in the skin. It may affect any part of the body, generally close to a previous apparent or unknown infected opening of the surface. Systemic symptoms are usually associated, such as fever, malaise, and symptoms of lymphangitis.

Local application of wet compresses:

Sodium bicarbonate 3% solution (add 8 teaspoonfuls to 1 liter of water),

Potassium permanganate, one 100-mg tablet, in 1 liter of water (warn about skin discoloration and staining of clothes),

are of good effect, but the patient will be treated systemically with antibiotics, to which the causative agent is sensitive. If the cause not known, use broad spectrum antibiotics.

Erysipelas. The course of erysipelas is similar to that of any acute infective disease, with fever, malaise, and digestive symptoms, and is soon characterized by the appearance of a painful spot in any location of the body (face, usually) that becomes a pink to red area sharply limited by a somewhat elevated boundary. The area included in the well-demarcated limits is swollen, and shiny. A few severe cases may have vesicles and even bullae.

Most strains of beta-hemolytic streptococci are sensitive to penicillin, which will be given to these patients, if they are not allergic to it (if they are, use an adequate substitute).

Penicillin (procaine), 600,000 units every 12 hours, intramuscularly.

The patient must rest in bed, with the head elevated. Hot packs may help; but acetylsalicylic acid, or similar drugs, will alleviate pain.

Acetylsalicylic acid, 600 mg, in tablets, repeated every 4 hours, preferably with some food.

Acetaminophen, 600 mg, by mouth, every 6 hours.

Abscesses. Abscesses are deep purulent painful tumors ordinarily leading to fluctuation, which is the characteristic sign. They may follow local infections (subcutaneous injections, osteomyelitis, suppurative lesions of the skin) or even visceral infections (kidney, prostate, rectum, appendix). Most abscesses present a characteristic picture, such as submammary, peritonsillar, retropharyngeal, anorectal, amebic, perinephritic, and some other abscesses.

Treat as carbuncle (q.v.).

Hidradenitis Suppurativa. A firm, painful tumor in the axilla (less frequently in the nipple or the anogenital region), it may be an infection of the sweat glands, that is, hidradenitis suppurativa. Furuncles are more painful and less firm than hidradenitis.

When localized in the axilla, pain is almost always annoying. Warm compresses may help, at the beginning; but when there is a collection of pus, only an incision with a small scalpel will control it. In more severe cases, the affected glands must eventually be removed surgically. While the lesions are painful, an analgesic may be somewhat helpful.

> Acetylsalicylic acid, 300 or 600 mg, in tablets, one every 4 hours, preferably with meals.

> Codeine, 60 mg, by mouth, every 4 hours.

Antibiotic therapy, if specific against sensitive germs, might be curative.

Herpes. Herpes, or herpes simplex, is characterized by one or more clusters of small, clear vesicles centered on inflammatory raised bases, which appear more frequently around the lips or the genitalia. They are painful when found on lips, nose, ears, etc.

Topical application of anesthetic ether has been claimed as effective in the treatment of herpes simplex, thus allaying pain, when present. Cold compresses will help, particularly if there is associated cellulitis. Also, other means of treatment have been advised (dusting with bismuth formic iodide; calamine or starch lotion; epinephrine, 1:100, locally; etc.).

> Bismuth formic iodide powder.

> Calamine lotion; apply three or four times a day.

> Starch lotion; apply twice a day.

> Epinephrine, 1% solution; apply twice a day, locally.

Herpes Zoster. Herpes zoster is exactly like herpes simplex, except that the eruption is frequently preceded by pain along a nerve path, and thereafter the vesicles also originate in the same region.

In the great majority of cases, pain has to be treated.

> Acetylsalicylic acid, 600 mg, in tablets, every 4 hours, preferably with meals.

> Codeine, 30 or 60 mg, by mouth, every 4 to 6 hours.

> Acetaminophen, 600 mg, by mouth, every 6 hours.

> Acetophenetidin, 300 mg, by mouth, every 4 hours.

> Propoxyphene hydrochloride, 65 mg, by mouth, every 4 hours.
>
> Meperidine, 100 mg, by mouth, every 4 to 6 hours.

Corticoids are also advised (not in herpes simplex), since relief is sometimes reported by both parenteral and oral use.

> Triamcinolone acetonide, 40 mg, suspension; inject into gluteal area.
>
> Prednisone, to start with 40 mg, a day, and rapidly decrease the dosage; but discontinuance has to be slow.

Local treatment may give some comfort. It can be carried out with the following:

> Sodium chloride, 1% solution, (2 teaspoonfuls to 1 liter of water) as wet compresses.
>
> Sodium bicarbonate, 3% solution, 8 teaspoonfuls to 1 liter of water, as wet compresses.
>
> Calamine lotion, apply locally and cover with cotton.

Persisting neuralgia after resolution of skin lesions may be annoying, but can be treated with triamcinolone acetonide (see above) and lidocaine infiltrating the painful area.

> Lidocaine, 1% solution, to use 1 to 3 ml, to anesthetize skin by infiltration.

Other Origin

Intertrigo. Inflamed opposing skin surfaces, intertrigo, become painful when rubbed one side against the other (beneath the breasts and in the axillae, the groins, the anal region, and even between the interdigital spaces).

The skin lesion has to be treated, since the only way to avoid discomfort is to prevent rubbing of the opposed skin surfaces. Wet dressings may help, in the acute stage.

> Sodium chloride, 1% solution (2 teaspoonfuls in a liter of water).
>
> Sodium bicarbonate, 3% solution, (8 teaspoonfuls in a liter of water).

Potassium permanganate, 100 mg, tablet, to be dissolved in 1 liter of water (warn against discoloration of the skin and staining of clothes).

Contact Dermatitis. When it reaches the state of red swelling and bullae formation, there is pain in addition to itching. There is a history of contact with a known allergenic substance, or at least the possibility of this contact. Tests can establish the sensitivity.

In chronic cases, advise a thorough cleansing of the area, using the above solutions, and keeping the lesion protected with drying powders.

Talcum powder.

Topical antibiotic powder.

Patients with severe acute contact dermatitis will receive corticoids.

Prednisone, 40 mg, to start, by mouth, in three divided doses (20, 10, 10) the first day; decrease by 5 mg, each following day; discontinue gradually over 6 days.

The use of local treatment is advisable, even for mild cases as only treatment; wet compresses will be applied on the lesions. Use the following:

Sodium bicarbonate, 3% solution (8 teaspoonfuls in 1 liter of water).

Erythema Nodosum. There are tender, red nodules often in the anterior aspect of the tibia; rarely, in the arms or other parts of the body. After a time, the red color changes to bluish and brown. Erythema nodosum may be an independent clinical entity (ordinarily, associated with systemic symptomatology) but may appear together with other diseases (streptococcal infections, rheumatic fever, endocarditis, tuberculosis, etc.).

The pain felt in the nodules may be helped with analgesics.

Acetylsalicylic acid, 600 mg, in tablets, every 4 to 6 hours, preferably with meals.

Codeine, 60 mg, by mouth, every 4 to 6 hours.

Patients should be hospitalized; if a known infection is present, it should be treated adequately; and if lesions need local help, use wet dressings.

Sodium bicarbonate, 3% solution (8 teaspoonfuls in 1 liter of water).

Erythema Multiforme. There are symmetrical lesions in the distal limbs, showing concentric rings; in severe cases they are combined with bullae on the mucosae. The Stevens-Johnson syndrome is a severe form of erythema multiforme invading all visible mucosae.

The initial painful lesions will be treated with wet dressings, as follows:

> Sodium chloride, 1% solution (2 teaspoonfuls in 1 liter of water).
>
> Sodium bicarbonate, 3% solution (8 teaspoonfuls in 1 liter of water).
>
> Neomycin, 0.1% solution, to use as such.

It seems advisable to use antibiotic therapy, with a tetracycline, or sulfapyridine; and corticoids in more resistant cases.

> Tetracycline, 250 mg, tablets, one every 6 hours, for 12 days.
>
> Sulfapyridine, 500 mg, every 6 hours, also for 12 days.
>
> Prednisone, 10 mg, every 12 hours the first 2 or 3 days; then 5 mg, every 12 hours for another 2 or 3 days; finally, decrease gradually to total stoppage in 3 days.

When there is an underlying disease (infection, rheumatism, lupus, ulcerative colitis, etc.), treat it vigorously also. Bed rest is imperative if there is fever.

Ulcers. When the skin loses its superficial layers and becomes ulcerated, pain is one of the most important associated symptoms. Ulcers may be due to trauma, to infective diseases, to circulatory insufficiency, to nervous ailments, or to cancer. Perhaps the most frequent form is the varicose ulcer in the legs, associated with evident varices and always pigmented. The diagnosis depends on the associated symptoms and signs.

Initial ulcers may improve by use of topical antibiotic preparations, preferably in powder form, under adhesive absorbent bandage. This will allay pain. Also provide a water or an air mattress. If needed, analgesics might be given.

> Codeine, 60 mg, by mouth, every 4 to 6 hours.
>
> Propoxyphene hydrochloride, 65 mg, by mouth, every 4 hours.

Chronic ulcers will be better evaluated by a surgeon, since cancer may be a possibility. Should a cancerous ulcer provoke pain, opiates of the type of morphine will be given.

> Morphine sulfate, 15 mg, by subcutaneous injection, as needed and tolerated.

> Methadone, 10 mg, by subcutaneous injection, as needed and tolerated.

Cancers had best be treated by specialists.

Gangrene. Gangrene is the necrosis of the tissues nourished by an obstructed artery. It occurs more frequently in the distal parts of the limbs. In gangrene the first symptoms are decrease in the variations in local temperature and in local warmth; and also some paresthesias. When fully developed, gangrene is severely painful in both of the two types: dry gangrene, which shows a dark, almost black mummified area; and moist gangrene, infected by putrefying bacteria, and showing sloughing of tissues and foul odor. Gangrene is due to arteriosclerosis (senile gangrene), diabetes, thromboangiitis obliterante, emboli, arteritis, ergotism, freezing, heating, electricity and other traumas, nervous disease, Reynaud's disease, and several other diseases.

The treatment is essentially surgical, and the patient has to be sent immediately to a specialist. In the meantime, to allay pain, which may reach great proportions, opiates must be given.

> Morphine sulfate, 15 mg, by subcutaneous injection, as needed and tolerated.

> Methadone, 10 mg, by subcutaneous injection, as needed and tolerated.

> Meperidine, 100 mg, by subcutaneous injection, every 4 hours, or as needed and tolerated.

Trauma. Any trauma will provoke pain in the skin: contusions, abrasions, lacerations, and wounds. The diagnosis is obvious in each instance.

When some sort of surgical repair has to be done, the patient will be referred to the specialist. Local anesthesia will suffice in most instances; and rarely analgesics are to be given thereafter.

> Procaine, 1% solution, 1 to 3 ml, to infiltrate the wounded area.

> Codeine, 30 or 60 mg, by mouth, every 4 to 6 hours.

> Propoxyphene hydrochloride, 65 mg, by mouth, every 4 hours.

Index

Abdomen
  acute, 187
  chronic pain, 223
  diffuse pain, 224
Abortion, 253
Abscess, 332
  hepatic, 186
  intracranial, 98
  kidney, 249
  perianal, 317
  perirenal, 203, 248
  peritonsillar, 129
  retropharyngeal, 129
  spinal, 160
  subdiaphragmatic, 186, 235
Accommodation, faulty, 117
Acetaminophen, 30
Acetophenetidin, 29
Acetylsalicylic acid, 23
  compounds, 25
Achilles' tendon contracture, 287, 309
Acids, poisoning, 219
Acidosis
  diabetic, 212, 246
  postsurgical, 216
Acne, 329
Acrodynia, 218, 269, 289
Acromegaly, 280
Acute abdomen, 187
Acute dilatation of the stomach, 199
Acute febrile respiratory diseases, *AFRI*, 82
Acute respiratory disease, *ARD*, 82
Adenitis, mesenteric, 211
Adrenal crisis, 213
Adrenal tumor, 252

Adnexitis, 205, 254
Alcohol, 47
Alcohol poisoning, 222
Alkalosis, 107
Alkaly poisoning, 219
Allergy, headache, 108
Alphaprodine, 16
Altitude, high, 102
Aminopyrine, 32
Ammonia (gas) poisoning, 257
Amyl nitrite, 57
Anal fissure, 317
Anal fistula, 317
Anal pain, 315
Anal trauma, 318
Analgesics, 1
  ideal, 1
  narcotic, 2
  not requiring narcotic prescription, 18
Anaphylactic shock, headache, 110
Anemia
  hemolytic, colic, 24
  pernicious, 274, 294
Anesthesia
  local, 41
  technic for use, 51
Aneurism
  aorta, 165, 175, 208, 244
  iliac arteries, 245
Angina pectoris, 170
Anileridine, 17
Anoxia, cerebral, 103
Antibiotics, 71
Antimalarials, 38
Antimony poisoning, 221

INDEX

Antipyrine, 31
Aorta, aneurism, 165, 175, 208
Aortitis, 175, 208
Aphthae, 126
Appendicitis, 199, 230, 236, 241
Aralen, 40
Arsenic poisoning, 220
Arteritis, 101
Articular pain, 261
Arthritis, 262, 280
   degenerative, 264, 283
   gouty, 262, 280, 299
   rheumatoid, 263, 282
   septic, 281
Aseptic meningitis, 83
Aspirin, 23
Atabrine, 40
Atelectasis, 180
Atophan, 34

Bacteremia, 86
Balanitis, 324
Barium poisoning, 221
Bartholinitis, 324
Benzene poisoning, 257
Benzocaine, 49
Biliary colic, 186, 189
Biliary lithiasis, 165, 186
Bismuth poisoning, 258
Bladder, diseases, 312
Blepharitis, 135
Bone
   cysts, 272, 293
   neoplasms, 275, 296
   tuberculosis, 272, 292
Bone pain
   face, 122
   limbs, 271
   traumatic, 271, 291
Brachial neuralgia, 275
Brain
   cysts, 97
   tumors, 97
Bromates, poisoning, 258
Bronchopneumonia, 178
Brucellosis, 90
Bursitis, 265, 277, 285, 308
Butamben picrate, 48
Butazolidin, 32
Butesin picrate, 48

Cachexia, pituitary, 214
Cadmium poisoning, 221
Caffeine poisoning, 258
Cancer, 92, 118, 127, 164, 182, 226, 235, 237, 242, 250, 321, 327
Cantharides, poisoning, 259
Carbon tetrachloride poisoning, 259
Carbuncle, 203, 329
Carisoprodol, 69
Carotid syncope, 209
Causalgia, 277, 299
Cellulitis, 331
   orbital, 136
Cervical ribs, 151, 158
Chills, 76
Chlorates, poisoning, 258
Chlormezazone, 69
Chlorobutanol, 50
Chloroguanide, 41
Chloroquine, 40
Chlorzoxazone, 70
Cholecystitis, 187, 229, 233
Chrohn's disease, 238
Chronic abdominal pain, 223
Cincophen, 34
Claudication, intermittent, 289
Climacterium, 279
Coal-tar derivatives, 29
Cocaine, 41
Codeine, 9
Colchicine, 36
   poisoning, 259
Colchicum derivatives, 36
   official preparations, 37
Colitis, 193, 230, 235, 237, 239, 241
Colorado tick fever, 83
Common cold, 81
Conjunctivitis, 131
Contact dermatitis, 335
Contracture of Achilles' tendon, 287, 309
Copper colic, 218
Cornea, ulcers, 133
Cortef, 64
Corticoids, 61
Cortisone, 63
Coxalgia, 284
Cramps, 267, 286, 307
Crural neuralgia, 297
Cryptitis, 319
Curare, 70

INDEX

Cushing's disease, 280
Cyclandelate, 57
Cystitis, 243

Dacryocystitis, 135
Darvon, 18
Decamethonium, 71
Degenerative arthritis, 264
Deltasone, 65
Demerol, 13
Dengue, 84
Dermatitis, contact, 335
Dexamethasone, 66
Diabetic acidosis, 212, 246
Dibucaine, 45
Diffuse abdominal pain, 224
Digitalis poisoning, 259
Dihydromorphinone, 7
Dihydroergotamine mesylate, 60
Dilatation of the stomach, 199
Dilaudid, 7
Diothane, 46
Dioxyline, 12
Diperodon, 46
Disk lesions, 167
Diverticulitis, 241
Dolophine, 14
Duodenal ulcer, 233
Dysmenorrhea, 204, 292, 322
Dysphagia, 145
    buccal, 145
    esophageal, 147
    pharyngeal, 146

Ecthyma, 331
Emotions, 94
Emphysema, 176
Encephalitis, 95
Endocranial hyperostosis, headache, 112
Endophthalmitis, 134
Enteritis, 239
Epididymitis, 326
Epilepsy, 98
Epiphysiolysis of the head of the femur, 292
Ergonovine maleate, 60
Ergotamine tartrate, 59
Ergotrate, 60
Erysipelas, 121, 332
Erythema multiforme, 336
Erythema nodosum, 335

Erythrityl tetranitrate, 57
Erythromelalgia, 269, 289
Esophagitis, 227
Esophagus
    cancer, 148
    diverticulosis, 148
    extrinsic compression, 149
    foreign bodies, 148
    ulcers, 147
    scar, 148
Ethoheptazine, 21
Ethylaminobenzoate, 49
Eugenol, 50

Face
    injury, 121
    pain, 117, 122
Familial Mediterranean fever, 200
Farcy (glanders), 89
Femur, epiphysiolysis of the head, 292
Fenidrone, 35
Fever
    and headache, 75
    neurological symptoms, 77
Fibrositis, 162, 304
Fluorides, poisoning, 223
Flushing of the skin, 77
Folliculitis, 329
Foot abnormalities, 302
Formaldehyde poisoning, 260
Fracture of the spine, 167
Furuncle, 120, 329
    external ear, 140

Gall bladder, perforation, 197
Gangrene, 270, 290, 337
Gasoline poisoning, 257
Gastric obstruction, 197
Gastritis, 228
Gastrointestinal diseases, headache, 111
Genital diseases, 169
Gingivitis, 124
Glanders (farcy), 87
Glaucoma, 137
    headache, 115
Glomus tumor, 277
Glossitis, 126
Gouty arthritis, 262, 280, 299
Growing pains, 303
Guaiacol, 49
Gynergen, 59

INDEX

Hay fever, 110, 170
Headache, 75
  acidosis, 107
  alkalosis, 107
  allergy, 108
  anaphylactic shock, 110
  aural, 96
  coffee, 104
  diabetes, 111
  endocranial hyperostosis, 112
  fever, 75
  gastrointestinal diseases, 111
  glaucoma, 115
  hay fever, 110
  heat, 114
  hepatic, 111
  histamine, 109
  hypoglycemia, 105
  intracranial calcifications, 113
  iritis and iridocyclitis, 116
  migraine, 108
  muscle strain, 113
  oral, 96
  ovaric, 106
  Paget's disease, 112
  strabismus and faulty accommodation, 117
  tea, 104
  tobacco, 144
  toxic, 104
  traumatic, 114
  treatment, metabolic and toxic, 105
  uremia, 105
  vapor (gas), 105
Heart failure, 100, 209
Heat headache, 114
Heel, painful, 302
Hematocele, 326
Hematoma
  subarachnoid, 98
  subdural, 97
Hemorrhoids, 315
Hemolytic anemia colic, 211
Hepatic congestion, 234
Hepatic headache, 111
Hepatitis, 234
Hepatomegalia, 230
Hernia
  diaphragmatic, 224
  hiatal, 227
  Petit's triangle, 169

Herpangina, 83
Herpes, 333
  zoster, 79, 333
    ophthalmic, 118
    otic, 141
Hiatal hernia, 227
Histamine headache, 109
Hordeolum 135
Hydradenitis suppurativa, 332
Hydrocele, 326
Hydrocortisone, 64
Hydronephrosis, 203, 248
Hydroxyphenylcinchoninic acid, 35
Hyperchlorhydria, 227
Hypertension, 100
Hypogastric pain, 243
Hypoglycemia, 212, 232, 246
Hypothyroidism, 213
Hypotension, 100
Hypoventilation, 102

Iliac fossa tumors, 256
Impetigo, 331
Indocin, 21
Indomethacin, 21
Infarction
  myocardial, 172, 208
  pulmonar, 179, 207
  spleen, 210
Infectious mononucleosis, 80
Influenza, 77, 154
Insecticides, poisoning, 220
Intercostal neuralgia, 185
Intermittent claudication, 289
Intertrigo, 334
Intestinal colic, 192
  obstruction, 197, 242
  perforation, 196
  tuberculosis, 224
Intracranial calcifications, headache, 113
Iritis and iridocyclitis, 133
  headache, 116
Isoxuprine, 58

Keratitis, interstitial, 132
Keratoconjunctivitis, 132
Kerosene poisoning, 257
Kidney
  abscess, 249
  cancer, 250
  colic, 187, 201

INDEX 343

diseases, 169
movable, 249
polycystic, 251
tuberculosis, 250
Klippel-Feil syndrone, 151, 159

Laryngitis, 130
Lead colic, 218
Leptospiroses, 92
Leritine, 17
Leukocytosis, 77
Leukopenia, 77
Lidocaine, 45
Lithiasis
biliary, 186
renal, 251
Liver congestion, 234
Local infections, 94
Low back pain, 153, 165, 168
Lymph nodes, enlarged, 77
Lymphogranuloma venereum, 94, 320

Malaria, 88
Malta fever, 70
Mammary gland diseases, 183
Mannitol hexanitrate, 57
Mastodynia, 182
Mastoiditis, 144
Measles, 80
Mediastinum
diseases, 176
tuberculosis, 164
tumors, 164
Meningitis, 94, 154
Meperidine, 13
Mephenesin, 69
Meprobamate, 68
Meralgia paresthetica, 297
Mercury, acrodynia, 218
Mesenteric adenitis, 211
vascular occlusion, 197, 209
Metatarsalgia, 301
Metaxalone, 70
Methadone, 14
Methocarbamol, 69
Methylhydromorphone, 6
Methylmorphine, 9
Methylprednisolone, 67
Methylsalicylate, 26
Metopon, 6

Migraine, 108
Milkman's disease, 274, 294
Morphine, 2
Mouth, trauma, 128
Multiple myeloma, 185, 274, 295
Multiple sclerosis, 298
Muscle pain, 76
Muscle relaxants, 68
Muscle strain, 113, 162
headache, 113
Myalgia, stress, 266, 285
Myelitis, 160
Myeloma, multiple, 185, 274, 295
Myocardial infarction, 172, 208
Myositis, 266, 285, 305
Myringitis, 142

Neck
cervical spine deformities, 151
pain, 149
rheumatism, 150
wry, 149, 163, 169, 304
Neocinchophen, 35
Neoplasm of the mouth, 127
Neuralgia
brachial, 275
crural, 297
feet, 301
intercostal, 185
suboccipital, 152, 161
Neuritis
optic, 134
retrobulbar, 134
Neurological symptoms and fever, 77
Neuroma, plantar, 302
Neurosis, 99
Nicotinic acid, 57
Nicotinil alcohol, 57
Nisentil, 16
Nitrates, 56
poisoning, 220, 298
Nitroglycerin, 56
Novocaine, 42
Numorphan, 8
Nupercaine, 45
Nylidrin, 58

Obstruction
gastric, 197
intestinal, 197, 242
pelvic arteries, 245

Oil of Wintergreen, 26
Ophthalmodynia, 131
Opium
  powdered, 6
  preparations, 6
Orchiepididymitis, 326
Orchitis, 326
Orphenadrine, 70
Osteitis, 255
Osteomalacia, 158, 273, 293
Osteomyelitis, 271, 292
Osteoporosis
  climacteric, 157
  senile, 157
Osteosis, 272, 293
Otalgia, 139
Otitis
  internal, 140
  media, 144
Otomycosis, 140
Ovarian cysts, 254
Ovulation pain, 204, 323
Oxinophen, 35
Oxymorphone, 8

Paget's disease, headache, 112
Pain in the face, 117
Pamaquine, 41
Pancreatic cancer, 235
Pancreatic colic, 191
Pancreatitis, 165, 191, 231, 238
Panophthalmitis, 134
Pantopon, 5
Papaverine, 10
Papillitis, 320
Paramethasone, 67
Paregoric, elixir, 6
Paronychia, 330
Paverll, 12
Pemphigus, 330
Penicillin, 71
Pentaerythritol tetranitrate, 57
Pentazocine, 19
Peptic ulcer, 165
Perforation, 195, 196, 197
Perianal abscess, 317
Pericarditis, 174
Perigastritis, 229
Perineal pain, 310
Periostitis, 255

Peritonitis, 194, 224
Pernicious anemia, 274, 294
Pharyngitis, 129
Phenacetin, 29
Phenazocine, 17
Phenoxybenzamine, 57
Phenylbutazone, 32
Phenylcinchoninic acid, 34
Phlebitis, 288
Phosphorus poisoning, 260
Phenol poisoning, 222
Phenyramidol, 70
Pituitary cachexia, 214
Plague, 89
Plantar neuroma, 302
Plantar warts, 302
Pleuritis, 155, 180, 206, 232
Pleurodynia, 84, 180, 206
Pneumonia, 178, 206
Pneumothorax, 181, 207
Poisoning, 217, 257
Poliomyelitis, 85
Polyarteritis nodosa, 268, 288, 316
Polycystic kidney, 251
Polycythemia vera, 294
Polyglobulia, 274
Polyneuritis, 276, 297
Pontocaine, 43
Porphyria, 214, 225
Postextraction pain, 127
Precordial pain, 170
Prednisolone, 66
Prednisone, 65
Pregnancy
  ectopic, 255
  rupture of ectopic, 205
Premenstrual tension, 322
Primadol, 17
Primaquine, 41
Procaine, 42
Proctitis, 318
Propoxyphene hydrochloride, 18
Prostatic lesions, 244, 311
Protrusion of intervertebral disks, 168
Psoitis, 169, 257, 307
Pulmonary infarction, 179, 207
Pustules, 330
Pyelitis, 247
Pyelonephritis, 202, 247
Pyramidon, 32

Pyrazolon derivatives, 31
Pyridium, 51
Pyrimethamine, 41

Q fever, 92
Quinacrine, 40
Quinine, 38

Rachialgia, 76
Radiculitis, 215, 232, 298
Rash, 76
Raynaud's disease, 270
Rectal cancer, 321
Rectal foreign bodies, 318
Rectal pain, 315
Rectal polyps, 320
Rectal prolapse, 318
Rectal spasm, 321
Rectal trauma, 318
Rectal tumors, 320
Recurrent fever, 92
Refraction errors, 139
Relapsing fever, 92
Renal abscess, 249
Renal cancer, 250
Renal colic, 187, 201
Renal diseases, 169
Renal lithiasis, 251
Renal tuberculosis, 250
Retrosternal pain, 170
Rheumatic fever, 264, 283
Rheumatoid arthritis, 263
Rheumatoid spondylitis, 156
Ribs
  cervical, 151, 158
  floating, 256
  thoracic, 184
Rickettsial diseases, 92
Rocky Mountain spotted fever, 92
Rubella, 80
Rubeola, 80
Rupture of ectopic pregnancy, 205
Rupture of the spleen, 210

Salicylamide, 27
Salicylates, 23
Salicylate, sodium, 25
Salicylsalicylic acid, 28
Salmonellosis, 87, 88
Scalenus anticus syndrome, 276

Scarlet fever, 87
Sciatica, 296
Seminal vesicle diseases, 312
Septicemia, 86
Sex organs
  cancer, 327
  foreign bodies, 325
  trauma, 325
Sigmoid cancer, 242
Sinus pain, 119
Sinusitis, 96
Skin pain, 329
Skin trauma, 337
Small pox, 77, 153
Sodium nitrite, 57
Spine
  bifida, 160
  epidural abscess, 160
  fracture, 167
  incurvations, 152, 159
  pain, 153
Spleen
  infarction, 210
  rupture, 210
Spondylitis, 155, 256
  hypertrophic, 157
  rheumatoid, 156
Sprain, acute, 166
Sternum, diseases, 184
Stiffness of neck, 77
Stomach, acute dilatation, 199
Stomatalgia, 123
Stomatitis, 124, 125
Strabismus, headache, 117
Strain, muscle, 113, 162, 304
Streptomycin, 72
Stress myalgia, 266, 285
Suboccipital neuralgia, 152, 161
Sulfas, 71, 72
Sweating, 77
Syncope, carotid, 209
Syphilis, 93
Systemic infections, 77

Tabes dorsalis, 215
Tachycardia, 76
Talwin, 19
Tamponade, cardiac, 175
Tarsitis, 301
Temperature curve, 75

Tennis elbow, 278, 309
Testes, torsion of the pedicle, 328
Tetany, 213, 268, 286, 306
Tetracaine, 43
Tetracyclines, 72
Thalium poisoning, 260
Thoracalgia, 184
Thoracodynia, 170
  chest pain, 178
  referred pain, 177
Thromboangiitis obliterans, 290, 327
Thrombosis of the pelvic veins, 246
Tolazoline, 57
Tonsillitis, 129
Tooth pain, 123
Torsion of a pedicle, 216, 217, 328
Torticollis, 149, 163, 169, 304
Trauma
  arms, 318
  bones, 271
  ear, 142, 143
  eye, 139
  mouth, 128
  rectum, 218
  sex organs, 325
  skin, 337
  spine, 166
Traumatic, headache, 114
Trench fever, 92
Triamcinolone, 67
Trichinosis, 163, 305
Trigeminal neuralgia, 118
Tuberculosis
  bones and joints, 272, 292
  intestinal, 224
  kidney, 250
  mediastinum, 164
  peritoneum, 224

Tularemia, 90
Turpentine oil poisoning, 261
Typhoid fever, 87, 201
Typhus, 92

Ulcerative colitis, 193
Ulcers, 336
  corneal, 133
  duodenal, 233
  peptic, 165, 188
Urethral diseases, 313
Urethritis, 325
Uterine diseases, 314

Vaginal diseases, 313
Vaginitis, 324
Valvular lesions, 173
Varicella, 78
Varices, 287
Varicocele, 327
Variola, 77, 153
Vasoconstrictors, 59
Vasodilators, 56
  peripheral, 57
Vertebrae, fusion, 151
Vesiculitis, spermatic, 327
Vincent's angina, 125
Viscus, perforation, 195
Vulvitis, 323

Warts, plantar, 302

Xylocaine, 45

Yellow fever, 91

Zactane, 21